Understanding Sleep

Application and Practice in Health Psychology

Andrew Baum and Margaret Chesney, Series Editors

Series Titles

Health-Promoting and Health-Compromising Behaviors Among Minority Adolescents
Edited by Dawn K. Wilson, James R. Rodrigue, & Wendell C. Taylor

Managing Chronic Illness: A Biopsychosocial Perspective
Edited by Perry M. Nicassio & Timothy W. Smith

Psychophysiological Disorders: Research and Clinical Applications
Edited by Robert J. Gatchel & Edward B. Blanchard

Understanding Sleep: The Evaluation and Treatment of Sleep Disorders
Edited by Mark R. Pressman & William C. Orr

Understanding Sleep
The Evaluation and Treatment of Sleep Disorders

Edited by
Mark R. Pressman, PhD
William C. Orr, PhD

American Psychological Association
Washington, DC

First printing May 1997
Second printing August 2000

Published by
American Psychological Association
750 First Street, NE
Washington, DC 20002

Copies may be ordered from
American Psychological Association
Order Department
P.O. Box 92984
Washington, DC 20090-2984

In the UK and Europe, copies may be ordered from
American Psychological Association
3 Henrietta Street
Covent Garden, London
WC2E 8LU England

Typeset in Palatino by Innodata Publishing Services Corporation, Halethorpe, MD
Printer: Data Reproductions Corp., Auburn Hills, MI
Cover Designer: Deborah Hodgdon, Boston, MA
Technical/Production Editor: Catherine R. Worth

Library of Congress Cataloging-in-Publication Data
Pressman, Mark R.
     Understanding sleep: the evaluation and treatment of sleep disorders / edited by Mark R. Pressman, William C. Orr.
       p.   cm.—(Application and practice in health psychology)
     Includes bibliographical references and index.
     ISBN 1-55798-747-5 (acid-free paper)
     1. Sleep disorders.   I. Pressman, Mark R.   II. Orr, William C.
III. Title.   IV. Series.
RC547.P74 1997
616.8'498—dc21

                                          97-1393
                                          CIP

British Library Cataloguing-in-Publication Data
A CIP record is available from the British Library

Printed in the United States of America

For my parents, Drs. Sylviette and Walter Pressman, my wife Rosalie, and my children Ariel David and Gabriel Aaron.
Mark R. Pressman, PhD

This book is dedicated to the memory of Harold L. Williams, PhD, whose insightful and incisive thinking inspired me and contributed greatly to the study of sleep as a scientific discipline.
William C. Orr, PhD

Contents

CONTRIBUTORS xi

SERIES FOREWORD xv
Andrew Baum and Margaret Chesney

INTRODUCTION 1

PART I: INTRODUCTION TO SLEEP DISORDERS 9

  1. The Basics of Sleep 11
     Max Hirshkowitz, Constance A. Moore, and Gisele Minhoto
  2. The Basics of Biological Rhythms 35
     Scott S. Campbell
  3. Introduction to Sleep Disorders 57
     Saul A. Rothenberg
  4. Psychophysiology of Sleep Deprivation
     and Disruption 73
     James K. Walsh and Scott S. Lindblom
  5. Public Policy and Sleep Disorders 111
     Mary A. Carskadon and Jennifer F. Taylor

PART II: DIAGNOSTIC METHODS AND TOOLS FOR THE
EVALUATION OF SLEEP DISORDERS 123

  6. The Diagnostic Interview and Differential Diagnosis
     for Complaints of Insomnia 125
     Arthur J. Spielman and Paul B. Glovinsky
  7. The Diagnostic Interview and Differential Diagnosis
     for Complaints of Excessive Daytime Sleepiness 161
     Jeanine L. White and Merrill M. Mitler
  8. The Polysomnogram 177
     Sonia Ancoli-Israel
  9. The Significance and Interpretation
     of the Polysomnogram 193
     Richard P. Allen

10. The Measurement of Daytime Sleepiness   209
    Sidney D. Nau

PART III: SLEEP DISORDERS AND THEIR TREATMENT   227

11. Delayed Sleep Phase Syndrome and
    Related Conditions   229
    Gary K. Zammit
12. Shift Work   249
    Timothy H. Monk
13. Obstructive Sleep Apnea: Natural History and
    Varieties of the Clinical Presentation   267
    William C. Orr
14. Obstructive Sleep Apnea: Treatment Options,
    Efficacy, and Effects   283
    Paul Saskin
15. Methods and Problems of Treatment Compliance
    in Obstructive Sleep Apnea   299
    Nancy Barone Kribbs
16. Behavioral Techniques and Biofeedback
    for Insomnia   315
    Richard R. Bootzin and Steven P. Rider
17. Hypnotics, Alcohol, and Caffeine:
    Relation to Insomnia   339
    Timothy Roehrs and Thomas Roth

PART IV: THE MEDICAL CONTEXT
OF SLEEP DISORDERS   357

18. Sleep and Sleep Disorders in
    Cardiopulmonary Diseases   359
    Joyce A. Walsleben
19. Sleep and Sleep Disorders in Noncardiopulmonary
    Medical Disorders   371
    *Mark R. Pressman, Stephen Gollomp, Robert L. Benz,
    and Donald D. Peterson*
20. Effects of Hospitalization, Surgery, and Anesthesia
    on Sleep and Biological Rhythms   385
    *Mark R. Pressman, Thomas J. Meyer, Donald D. Peterson,
    Lee W. Greenspon, and William G. Figueroa*

21. Sleep Deprivation and the Immune System   401
    Carol A. Everson

PART V: SLEEP DISORDERS ACROSS THE LIFE SPAN   425

22. Children and Sleep   427
    Jodi A. Mindell
23. Sleep and Aging   441
    Donald L. Bliwise
24. Sleep and Pregnancy   465
    Gila Hertz

PART VI: PSYCHOLOGICAL DISORDERS AND SLEEP   481

25. Sleep in Depression and Anxiety   483
    J. Catesby Ware and Charles M. Morin

Appendix A: The International Classification
             of Sleep Disorders   505

Appendix B: Diagnostic and Statistical Manual
             (DSM-IV) Sleep Disorder Codes   509

Appendix C: ICD-9-CM Sleep Disorder Codes   511

Appendix D: CPT (Procedure) Codes for Sleep
             Laboratory Studies   513

Appendix E: Requirements, Eligibility, and Examination
             Process for Certification as a Clinical Sleep
             Specialist by the American Board of
             Sleep Medicine   515

AUTHOR INDEX   521

SUBJECT INDEX   547

ABOUT THE EDITORS   565

Contributors

Richard P. Allen, PhD, Assistant Professor of Neurology, Johns Hopkins School of Medicine and Co-Director, John Hopkins Sleep Disorders Center, Johns Hopkins Bayview Medical Center, Baltimore, MD

Sonia Ancoli-Israel, PhD, Professor of Psychiatry, University of California, San Diego, and Director, Sleep Disorders Clinic, Veterans Affairs Medical Center, San Diego

Robert L. Benz, MD, Clinical Professor of Medicine, Jefferson Medical College, Philadelphia, PA, and Chief, Division of Nephrology, Department of Medicine, The Lankenau Hospital and Medical Research Center Wynnewood, PA

Donald L. Bliwise, PhD, Associate Professor of Neurology, Emory University School of Medicine, and Director, Sleep Disorders Center, Emory University Medical School, Atlanta, GA

Richard R. Bootzin, PhD, Professor of Psychology, Department of Psychology, University of Arizona, Tucson

Scott S. Campbell, PhD, Laboratory of Human Chronobiology, Department of Psychiatry, Cornell University Medical College, and Institute for Circadian Physiology, White Plains, NY

Mary A. Carskadon, PhD, Professor of Psychiatry and Human Behavior, Brown University School of Medicine, and Director, Chronobiology and Sleep Research Laboratory, E.P. Bradley Hospital, East Providence, RI

Carol A. Everson, PhD, Senior Fellow, Clinical Psychobiology Branch, National Institute of Mental Health, National Institutes of Health, Bethesda, MD, and Department of Physiology and Biophysics, College of Medicine, The University of Tennessee, Memphis, The Health Science Center

William G. Figueroa, MD, Clinical Professor of Medicine, Jefferson Medical College, Philadelphia, PA, and Division of Pulmonary and Critical Care Medicine, Department of Medicine, The Lankenau Hospital and Medical Research Center, Wynnewood, PA

Paul B. Glovinsky, PhD, Department of Psychology, City College of New York and The Insomnia Treatment Center, New York

Stephen Gollomp, MD, Clinical Assistant Professor of Neurology, University of Pennsylvania School of Medicine, Philadelphia, and

Division of Neurology, Department of Medicine, The Lankenau Hospital and Medical Research Center, Wynnewood, PA

Lee W. Greenspon, MD, Clinical Associate Professor of Medicine, Medical College of Pennsylvania, Philadelphia, and Director, Intensive Care Units and Division of Pulmonary and Critical Care Medicine, Department of Medicine, The Lankenau Hospital and Medical Research Center, Wynnewood, PA

Gila Hertz, PhD, Clinical Associate Professor of Psyciatry and Behavioral Sciences, State University of New York, Stoneybrook, and Director, Center for Insomnia and Sleep Disorders, Huntington, NY

Max Hirshkowitz, PhD, Associate Professor of Psychiatry, Baylor College of Medicine, and Director, Sleep Research Center, Veteran's Affairs Medical Center, Houston, TX

Nancy Barone Kribbs, PhD, Adjunct Assistant Professor of Psychiatry, University of Pennsylvania School of Medicine, Philadelphia, and Cephalon Inc., Westchester, PA

Scott S. Lindblom, MD, Clinical Fellow, Sleep Medicine and Research Center, and Fellow, Division of Pulmonary and Critical Care Medicine, Washington University School of Medicine, St. Louis, MO

Thomas J. Meyer, MD, Clinical Assistant Professor of Medicine, Jefferson Medical College, Philadelphia, and Division of Pulmonary and Critical Care Medicine, Department of Medicine, The Lankenau Hospital and Medical Research Center, Wynnewood, PA

Jodi A. Mindell, PhD, Associate Professor of Psychology, St. Joseph's University, Philadelphia, and Allegheny University of the Health Sciences, PA

Gisele Minhoto, MD, Research Fellow, Sleep Research and Diagnostic Centers, Veterans Affairs Hospital Center, Houston, TX

Merrill M. Mitler, PhD, Professor of Neuropharmacology, Scripps Research Institute, La Jolla, CA

Timothy H. Monk, PhD, Professor of Psychiatry, University of Pittsburgh School of Medicine, and Director, Laboratory of Human Chronobiology, Western Psychiatric Institute and Clinic, Pittsburgh, PA

Constance A. Moore, MD, Director, Sleep Diagnostic Center, Veteran Affairs Medical Center, Houston, TX

Charles M. Morin, PhD, Associate Professor of Psychology and Psychiatry, Universite Laval, Ecole de Psychologie, Ste-Foy, Quebec, Canada

Sidney D. Nau, PhD, Director, Sleep Disorders and Research Center, Deaconess Incarnate Word Health System, St. Louis, MO

William C. Orr, PhD, Adjunct Professor of Psychiatry and Behavioral Sciences, University of Oklahoma Health Sciences Center, Oklahoma City, and President and Chief Operating Officer, Thomas N. Lynn Institute for Healthcare Research, Integris-Baptist Medical Center, Oklahoma City

Donald D. Peterson, MD, Clinical Associate Professor of Medicine, Jefferson Medical College, Philadelphia, and Chief, Sleep Disorder Center, Division of Pulmonary and Critical Care Medicine, Department of Medicine, The Lankenau Hospital and Medical Research Center, Wynnewood, PA

Mark R. Pressman, PhD, Clinical Associate Professor, Jefferson Medical College, Philadelphia, and Associate Director, Sleep Disorders Center, The Lankenau Hospital and Medical Research Center, Wynnewood, PA

Steven P. Rider, MA, Department of Psychology, University of Arizona, Tucson

Timothy Roehrs, PhD, Adjunct Professor, Department of Psychiatry, Wayne State University School of Medicine, and Director of Research, Sleep Disorders and Research Center, Henry Ford Sleep Center, Detroit, MI

Thomas Roth, PhD, Clinical Professor of Psychiatry, University of Michigan School of Medicine, Ann Arbor, and Head, Sleep Disorders and Research Center, Henry Ford Sleep Center, Detroit, MI

Saul A. Rothenberg, PhD, Clinical Instructor of Neurology, Albert Einstein College of Medicine, Bronx, and Sleep/Wake Disorders Center, Montefiore Medical Center, Bronx, NY

Paul Saskin, PhD, Clinical Director, Regional Center for Sleep Disorders, Columbia Sunrise Health Strategies, Las Vegas, NV

Arthur J. Spielman, PhD, Director, Sleep Disorders Center, and Professor of Psychology, Department of Psychology, City College of New York

Jennifer F. Taylor, PhD, Postdoctoral Research Fellow, Department of Psychiatry and Human Behavior, Brown University School of Medicine, East Providence, RI

James K. Walsh, PhD, Clinical Associate Professor, Department of Psychiatry, St. Louis University School of Medicine, St. Louis, and Executive Director and Senior Scientist, Sleep Medicine and Research Center, St. Luke's Hospital, Chesterfield, MO

Joyce A. Walsleben, RN, PhD, Research Assistant Professor, New York University School of Medicine, and Director, New York University/Bellevue Hospital Sleep Disorders Center, Department of Pulmonary and Critical Care Medicine, New York University Medical Center

J. Catesby Ware, PhD, Professor of Psychiatry and Behavioral Sciences, Eastern Virginia Medical School, Norfolk, and Director, Sleep Disorders Center, Sentara Norfolk General Hospital, Norfolk, VA

Jeanine L. White, PhD, Associate Faculty, Department of Psychology, National University, La Jolla, CA

Gary K. Zammit, PhD, Assistant Professor of Clinical Psychology in Psychiatry, Columbia University College of Physicians and Surgeons, and Director, Sleep Disorders Institute at St. Luke's-Roosevelt Hospital Center, New York

Foreword

The Division of Health Psychology (Division 38) of the American Psychological Association presents the fourth volume in its series highlighting the application and practice of health psychology. One of the driving forces behind the establishment of the division was interest in health promotion and disease prevention and treatment through the application of principles and procedures that were emerging in the research arena. The vitality of health psychology depends on an active dialogue between its researchers and practitioners. One of the important goals of the series is to further expand this dialogue. Attempts to translate research findings into applications and interventions, to test and evaluate the efficacy of these interventions, and to denote important clinical experiences and research needs of the practice of health psychology are the focus of these volumes. Transfer of knowledge; feedback to researchers regarding needs, failures, and successes of clinical interventions; and facilitation and expansion of necessary dialogue between scientist and practitioner are the objectives.

Toward these aims, the volumes in this series are meant to function as vehicles for translating research into practice, with an analysis of issues related to the evaluation, prevention, and treatment of health behaviors and health problems. These goals are met by treating clinical or applied health psychology as broadly as possible, including community and public health assessment and intervention methods and problems of health care use. Issues are considered across a variety of settings, including hospitals, the practitioner's office, community clinics, work-site settings, schools, and managed care settings. Each volume provides direction in areas of need and populations to be served by health psychology intervention; critically examines issues and problems involved in clinical evaluation, prevention, and treatment of specific disorders; and illustrates the effectiveness of novel clinical approaches to diagnosis and treatment that may guide future research and innovation. Each volume focuses on a topic, such as this book's emphasis on sleep disorders, and synthesizes research on a range of topics to reinforce the theoretical and scientific rationale for the practice of health psychology and to identify critical issues in the prevention, assessment, and management of health problems.

Andrew Baum
Margaret Chesney

Introduction

Mark R. Pressman and William C. Orr

For centuries the phenomenon of sleep was considered the province of poets and philosophers. The psychoanalytic revolution brought the issue of sleep—dreams, in particular—into the province of psychology and psychiatry. Although descriptions of sleep-related brain-wave activity as seen on electroencephalography (EEG) were published in the decades of the 1930s and 1940s, the discovery of the relationship between dreaming and a specific stage of sleep (i.e., rapid eye movement sleep) catapulted sleep into the realm of scientific psychobiological investigation. The promise of some biological relationship between the "psychosis of sleep" (i.e., dreaming) and a distinct physiological entity such as rapid eye movement (REM) sleep stimulated a rather remarkable burgeoning of research into the biology and psychology of sleep in academic departments of psychiatry and psychology during the 1960s. As research into the physiology of sleep progressed, researchers in departments of basic sciences such as pharmacology and physiology began to study the neural mechanisms of sleep.

The great excitement and promise of sleep as a link to the biology of mental illness has led to some disappointment, but the intensive investigation into the basic physiology and neural biology of sleep has resulted in clinical applications of sleep physiology far beyond even the boldest predictions of 20 years ago. The specific discovery of a sleep-related breathing disorder (i.e., sleep apnea) and epidemiological studies documenting its ubiquity in the population have resulted in a proliferation of interest in the application of sleep physiology to clinical medicine. The natural consequence has been a "reawakening" of interest in sleep in its broadest manifestations to include the psychological as well as organic causes of disturbed sleep.

This increased interest in sleep is manifested in thousands of peer-reviewed journal articles published in the last few years, along with dozens of volumes devoted to sleep, biological rhythms, and sleep disorders. Competing nosologies of sleep disorders have appeared. Over 2,000 individuals attend the national clinical and sleep research meetings each year. Over 200 sleep disorders centers—tertiary diagnostic and treatment facilities—have been set up in the last 20 years. A process exists for accrediting these facilities. Hundreds of physicians and psychologists have taken and passed the certification test for sleep specialists given by the American Board of Sleep Medicine. The American Medical Association now lists four procedure codes for the performance of sleep studies. Perhaps the ultimate marker of the maturity of the field is that tens of thousands of sleep studies and sleep disorder evaluations are conducted each year, paid for by the patient's medical insurance. This volume is intended to distill what has been learned over the past 20 years so that those who make the frontline contacts with patients complaining of sleep problems (e.g., psychologists, psychiatrists, physicians, nurses) may become more proficient at both the detection and the treatment of these debilitating disorders.

What Is Known About Sleep

In many ways, sleep research has not maintained an equal pace with the rapidly expanding field of clinical sleep disorders medicine and psychology. Sleep research has suffered like all other research areas owing to the shrinking research dollar. Nevertheless, new and exciting research continues to appear. Sleep research is a sufficiently young field that most of the major questions about sleep (e.g., Why do we sleep? What are the brain mechanisms regulating sleep?) have not yet been answered.

Sleep researchers do know that the sleeping brain is not "asleep" in the generic sense; physiologically, it can be as active during sleep as it is during wakefulness. This concept has its roots in the initial publications of the results of modern sleep research starting in the early 1930s. Soon after electroencephalography was invented, brain researchers were studying sleep. Even with the primitive equipment of the day, it was clear that sleep is a complicated process with a wide variety of brain-wave activity present in a single night of sleep. The father of modern sleep research, Nathaniel Kleitman, a University of Chicago physiologist, published the first major volume on sleep in 1939. In 1957 REM sleep was described for the first time and its relationship to dreaming established. The modern clinical specialty of sleep medicine, which includes the psychological treatment of sleep disorders, took root in the 1960s. Before that time, some sleep disorders had been described, such as insomnia and narcolepsy, but diagnosis and treatment were unsophisticated by today's standards. Most sleep disorders were treated symptomatically with alerting or sedating medication. With the advent of techniques to study human physiology during sleep and the description and quantification of sleep stages, the mechanisms of sleep pathology could be more fully elucidated. As a result, new diagnostic and treatment techniques were developed.

The Psychological and Physical Roots of Sleep Disorders

Sleep specialists have now identified over 80 different sleep disorders with a variety of causes. Some are purely physiological in origin, such as those caused by disruptive breathing or involuntary leg movements, whereas others are psychological in origin, related to stress, anxiety, or depression. Still others do not fall clearly into either category, and some fall into overlapping categories. Some individuals have more than one sleep disorder. Additionally, coping with a sleep disorder of physiological origin may provoke a psychological response that further disrupts sleep.

The cause of a sleep disorder may be determined only by taking a broad approach to diagnosis. All factors that may result in changes in the quantity, quality, and timing of sleep must be considered. Clinical sleep specialists must be trained to recognize the signs and symptoms of all sleep problems whether they be physiological (medical) or psychological. Many sleep disorders of physiological origin manifest symptoms only during sleep. A patient may show no signs of abnormality on pulmonary function tests or an electrocardiogram taken during the day but may have grossly abnormal breathing or even life-threatening cardiac arrhythmias during sleep. The modern sleep specialist must be able to detect the subtle signs and symptoms in the patient's history that point to pathology whether it is physiological, psychological, or a combination of both.

Modern sleep specialists also deal with a much broader scope of problems than in the past. Not only must they deal with the traditional problems of patients who have difficulty falling asleep or staying asleep, but also they must assist patients who awaken feeling unrefreshed and feel sleepy during the day. Patients who fall asleep at inappropriate times such as while driving are increasingly referred to sleep specialists for diagnosis and treatment. Patients may feel drowsy or fall asleep inappropriately for all the commonly understood reasons; however, the sleepy patient may be found to have an easily diagnosable sleep disorder. There are at least 20 sleep disorders that can result in severe daytime sleepiness (fatigue). The causes of such sleepiness range from the usual suspects, such as insufficient sleep, to organic sleep disorders, such as sleep apnea, to disorders of intrinsic biological rhythms. Psychological disorders may also limit or disrupt sleep-producing symptoms of sleepiness or fatigue.

Psychologists, physicians, and other health professionals all may function as clinical sleep specialists. However, to do this they must be knowledgeable about sleep disorders that often are well outside their original specialties or subspecialties. Sleep medicine or sleep psychology is clearly a new subspecialty.

This Volume

To provide an overview of sleep and sleep disorders, this book is organized into several parts. The first part provides an introduction to concepts and terminology that are important to the field and essential for the understanding of material presented later. Other parts deal with diagnostic methods and tools for the evaluation of sleep disorders, selected sleep disorders and their treatment, the medical context of sleep disorders, changes in sleep with age, and psychological disorders of sleep.

In the first part, in chapter 1, Hirshkowitz, Moore, and Minhoto describe the basics of sleep including its composition, organization, and possible functions. In chapter 2, Campbell puts sleep and wakefulness in perspective with a description of circadian (24-hr) rhythms. Sleep and wakefulness cannot be viewed or studied in isolation. Wakefulness clearly affects sleep, and sleep affects wakefulness. Additionally, some physiological and psychological functions vary over the 24 hours without regard to the presence of sleep or wakefulness. The science of circadian rhythms, or chronobiology, provides essential information for the understanding of sleep and wakefulness. Rothenberg introduces modern concepts of sleep disorders in chapter 3 and includes a discussion of the various sleep disorders nosologies. Brief descriptions of many common sleep disorders are provided. Sleep deprivation is central to many sleep disorders and their consequences; it has been a major topic of psychological research for more than 100 years regarding its effects on cognition and performance. Walsh and Lindblom present a state-of-the-art review of the different types of sleep deprivation and their consequences in chapter 4. Sleep deprivation and sleep disorders not only affect individuals but also impact society as a whole. Sleep disorders lead to reduced productivity and increased numbers of accidents and incur a tremendous cost to society. In 1990 the National Commission on Sleep Disorders Research was appointed by the U.S. Congress to investigate the social and economic effects of sleep disorders. The report of this commission forms the basis of the introduction to public policy issues related to sleep disorders and sleep deprivation by Carskadon and Taylor presented in chapter 5.

Part II of the book is devoted to clinical issues of evaluating patients with sleep disorders. In chapter 6, Spielman and Glovinsky provide a state-of-the-art review of the diagnosis of patients with complaints of insomnia. They provide a thorough discussion of the course of insomnia as well as its varying determinants. A unique feature of this chapter is the detailed instruction in the use of sleep logs, an innovation that allows the different forms of insomnia to be more easily diagnosed. In chapter 7, White and Mitler discuss in detail the basics of evaluating a patient who presents with a complaint of daytime sleepiness or fatigue. All too often, it is assumed that a patient is sleepy owing to insufficient sleep, excessive physical activity, or depression. However, many sleep disorders can produce profound daytime sleepiness.

Evaluation of sleep disorders frequently requires use of objective diagnostic tests. In chapter 8, Ancoli-Israel describes and discusses the use of the polysomnogram (sleep study), both in the sleep laboratory and in other settings, as well the use of ambulatory equipment. Allen in chapter 9 reviews the basics of interpreting sleep study data. In addition to nocturnal sleep studies, other tests have been developed for the assessment of alertness and sleepiness; these tests have both clinical and research uses. Nau provides a review of the most common techniques for assessing alertness and sleepiness in chapter 10.

Part III deals with selected sleep disorders and their treatment. In chapter 11, Zammit discusses how disturbances of biological rhythms produce sleep disorders. Biological rhythm disorders are often misdiagnosed as insomnia and do not respond to the usual insomnia treatments. In chapter 12, Monk discusses the most common cause of biological rhythm disturbance, shift work, which affects millions of Americans. Orr reviews the different presenting symptoms for sleep apnea syndrome, one of the most common and serious organic sleep disorders, in chapter 13. Sleep apnea syndrome was recently described in the *New England Journal of Medicine* as a major public health problem. Saskin describes the state-of-the-art treatments for sleep apnea in chapter 14. One of the most common treatments for sleep apnea has a high success rate but may be poorly tolerated by the patient. Compliance to recommendations thus becomes a major issue in the successful treatment of sleep apnea. Kribbs in chapter 15 describes the research on patient treatment compliance that has been done to date. Most Americans who receive treatment for insomnia are willing to take a sleeping pill or other sedating substance. However, nonpharmacological treatments can be more efficacious and long lasting. In chapter 16, Bootzin and Rider review the latest behavioral and biofeedback techniques for treating insomnia. In chapter 17, Roehrs and Roth review the effects of common sleeping pills plus alcohol and caffeine on sleep and sleep disorders.

Many common medical conditions are associated with or made worse by sleep disorders; this subject is the concern of Part IV. In chapter 18, Walsleben reviews changes in sleep and sleep disorders that occur in cardiopulmonary diseases. In chapter 19, Pressman and colleagues review changes in sleep and sleep disorders in a variety of noncardiopulmonary sleep disorders such as occur with stroke and kidney failure. Pressman and colleagues further look at what happens to sleep and sleep disorders in hospitalized patients in chapter 20. What effect do the hospital environment, surgery, and anesthesia have on the patient's quality and quantity of sleep? How do sleep problems affect the course of the patient's hospitalization and recovery? Everson takes a more basic approach to the issue of the effect of sleep disorders on health in her review of the relationship between sleep deprivation and immune function in chapter 21.

In Part V of the book changes in sleep and sleep disorders across the life span are reviewed. It is well known that the overall quality and quantity of sleep change with age. However, different types of sleep disorders may also appear as a function of normal aging. In chapter 22, Mindell discusses the wide variety of sleep problems that can occur in children, and in chapter 23, Bliwise reviews sleep changes and sleep disorders that occur with aging. Hertz reviews the effects of pregnancy on sleep and sleep disorders in chapter 24.

The subject of psychological disorders and sleep was intentionally left for the last—Part VI. Although anxiety and depression are major causes of insomnia and related sleep disorders, they are clearly not only causes of sleep problems. In a society in which is often assumed that a sleep problem must be stress-or depression-related, the well-educated and trained clinician must first rule out the many organic causes of sleep disorders. Once the differential diagnosis has been successfully completed and anxiety or depression is identified as the most probable cause of the sleep disorder, appropriate psychological evaluation and treatment may be initiated. Ware and Morin provide a state-of-the-art review of the interaction of sleep and psychological disorders.

Ben Franklin said, "Early to bed and early to rise, makes a man healthy, wealthy, and wise." It should only be so simple! An understanding of sleep and its many disorders requires psychologists and other health professionals to leave the narrow confines of their specialties and subspecialties and take a more global view of the interaction of sleep with every other aspect of human life. Familiarity with both physiological and psychological symptoms of sleep disorders is essential. This book represents a starting point for learning about sleep disorders, and we hope it will be a useful resource for the health care community.

I

Introduction to Sleep Disorders

The Basics of Sleep

Max Hirshkowitz, Constance A. Moore,
and Gisele Minhoto

What Is Sleep?

Sleep is universal and essential for survival. Clinicians interested in human sleep must recognize its three most basic characteristics: (a) sleep is a brain process, (b) it is an active process, and (c) it is not a single process. In this chapter, the characteristics of the different sleep processes, the basic factors regulating sleep, and the importance of sleep are discussed.

The behavioral inactivity during sleep biases observers toward believing that mental activity ceases during sleep. When asked how they know they have slept, many people deduce an answer on the basis of two impressions: First, they feel refreshed, and second, they are unable to recall thoughts and events from the interval between first going to bed and arising. Sleep can produce amnesia. People may mistakenly interpret the sleep-related process of forgetting (or failing to store information in long-term memory) as mental inactivity. By contrast, we have no difficulty accepting that mental activity occurs during dreams, essentially because we occasionally remember dreams.

Electroencephalographic Correlates of Sleep and Wakefulness

Because sleep is a brain process, researchers commonly study it by recording brain electrical activity. Traditional laboratory studies of

11

human sleep rely mainly on electroencephalography (EEG). EEG involves inspecting wavelike tracings produced by ink pens on moving chart paper or computer screens. EEG activity is characterized by both the frequency and the amplitude of the waves. *Frequency* refers to how many times the waves appear per second, often referred to as *cycles per second* (cps) or *hertz* (Hz). The more cycles per second, the faster the EEG frequency. *Amplitude* refers to how high the waveform is on the paper tracing. Because these waveforms reflect electrical activity of the brain, they are usually measured in microvolts (μV). EEG activity is generally divided into the following four categories according to ranges of frequency from slowest to fastest: delta 0.5–3 cps, theta 4–7 cps, alpha 8–13 cps, and beta (14–25 cps). Other EEG characteristics, reviewed in the next sections, are also important for describing sleep.

In most individuals, wakeful relaxation with eyes closed is associated with an EEG activity called the *alpha rhythm*. In adults, the alpha rhythm has a frequency of 8–13 cps, has an amplitude that is usually below 50 microvolts μV, and is most prominent over the rear portion of the scalp (parietooccipital cortex) when eyes are closed. Eye opening, strenuous mental activity, and arousing stimuli block the alpha rhythm.

Hans Berger, known as the father of EEG, is widely recognized for discovering and describing the alpha rhythm (see Berger, 1929). It is less well known that Berger also made the first EEG recordings of human sleep. He correlated sleep with alpha rhythm disappearance, a phenomenon still recognized as the most robust polygraphic marker of sleep onset. However, some individuals have little or no alpha activity. When Loomis, Harvey, and Hobart (1937) made the first continuous, all-night recordings of sleep EEG, they noted difficulty differentiating wakefulness from sleep in "non-alpha-type" individuals. However, they noted slow, rolling eye movements appearing at sleep onset, enabling them to refine EEG scoring criteria for sleep onset. Current, multichannel polygraphic criteria correlate sleep onset with (a) alpha reduction, slowing, and finally disappearance; (b) appearance of fast, sharp-looking waves at the top of the scalp (vertex sharp transients); (c) disappearance of rapid eye movements, eyelid movement activity, and blinking; (d) appearance of slow, rolling eye movements; and (e) a decrease in chin muscle activity (submental electromyographic activity; see Figure 1). However, not all of these correlates necessarily appear at sleep onset in any given recording (Rechtschaffen & Kales, 1968).

Sleep onset may be abruptly followed by an awakening. Called *microsleeps*, such episodes last from 3 to 15 seconds. During microsleep,

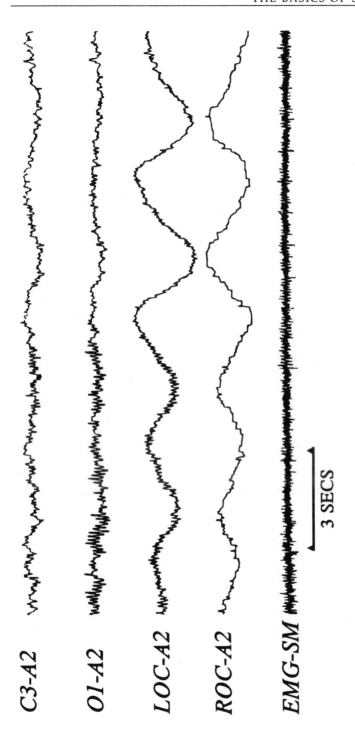

C3-A2

O1-A2

LOC-A2

ROC-A2

EMG-SM

3 SECS

Figure 1. Sleep onset with electroencephalographic (EEG) alpha disappearance and slow eye movements present. The two top tracings show central (C3) and occipital (O1) EEG activity electrically referenced to the mastoid (A2). Similarly referenced left outer canthus (LOC) and right outer canthus (ROC) provide tracings of eye-movement activity. Finally, muscle tone is monitored from electrodes placed under the chin to record submental electromyographic activity (EMG-SM).

responsiveness to environmental stimuli is impaired or absent. These episodes may occur with eyes open or closed, and they may occur without warning in sleep-deprived individuals. At highway speed, a car traverses a distance equivalent to the length of a football field during a 3- to 4-second microsleep.

The EEG of Human Sleep and Polysomnography

A standard sleep recording, called a *polysomnogram*, is a continuous, all-night tracing of electroencephalographic (brain-wave), electrooculographic (eye movement), and submental electromyographic (chin muscle) events. In clinical practice, sleep-related breathing, cardiac rhythm, and leg muscle activity are also recorded. This wealth of data presents the sleep specialist, or polysomnographer, with the major task of data reduction. Before inexpensive digital computer systems were available, it was impractical routinely to count and measure each relevant EEG waveform. Therefore, a system was needed to summarize data.

Current standards for categorizing different sleep stages are described in a manual published by the National Institutes of Health (Rechtschaffen & Kales, 1968). This manual resulted from the combined efforts of leading sleep researchers throughout the world who formed an ad hoc standardization committee, chaired by Allan Rechtschaffen and Anthony Kales. The project's success in no small measure derived from the chairmen's insistence on consensus. The manual describes and illustrates a wide variety of sleep-related brain electrical events. It is essential reading for anyone interested in the electrophysiology of human sleep. The "R & K system," as it is often called, remains the standard for recording and classifying sleep stages in humans.

Initial data reduction entails summarizing waveform activity over a specified time frame, called an *epoch*. Each polygraphic epoch is classified as Stage Wake (or W0), 1, 2, 3, 4, rapid eye movement REM sleep or movement time (when tracing is obscured by muscle artifact) according to electrophysiological criteria. Table 1 shows EEG characteristics for the different sleep stages. Although some laboratories use 1-minute epochs and others use 20-second epochs, the most common epoch duration is 30 seconds. It is convenient that recordings made with paper speeds of 10 mm per second produce one 30-second epoch per polygraph page (Carskadon & Rechtschaffen, 1994).

The sleep-stage scoring system has proved remarkably useful and has greatly facilitated the understanding of sleep. With it one can

Table 1

Electrophysiological Characteristics of Sleep Stages

Stage of sleep	Predominant EEG Activity	EOG characteristics	EMG activity
1	Low voltage, mixed frequency	Slow	Decreased from awake
2	Sleep spindles and K complexes	None	Decreased from awake
3	Sleep spindles and slow waves	None	Decreased from awake
4	Mostly slow waves	None	Decreased from awake
REM	Low voltage, mixed frequency	Rapid	Nearly absent

Note. EEG = electroencephalographic; EOG = electrooculographic; EMG = electromyographic; REM = rapid eye movement. Derived from information in *A Manual of Standardized Terminology, Techniques, and Scoring System for Sleep Stages of Human Subjects*, by A. Rechtschaffen and A. Kales, 1968, National Institutes of Health Publication No. 204, Washington, DC: U.S. Government Printing Office.

describe the progression of sleep, compare the patterns recorded in patients with those derived from normal controls, and investigate sleep alterations by experimental manipulation. The system's weaknesses constitute the inherent trade-off made when generalization is adopted. The detail is lost, and individual polygraphic events become invisible. For example, a single epoch (recorded page of sleep) may contain any number of sleep-stage-defining polygraphic waveforms. Regardless of whether it contains one event (such as an eye movement) or a dozen, the stage classification remains the same. Therefore, potentially useful information concerning sleep-related brain processes may be overlooked.

   Delta waves and slow wave sleep (sleep stages 3 and 4). Delta activity is the slowest EEG activity to occur during sleep and may be the most salient sleep-related EEG feature in humans (see Figure 2). Delta wave

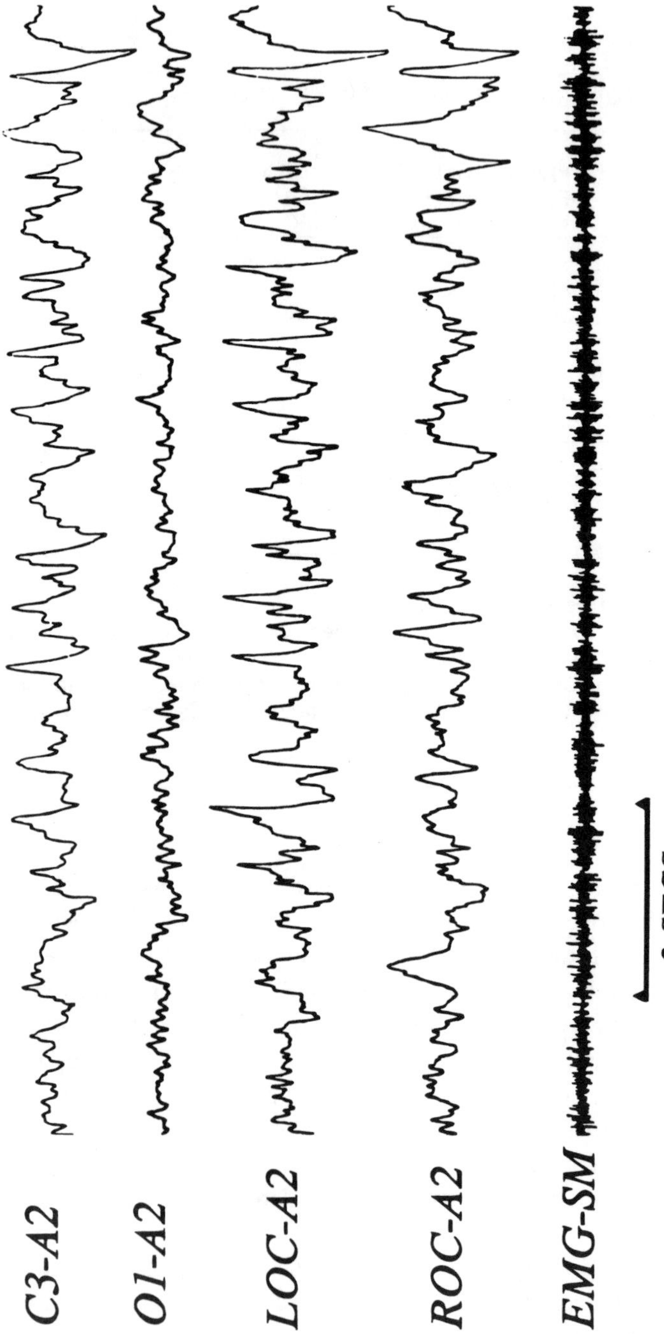

Figure 2. EEG delta activity during slow wave sleep in an adult. Slow wave activity is prominent in central EEG (C3-A2), occipital EEG (O1-A2), and both left and right electrooculogram (LOC-A2 and ROC-A2) channels. Submental electromyogram is also shown (EMG-SM).

frequency is less than 4 cps, usually ranging between 0.1 and 3.5 cps. Slow waves, the subset of delta activity of interest to sleep specialists, have a frequency of 2 cps or less. For slow waves, standard scoring requires a minimum amplitude of 75 µV; however, many laboratories relax this criterion for the elderly. These high-voltage (relative to other brain electrical activities) waves are "synchronized," meaning each delta wave from different areas of the brain is in phase with others. Delta EEG amplitude is much higher in children than adults and usually declines even further with advancing age.

Although data suggest that slow waves originate in the cerebral cortex, thalamic neurons appear also to be involved in generating delta activity (Steriades, 1994). Delta waves are maximal over frontal and central cortex recording sites; however, they occur prominently across the entire scalp surface during slow wave sleep. Delta activity is the defining characteristic of Stages 3 and 4 sleep, commonly referred to collectively as slow wave sleep (SWS). When slow waves make up 50% or more of an epoch, the epoch is classified as Stage 4 sleep. Stage 3 sleep is scored when delta occupies between 20 and 50% of a recording epoch (Rechtschaffen & Kales, 1968).

Sleep spindles, K-complexes, and Stage 2 sleep. Sleep spindles are EEG waveform bursts with a mean frequency of 11.5 to 16 cps and a duration of 0.5 seconds or more. The sleep spindle typically has a waxing and waning "spindle" shape, hence the name (see Figure 3). Amplitude seldom exceeds 50 mV in adults. When recorded from the scalp, spindles are usually bilaterally symmetrical. However, they originate through interaction between thalamic nucleus reticularis neurons (the spindle pacemaker) and thalamocortical neurons. It is interesting that athalamic animals continue to have slow waves; however, cortical spindles disappear (McCarley, 1994; Steriades, 1994). Therefore, spindles represent a sleep-related brain process different from that signified by slow wave activity. Spindle incidence and duration often increase in response to administration of benzodiazepines (a pharmacological class of drugs used as sleeping pills and antianxiety medication), presumably through stimulation of the spindle pacemaker's GABA-ergic (gamma-aminobutyric acid) neurons.

The K complex is a high-voltage waveform that can be either slow or sharply contoured but is typically less than one-half of a second in duration. In standard recordings, it is recognizable by a well-delineated negative (upward) sharp wave, followed by a positive (downward) component (see Figure 3). Sleep spindles often follow a K complex. The

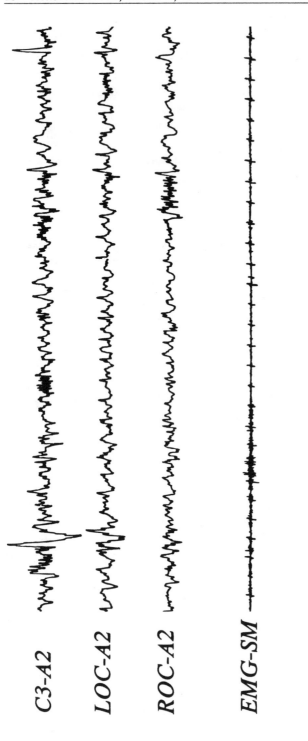

Figure 3. K-complex activity and sleep spindle activity. This recording segment illustrates a K complex preceded by a spindle (in the first 3 sec of recording) and several sleep spindles (at approximately 7 and 12 sec). C3-A2 is monopolar central EEG; LOC-A2 is left electrooculogram, ROC-A2 is right electrooculogram, and EMG-SM is submental electromyogram.

K-complex is generally maximal at or near the vertex (top of the scalps, Carskadon & Rechtschaffen, 1994). K complexes occur either spontaneously or in response to external stimuli. Arousals are more likely within several minutes following a K complex than before; K-alpha activity has been implicated with arousal (Sassin & Johnson, 1968; Naitoh, Antony-Baas, Muzef, & Ehrhart, 1982). Some drugs (e.g., benzodiazepines) and aging reportedly reduce K-complex activity (Anch, Browman, Mitler, & Walsh, 1988). The presence of spindles and K complexes in the absence of significant slow wave activity (20% of the epoch) essentially defines Stage 2 sleep (Rechtschaffen & Kales, 1968).

Rapid eye movements and Stage REM sleep. If an epoch neither meets criteria for wakefulness nor contains significant delta activity, sleep spindles, or K complexes, it is classified as either Stage 1 or REM sleep, depending on characteristics of eye movement activity. If rapid eye movements are present, REM sleep is scored. The EEG in both Stage 1 and REM sleep is marked by low-voltage (low-amplitude), mixed-frequency activity. This activity is thought to reflect generally increased cerebral activation. During REM sleep, theta waves (4–7 cps) with a distinctive notched appearance (sawtooth waves) may be present (see Figure 4).

The saccadic eye movements of REM sleep can appear in bursts or in isolation. Standard technique for eye-movement recording involves electrodes placed slightly lateral to each eye and referenced to an electrically neutral site (either mastoid or earlobe). Separate recording channels for each eye facilitate eye-movement recognition; on the tracing, one typically sees out-of-phase potentials between the left and right electrooculograms.

REM sleep is also characterized by a general loss of voluntary muscle tone. During REM, the sleeping individual is unable to move. Involuntary muscles of the heart, lungs, and other organs continue to function, but for all intents and purposes, the individual is paralyzed during REM sleep. The function of this type of muscle inhibition is unknown, but the characteristic may serve a safety function by preventing the dreaming individual from physically acting out a dream. Surgical lesioning of the area of the brain responsible for this inhibition of muscle tone in cats produced dreaming animals who pounced on imaginary prey. This muscle inhibition is also absent in some humans who suffer from REM sleep behavior disorder. These individuals attempt to act out their dreams, sometimes injuring themselves and their spouses.

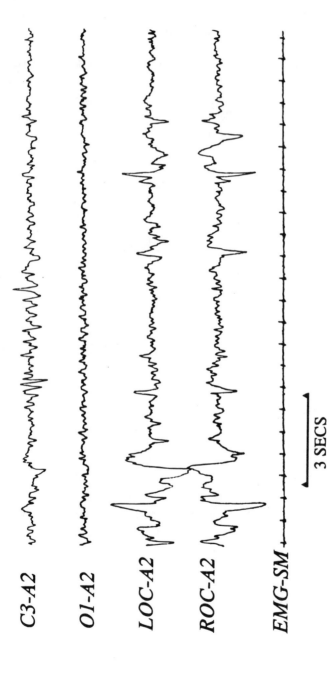

Figure 4. REM sleep with sawtooth EEG theta activity. This partial epoch begins with a burst of rapid eye movements (REMs) apparent from out-of-phase pen deflections recorded on the LOC-A2 and ROC-A2 channels (left and right outer canthi, respectively, referenced to the mastoid). Other REMs, with less burst intensity, continue to occur. Central EEG (C3-A2) but not occipital (O1-A2) shows a well-formed train of sawtooth theta activity approximately in the center of this tracing. Submental electromyogram (EMG-SM) shows the typical near absence of activity (except for a pulse artifact) associated with REM sleep.

The discovery of REM sleep and its association with dreaming (Aserinsky & Kleitman, 1953) produced great excitement in the psychiatric community. In the original study, dreams were reported 20 out of 27 times when participants were awakened from REM sleep. By contrast, awakenings from non-REM (NREM) sleep stages yielded dream reports on only 4 of 23 trials. The discovery of an identifiable physiological state associated with dreaming opened a floodgate of dream research. Freud characterized dreams as "the royal road to the unconscious," and many researchers believed that sleep studies could unlock the mind's elusive mysteries.

Laboratory studies of dreaming have produced a wide assortment of interesting facts and have answered some basic questions about dreaming. For example, people usually dream in color; most dreams are not especially remarkable; we appear to dream in real time; we often dream about recent events; and people sleeping in the laboratory frequently dream about sleeping in the laboratory (Ellman & Antrobus, 1991). Later investigations revealed that REM sleep eye movements correspond to directions of gaze during dreams (Herman et al., 1984). Dream research generally supports such psychoanalytic concepts as *daytime residue, continuity, condensation*, and *repressed wish* (Freud, 1950). However, a unified theory of dreaming has not emerged from the research. The basic understanding of dream process remains fragmented, and assertions concerning the meaning of dreams continue to be primarily theoretical.

A neurophysiologically based theory of dreaming posits that dreams are created by the cortex in an attempt to make sense of and organize random incoming pontine activity (Hobson & McCarley, 1977). The "activation-synthesis hypothesis" views the dream as epiphenomenological and without purpose. Nonetheless, because the dream narrative is created and its meaning is attributed, it is clear that the dream expresses an individual's current concerns and preoccupations. In this way, neurophysiological findings agree with this basic premise of Calvin Hall's (1953) theoretical framework.

Slow eye movements and Stage 1 sleep. If a recording epoch does not meet criteria for wakefulness or sleep Stages 4, 3, 2, or REM, then by default, Stage 1 sleep is scored. Stage 1 sleep, like REM sleep, is characterized by low-voltage, mixed-frequency EEG activity. However, slow eye movements (SEMs) are sometimes present, particularly at sleep onset. SEMs are characteristically slow, pendular swings of the eyeballs from one side of the orbit to the other (see Figure 1). An excursion, once started, continues smoothly and without interruption through a relatively wide arc. Most SEMs are horizontal.

Sleep stage smoothing rules and the normal sleep pattern. Sleep stage scoring also includes a number of smoothing rules designed to enhance continuity of sleep stage progressions (for details, see Rechtschaffen & Kales, 1968). When sleep stages are plotted as a function of time, distinct patterns emerge (see Figure 5). The most obvious pattern is an alternation of NREM and REM sleep stages, occurring approximately every 90–120 minutes. Furthermore, most SWS occurs in the first third of the night, and most REM sleep is in the second half of the night. Sleep normally begins with a progression through NREM sleep stages, followed afterward by REM sleep. Finally, REM sleep occurs in four to six discrete episodes each night (Carskadon & Dement, 1994; Williams, Karacan, & Hursch, 1974).

Nightly summary measures and sleep architecture. Overall, in normal young adults, approximate nightly percentages of each stage are as follows: less than 5% awake time, 2–5% Stage 1, 45–55% Stage 2, 3–8% Stage 3, 10–15% Stage 4, and 20–25% Stage REM sleep (Hirshkowitz, Moore, Hamilton, Rando, & Karacan, 1992; Williams et al., 1974).

Important nightly summary measures include sleep period time (the duration between sleep onset and the final awakening), total sleep time, latency to sleep, latency to persistent sleep, the number of awakenings and the number of awakenings per hour of sleep, wakefulness duration after sleep onset, total wakefulness time, sleep efficiency (total sleep time divided by time in bed), number of sleep stage changes, minutes and percentages of each sleep stage, latencies to each sleep stage from sleep onset, REM sleep cycle length, and REM sleep fragmentation. Many other measures can also be derived.

How Does Sleep Change as a Function of Age?

Sleep patterns change over the life span (see Figure 6). At birth, an infant sleeps twice as much as an adult. However, as parents are keenly aware, infants do not sleep according to the same schedule as adults. Sleep and awake episodes occur many times during the 24-hour period, and the cycle may be erratic. Furthermore, REM sleep may occur at sleep onset and constitutes approximately 50% of the sleep period. The percentage of REM sleep declines until adolescence and then stabilizes

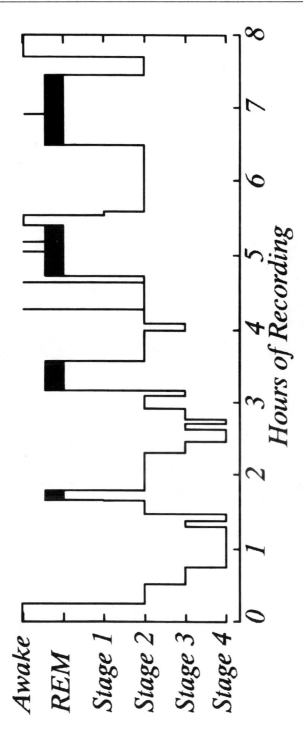

Figure 5. The normal sleep pattern of a young adult.

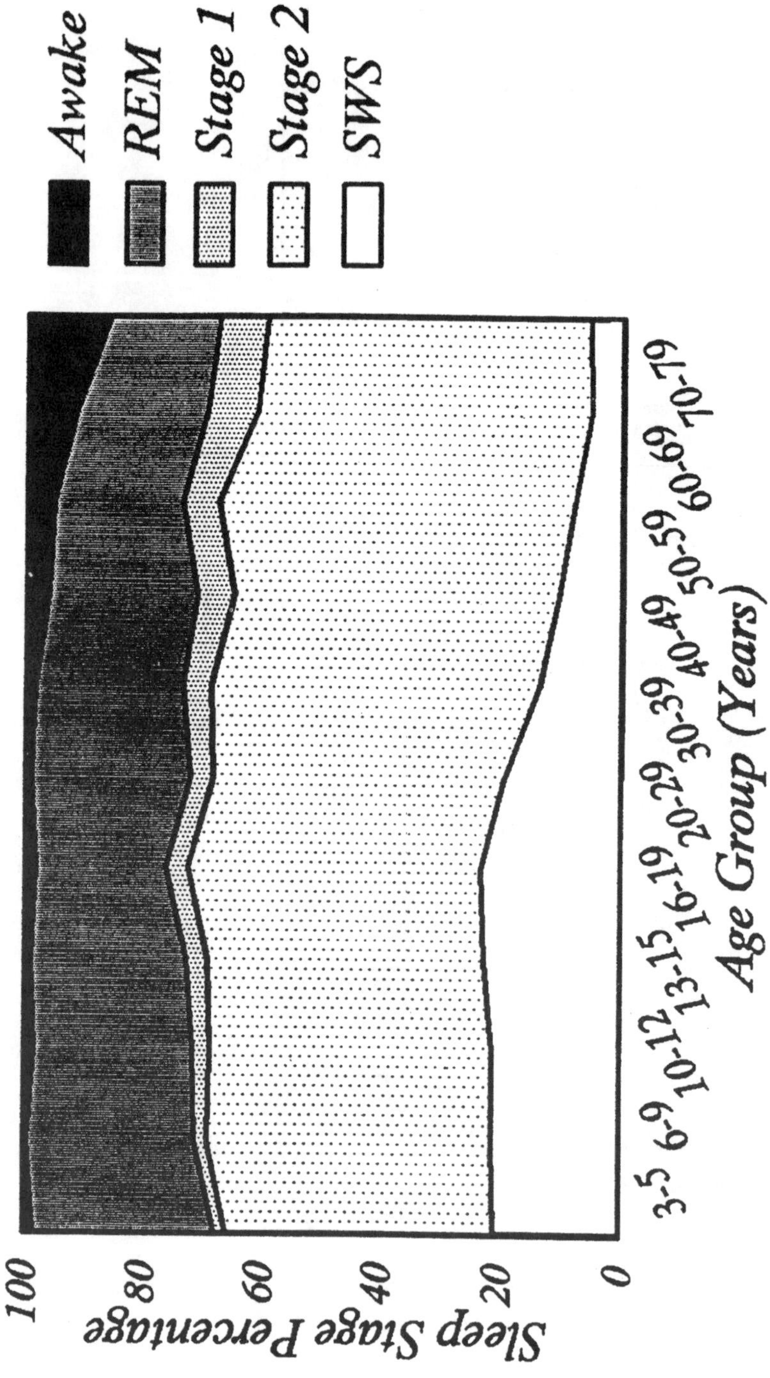

Figure 6. Changes in sleep stage percentages as a function of age. Stage W (awake), rapid eye movement sleep, Stage 1, Stage 2, and slow wave sleep characteristically associated with aging are illustrated.

at adult levels. Sex differences in sleep pattern are minimal, especially in younger age groups. After adolescence, SWS begins to decline and may eventually disappear with advancing age (Hirshkowitz et al., 1992; Miles & Dement, 1980; Roffwarg, Muzio, & Dement, 1966; Williams et al., 1974).

Total sleep time declines throughout the life span, and after middle age, wakefulness intermixed with sleep (fragmentation) begins to increase in many individuals. Sleep fragmentation may arise secondary to other medical disorders, as a side effect of medication, or specifically as a result of a sleep disorder. Common dyssomnias afflicting the elderly include various insomnias, sleep-disordered breathing, and sleep-related movement disorders. Aging can exaggerate sleep pattern differences between women and men. These differences may relate to general health issues and the differential sex ratio for some sleep disorders (Ancoli-Israel, Kripke, Mason, & Messin, 1981; Webb, 1974).

How is Sleep Regulated?

There are significant nonpathological individual differences in sleep. Some people are naturally long sleepers, whereas others are short sleepers. Although sleep requirement does not appear to correlate with intelligence, several investigators have reported personality differences between long and short sleepers (Hartmann, Baekeland, & Zwilling, 1972). In general, long sleepers tend to be more introverted and creative, whereas short sleepers are more extroverted and concrete. The reason some people require less sleep than others remains unclear. However, differences likely stem from an interplay of the three principal factors coordinating sleep and wakefulness: autonomic nervous system balance, homeostatic drive for sleep, and circadian rhythm.

Autonomic Nervous System Balance

Sleep is associated with an overall change in autonomic nervous system (ANS) balance toward parasympathetic dominance. Whereas parasympathetic activation increases, sympathetic outflow mostly declines (Parmeggiani, 1994). Experimental anterior hypothalamic and preoptic area stimulation produces parasympathetic signs, including decreased heart rate, decreased blood pressure, and pupillary miosis.

Stimulation of these parasympathetic centers in animals also produces electroencephalographic and behavioral signs of sleep. The opposite activity constellation results from stimulation of the sympathetic regulatory centers of the midbrain reticular formation and posterior hypothalamus. In discussing autonomic activity in sleep, Parmeggiani (1994) declared that "a prevalence of parasympathetic activity is the autonomic hallmark of the state."

Increases in sympathetic outflow carry a potential for disturbing sleep. It does not seem to matter whether these increases arise from endogenous or exogenous sources. Common endogenous causes of sleep disruption include fear, anxiety, worry, muscle tension, and pain. Exogenous sleep-disturbing sympathetic influences include ingestion of stimulants, excessive heat, and sudden or intrusive noise.

Two important characteristics of ANS activity are particularly relevant to sleep disruption. First, many autonomically mediated responses are amenable to classical conditioning. Pairing a stimulus cue with a stimulus that automatically evokes a response leads to conditioned reactivity to the stimulus cue. Just as Pavlov's dog salivated to a bell after the sound was paired with food, humans can react autonomically to stimuli present in the bedroom environment. For example, if the bed is repeatedly associated with frustrating, anxiety-provoking, and unsuccessful attempts to sleep, insomnia may become conditioned (Hauri & Fisher, 1986).

The second ANS characteristic especially relevant to sleeplessness is related to the long refractory period following sympathetic nervous system activation. An evoked sympathetic response does not immediately dissipate when the threat is removed. The classic example is the response produced in a bystander when someone nearby unexpectedly pulls out a gun for no apparent reason. The evoked autonomic arousal does not vanish rapidly even when the gun is shown to be merely a plastic toy. Once sympathetic arousal has occurred, it may take a while before the sleep-promoting autonomic balance returns.

Homeostatic Drive for Sleep

Prolonged wakefulness produces sleep debt. In general, the longer individuals remain awake, the sleepier they become (Carskadon & Dement, 1981). Hypothalamic regulation of sleepiness is similar to that for thirst, hunger, and sex. These motivational states direct behavioral systems to perform actions to reduce drive. Drive reduction should not be misinterpreted as indicating function. The purpose of sleep is not to relieve sleepiness, just as the purpose of eating is not to relieve hunger. The drive state serves to mobilize a behavior that will satisfy underlying requirements. In the case of sleepiness, the behavior is to cease activity.

Homeostatic mechanisms help regulate both sleep in general and the specific stages of sleep. When an individual is selectively deprived of REM sleep, an "REM debt" accrues. If a person is given the opportunity subsequently to sleep without disturbance, REM sleep rebounds above normal levels (Dement, 1960). SWS has a similar compensatory response to selective deprivation. These findings suggest that there are specialized functional brain requirements for different types of sleep.

When one attempts continuous, uninterrupted wakefulness, sleep eventually becomes irresistible. However, during a prolonged vigil, sleepiness waxes and wanes. Sometimes after staying up all night, the chronobiological self-abuser notes a surge of energy at daybreak. This exception to the homeostatic mechanism of a continually increasing sleep debt is due to the presence of another factor regulating sleep and wakefulness: the circadian rhythm.

Circadian Rhythm

The circadian rhythm is superimposed on the homeostatic effects produced by sustained wakefulness. The term *circadian* derives from the Latin *circa*, meaning "approximately" and *dian* meaning "day." The oscillatory period of the circadian pacemaker is usually between 24 and 26 hours (Moore-Ede, Sulzman, & Fuller, 1982; Webb, 1982). The circadian pacemaker is one of the many biological clocks regulating physiological activity and behavior. Currently, the seat of the circadian timekeeping is thought to be located in the suprachiasmatic nucleus (Sleep Research Society, 1993). The firing patterns of this nucleus also correlate with daily fluctuation in core body temperature. It is interesting that the nucleus firing patterns persist even in physiologically isolated brain preparations.

Temperature cycle is often used as a marker of circadian rhythm. Studies of the temperature rhythm have indicated that maximum alertness occurs near the peak. When temperature starts to fall, drowsiness ensues, and when it reaches nadir, sleepiness can be overwhelming. As temperature starts to rise, sleepiness decreases and alertness increases. The cycle begins again when temperature again reaches maximum.

Lack of synchrony between this biological rhythm and the scheduled bedtime can impair nocturnal sleep (sometimes producing insomnia) and diurnal alertness (sometimes causing hypersomnolence). Under extreme conditions in which individuals are deprived of cues indicating time of day, the sleep–wake cycle and the temperature rhythm dissociate. Studies performed in caves, bunkers, and chronobiology research laboratories also have indicated that most adults exhibit features of a delayed sleep phase. The sleep–wake cycle, in the absence of time cues, drifts to a later and later period on each successive day. These data present a riddle. If the circadian pacemaker usually runs slow, how can it maintain accurate timing?

Recent work suggests that, under normal circumstances, the human circadian rhythm is reset daily by bright light. Moreover, the biological clock can be stopped and reset with precise timing of bright light exposure. The use of bright light exposure to overcome desynchrony between environmental and biological clocks produced by *jet lag*, shift work, and space travel represents an intriguing frontier in sleep research (Czeisler et al., 1986).

In addition to the sleep–wake circadian cycle, many other biological rhythms exist. Some are circadian, and some are ultradian (cycling faster than 24 hr); some are sleep-state-dependent, and others are sleep-state-independent. Neuroendocrine rhythms have been studied, and their secretory patterns differ (Anch et al., 1988; Mendelson, 1987; Orem & Barnes, 1980). Growth hormone release is strikingly sleep-state-dependent and, under normal circumstances, is tightly coupled to SWS (Takahashi, Kipnis, & Daughaday, 1968). Human growth hormone release peaks early in the night and rises in conjunction with, and depends on, the occurrence of SWS. By contrast, plasma cortisol and adrenocorticotropic hormone release are sleep-state-independent daily rhythms; these levels drop throughout the day and are suppressed in the first hour or more of sleep. Approximately 3–5 hours after sleep onset an increase occurs, and levels may rise until awakening. Prolactin levels rise 60–90 minutes after sleep onset and peak in the last 1–2 hours of the sleep period. Prolactin release appears to be sleep-dependent and shifts when sleep stages shift. Testosterone levels are also stage-specific. In men, testosterone levels peak several times during the night. Peak values occur proximal to the onset of REM sleep episodes.

Why Do We Sleep?

Sleep is necessary to sustain life. Laboratory animals deprived of sleep die (Rechtschaffen, Bergmann, Everson, Kushida, & Gilliland, 1989) and, presumably, so would humans. Many sleep disorders are life threatening, either directly (as in fatal familial insomnia and obstructive sleep apnea) or indirectly (as a result of sleep-related motor vehicle accidents).

The 1959–1960 American Cancer Society survey of more than 1 million Americans included several questions related to sleep habits. Results revealed increased mortality rates for individuals who habitually sleep significantly more or less than a norm of 7–8 hours per night. For example, men who were 30 years or older and slept less than 4 hours per night had a 6-year follow-up death rate 2.8 times higher than those who slept 7–8 hours per night. For women, the comparable short-sleeper 6-year mortality ratio was 1.5 (Kripke, Simons, Garfinkel, & Hammond, 1979). Early studies were criticized because fatal diseases commonly produce insomnia. Wingard and Berkman (1983) conducted a 9-year follow-up evaluation in 4,713 individuals, with disease and age controlled. They found a similar pattern. Rates adjusted for age and comorbidity showed that persons sleeping 6 hours or less or 9 hours or more per night had a 30% higher death rate than those sleeping 7–8 hours per night. Even in subgroups reporting no health problems, short-sleeper death rates were 1.8 times higher than death rates for normal sleepers. However, knowing what happens when people do not sleep does not mean scientists can explain the function of sleep.

Even if one accepts the overarching role of sleep in sustaining life, the manner by which it accomplishes this feat remains an unanswered question. The debate concerning the purpose of sleep is ongoing and has spawned several theories. Each theory weaves an explanation of the function of sleep from common observations and research findings. However, no single model explains enough data to be truly satisfying. When carefully considered, the reasons for this lack are readily apparent. First, sleep research is a field in its infancy. Furthermore, the function of any behavior, cognition, or emotion is difficult to prove scientifically, and sleep is no exception. Research tends toward converging reductionism, whereas the question of function is divergent. Until the last quarter of this century, few tools were available to investigate brain functions rigorously. Advances in neurophysiology, neuropharmacology, and imaging techniques will facilitate answering many basic questions. Finally, a theory concerning the function of any dynamic process must satisfactorily integrate multiple internal and external influences. Notwithstanding these obstacles, several prominent theories exist; they are briefly summarized in the paragraphs that follow.

The *adaptive theory* proposes that sleep increases an animal's survival probability (Meddis, 1977; Webb, 1975). Survival encompasses feeding, other predatory behaviors, and avoiding danger. Support for this theory derives from the observation that species differ with respect to their sleep–wake cycle and that each cycle seems, at face value, adaptive for the species' biological niche. For example, visually oriented creatures without highly adapted night vision become relatively immobile when the sun goes down; otherwise, they may become food.

The *energy conservation theory* emphasizes overall decreased metabolism during sleep. Zeplin and Rechtschaffen (1974) described a relationship between metabolic rate and sleep duration. Animals with high metabolic rates sleep longer than those that burn energy more slowly. These same authors pointed out, however, that a 200-pound individual achieves an approximate net savings of merely 120 calories by sleeping 8 hours rather than remaining in a state of relaxed wakefulness (Zeplin, 1994). The major challenge of the energy conservation theory, therefore, is to explain how such an inefficient process evolved.

The *restorative theory of sleep* forwards perhaps the most intuitive explanation of sleep's function. Indeed, Shakespeare called sleep "the great restorer." Although researchers argue over details, the idea that sleep plays a critical role in revitalization is seldom doubted. Neural mechanisms suggested to underlie sleep-related restoration include neutralization of accumulated neurotoxins, responses to increased wakefulness-related sleep-inducing substances, neurochemical synthesis, and redistribution of brain chemicals (Drucker-Colin, 1979; Hartmann, 1973; Kleitman, 1963). Furthermore, different restorative functions have been advanced for SWS and REM sleep.

The belief that tissue restitution occurs during slow wave sleep derives from several sources (Adam & Oswald, 1977). It has been reported that increased tissue synthesis, cell division, and growth hormone release occur during SWS. Also, some data show that athletes have increased SWS. SWS-related declines in oxygen consumption suggest decreased catabolism. Starvation is followed by increased SWS, suggesting a compensatory mechanism. Patients with hyperthyroidism have increased SWS (Dunleavy, Oswald, Brown, & Strong, 1974), whereas patients with hypothyroidism have reduced SWS (Kales, et al., 1967). Finally, SWS is high during children's peak developmental years and declines (or can even disappear) with advancing age.

Even before the discovery of REM sleep, Hughlings Jackson proposed that sleep both clears unimportant information from memory and consolidates more important experience. The modernized version of this conceptualization is called the *programming–reprogramming hypothesis* (Dewan, 1968). This theory receives support from the fact that infants, whose brains are presumably engaged in intense programming during early development, have more than twice as much sleep as adults, a large proportion of which is REM sleep. Recent theories focus more sharply on the possibility that REM sleep restoration subserves memory and intellectual functions. In adults, studies indicate an increase in REM sleep during periods associated with intense learning (Smith & Lapp, 1991). Additionally, decreased creative problem solving accompanies REM sleep deprivation, suggesting a role for REM sleep in higher cortical function, particularly divergent thinking (Horne, 1988).

Horne (1988) critically reviewed the evidence on which the tissue restitution theory is built. He argued that adequate food intake and rest, not sleep, are critical for growth and repair. Moreover, he concluded that interpretations of increased cell division and growth hormone release are misleading, noting also that sleep deprivation does not cause physical illness. Nonetheless, he endorsed the core concept that the cerebrum needs sleep. Webb (1988) also critiqued sleep function hypotheses, offering a hybrid adaptive–restorative–behavioral conceptualization. The behavioral portion of this model postulates that an individual may modify sleep time, duration, or both, according to changing environmental and endogenous factors.

Conclusion

The brain requires sleep to function properly. The importance of sleep is poorly recognized by the general public. The National Commission on Sleep Disorders Research (1993) reported to Congress that more than 100 Americans die on the nation's highway each day from sleep-related motor vehicle accidents. The direct yearly cost of sleep disorders to the taxpayer is estimated at $15.8 billion. Investigations have linked many major industrial catastrophes to sleeplessness and consequent sleepiness. Excessive sleepiness is a serious, potentially life-threatening condition that affects not only individuals but also families, coworkers, and society in general.

Unfortunately, the clinical community, like the general public, is uninformed about sleep and sleep disorders. Although individuals afflicted with sleep problems may desperately seek help, they commonly meet with ignorance, indifference, or both. A study conducted by the National Commission on Sleep Disorders Research (Rosen, Rosekind, Rosevear, Cole, & Dement, 1993) indicated that medical students receive, on average, less than 2 hours of training in sleep medicine. Additionally, less than 1 hour of training was provided by more than half of the medical schools surveyed. This pattern of neglect requires correction. Understanding sleep psychology, physiology, and pathophysiology is clinically relevant, useful, and important for all health care practitioners.

REFERENCES

Adam, K., & Oswald, I. (1977). Sleep is for tissue restoration. *Journal of the Royal College of Physicians, 11*, 376–388.

Anch, A. M., Browman, C. P., Mitler, M. M., & Walsh, J. K. (1988). *Sleep: A scientific perspective.* Englewood Cliffs, NJ: Prentice-Hall.

Ancoli-Israel, S., Kripke, D. F., Mason, W., & Messin, S. (1981). Sleep apnea and nocturnal myoclonus in a senior population. *Sleep, 4*, 349–358.

Aserinsky, E., & Kleitman, N. (1953). Regularly occurring periods of eye motility, and concomitant phenomena during sleep. *Science, 118*, 273–274.

Berger, H. (1929). Ueber das elecktroenkephalogramm des menschen. *Arch Psychiatr Nervenber, 87*, 527–570.

Carskadon, M. A., & Dement, W. C. (1981). Cumulative effects of sleep restriction on daytime sleepiness. *Psychophysiology, 18*, 107–113.

Carskadon, M. A., & Dement, W. C. (1994). Normal human sleep: An overview. In M. H. Kryger, T. Roth, & W. C. Dement (Eds.), *Principles and practice of sleep medicine* (pp. 16–25). Philadelphia: Saunders.

Carskadon, M. A., & Rechtschaffen, A. (1994). Monitoring and staging human sleep. In M. H. Kryger, T. Roth, & W. C. Dement (Eds.), *Principles and practice of sleep medicine* (pp. 943–960). Philadelphia: Saunders.

Czeisler, C. A., Allan, J. S., Strogatz, S. H., Ronda, J. M., Sanchez, R., Rios, C. D., Freitag, W. O., Richardson, G. S., & Kronauer, R. E. (1986). Bright light resets the human circadian pacemaker independent of the timing of the sleep-wake cycle. *Science, 233*, 667–671.

Dement, W. (1960). The effect of dream deprivation. *Science, 131*, 1705–1707.

Dewan E. (1968). The P (programming) hypothesis for REMS. *Psychophysiology, 5*, 365–366.

Drucker-Colin, R. (1979). Protein molecules and the regulation of REM sleep: Possible implications for function. In R. Drucker-Colin, M. Shkurovich, & M. B. Sterman (Eds.), *The functions of sleep* (pp. 99–111). New York: Academic Press.

Dunleavy, D. L. F., Oswald, I., Brown, P., & Strong, J. A. (1974). Hyperthyroidism, sleep and growth hormone. *Electroencephalography Clinical Neurophysiology, 36,* 259–263.

Ellman, S. J., & Antrobus, J. S. (1991). *The mind in sleep.* New York: Wiley.

Freud, S. (1950). *The interpretation of dreams.* New York: Random House.

Hall, C. S. (1953). *The meaning of dreams.* New York: Harper & Row.

Hartmann, E. (1973). *The functions of sleep.* New Haven, CT: Yale University Press.

Hartmann, E., Baekeland, R., & Zwilling, G. (1972). Psychological differences between long and short sleepers. *Archives of General Psychiatry, 26,* 463–468.

Hauri, P., & Fisher, J. (1986). Persistent psychophysiologic (learned) insomnia. *Sleep, 9,* 38–53.

Herman, J. H., Erman, M., Boys, R., Peiser, L., Taylor, M. E., & Roffwarg, H. P. (1984). Evidence for a directional correspondence between eye movements and dream imagery in REM sleep. *Sleep, 7,* 52–63.

Hirshkowitz, M., Moore, C. A., Hamilton, C. R., Rando, K. C., & Karacan, I. (1992). Polysomnography of adults and elderly: Sleep architecture, respiration, and leg movements. *Journal of Clinical Neurophysiology, 9,* 56–63.

Hobson, J. A., & McCarley, R. W. (1977). The brain as a dream state generator: An activation-synthesis hypothesis of the dream process. *American Journal of Psychiatry, 134,* 1335–1348.

Horne, J. (1988). *Why we sleep.* Oxford, England: Oxford University Press.

Kales, A., Heuser, G., Jacobson, A., Kales, J. D., Hanley, J., Zweizig, J. R., & Paulson, M. M. (1967). All-night sleep studies in hypothyroid patients before and after treatment. *Journal of Clinical Endocrinology, 27,* 1593–1599.

Kleitman, N. (1963). *Sleep and wakefulness* (Rev. ed.). Chicago: University of Chicago Press.

Kripke, D. F., Simons, R. N., Garfinkel, L., & Hammond, E. C. (1979). Short and long sleep and sleeping pills: Is increased mortality associated? *Archives of General Psychiatry, 36,* 103–116.

Loomis, A. L., Harvey, E. N., & Hobart, G. A. (1937). Cerebral states during sleep, as studied by human brain potentials. *Journal of Experimental Psychology, 21,* 127–145.

McCarley, R. W. (1994). Neurophysiology of sleep: Basic mechanisms underlying control of wakefulness and sleep. In S. Chokroverty (Ed.), *Sleep disorders medicine: Basic science, technical considerations, and clinical aspects* (pp. 17–36). Boston: Butterworth-Heinemann.

Meddis, R. (1977). *The sleep instinct.* London: Routledge & Kegan Paul.

Mendelson, W. B. (1987). *Human sleep: Research and clinical care.* New York: Plenum Press.

Miles, L. E., & Dement, W. C. (1980). Sleep and aging. *Sleep, 3,* 119–220.

Moore-Ede, M. C., Sulzman, F. M., & Fuller, C. F. (1982). *The clocks that time us.* Cambridge, MA: Harvard University Press.

Naitoh, P., Antony-Baas, V., Muzet, A., & Ehrhart, J. (1982). Dynamic relation of sleep spindles and K-complexes to spontaneous phasic arousals in sleeping human subjects. *Sleep, 5,* 58–72.

National Commission on Sleep Disorders Research. (1993). Wake up America: A national sleep alert: Vol. 1. Executive summary and executive report. Washington, DC: Author.

Orem, J., & Barnes, C. D. (Eds). (1980). *Physiology in sleep.* New York: Academic Press.

Parmeggiani, P. L. (1994). The autonomic nervous system in sleep. In M. H. Kryger, T. Roth, & W. C. Dement (Eds.), *Principles and practice of sleep medicine* (pp. 194–203). Philadelphia: Saunders.

Rechtschaffen, A., Bergmann, B. M., Everson, C. A., Kushida, C. A., & Gilliland, M. A. (1989). Sleep deprivation in the rat: X. Integration and discussion of the findings. *Sleep, 12,* 68–87.

Rechtschaffen, A., & Kales, A. (1968). *A manual of standardized terminology, techniques, and scoring system for sleep stages of human subjects* (National Institutes of Health Publication No. 204). Washington, DC: U.S. Government Printing Office.

Roffwarg, H. P., Muzio, J. N., & Dement, W. C. (1966). Ontogenetic development of the human sleep-dream cycle. *Science, 152,* 604–619.

Rosen, R. C., Rosekind, M., Rosevear, C., Cole, W. E., & Dement, W. C. (1993). Physician education in sleep and sleep disorders: A national survey of U.S. medical schools. *Sleep, 16,* 249–254.

Sassin, J. F., & Johnson, L. C. (1968). Body motility during sleep and its relation to the K-complex. *Experimental Neurology, 22,* 133–144.

Sleep Research Society. (1993). *Basics of sleep behavior.* Los Angeles: UCLA and the Sleep Research Society.

Smith, C., & Lapp, L. (1991). Increases in number of REMS and REM density in humans following an intensive learning period. *Sleep, 14,* 325–330.

Steriades, M. (1994). Brain electrical activity and sensory processing during waking and sleeping states. In M.H. Kryger, T. Roth, & W.C. Dement (Eds.), *Principles and practice of sleep medicine* (pp. 105–124). Philadelphia: Saunders.

Takahashi, Y., Kipnis, D., & Daughaday, W. (1968). Growth hormone secretion during sleep. *Journal of Clinical Investigation, 47,* 2079–2090.

Webb, W. B. (1975). *Sleep: The gentle tyrant.* Englewood Cliffs, NJ: Prentice-Hall.

Webb, W. B. (1982). Sleep in older persons: Sleep structure of 50- to 60-year-old men and women. *Journal of Gerontology, 37,* 581–586.

Webb, W. B. (1988). An objective behavioral model of sleep. *Sleep, 11,* 488–496.

Williams, R. L., Karacan, I., & Hursch, C. J. (1974). *EEG of human sleep: Clinical applications.* New York: Wiley.

Wingard, D. L., & Berkman, L. F. (1983). Mortality risk associated with sleeping patterns among adults. *Sleep, 6,* 102–107.

Zeplin H. (1994). Mammalian sleep. In M. H. Kryger, T. Roth, & W. C. Dement (Eds.), *Principles and practice of sleep medicine* (pp. 69–80). Philadelphia: Saunders.

Zeplin, H., & Rechtschaffen, A. (1974). Mammalian sleep, longevity, and energy conservation. *Brain, Behavior and Evolution, 10,* 425–470.

2

The Basics
of Biological Rhythms

Scott S. Campbell

B iological rhythms are the events within a biological system that recur at more or less regular intervals (Aschoff, 1981). A common way to classify such rhythms is by the frequency of their recurrence, which can range from several cycles per second to one cycle per several years. It is not surprising that the most predominant biological rhythms are those that occur in coincidence with the geophysical cycle of day and night: the circadian rhythms (*circa* = "about," *dies* = "day").

In response to the natural alternation of light and darkness, most species have developed endogenously mediated rhythms with frequencies close to 24 hours. The pervasive nature of such rhythmicity in physiology and behavior suggests that this circadian (Halberg, 1959) temporal organization is vital to the overall well-being of the organism. Among the numerous systems and functions mediated by the circadian timing system are hormonal output, body core temperature, rest and activity, sleep and wakefulness, and motor and cognitive performance. In all, literally hundreds of circadian rhythms in mammalian species have been identified (e.g., Aschoff, 1981; Conroy & Mills, 1970). Aschoff (1965) noted that "there is apparently no organ

Acknowledgments: This work was supported in part by National Institute of Mental Health Grants (R01 MH45067, K02 MH01099, and P20 MH49762) and a grant from the Tolly Vinik Trust.

and no function in the body which does not exhibit a similar daily rhythmicity" (p. 1427).

Because of the predominance of rhythms that recur about once a day, biological rhythms with longer or shorter frequencies have typically been classified separately; they are called *infradian* or *ultradian* rhythms, respectively. An example of an infradian rhythm is the human menstrual cycle. An example of an ultradian rhythm is the recurrence of REM sleep about every 90 minutes throughout a normal night's sleep. It is rhythms in the circadian range and, to a lesser extent, the ultradian range that are of primary relevance to the topic of this chapter, because the human sleep–wake cycle is primarily a circadian system but with important ultradian components.

This chapter begins with a description of methodology and terms employed in human chronobiological research. Brief overviews of the history of human circadian rhythms research and their biological basis are then presented. The chapter concludes with a discussion of some of the basic principles of chronobiology that have been exploited in the examination and treatment of sleep disturbance in humans.

Measurement and Terminology

Like all subdisciplines within psychology, the study of human biological rhythms has its own language and means of assessment. A fundamental part of understanding human circadian rhythms is becoming familiar with these terms and measurement techniques. Figure 1 illustrates several of the most frequently used terms as they apply to the most commonly measured circadian variable, body core temperature. Why body core temperature? As can be seen from the figure, body temperature is characterized by a robust 24-hour variation. In addition, this is a variable for which it is relatively easy to obtain continuous, sensitive measurement across the 24-hour day. As such, the 24-hour variation in body temperature and its relationship to various aspects of sleep have been topics of investigation for over a century.

Typically, the raw temperature curve obtained across a 24-hour (or longer) period is smoothed using some form of mathematical curve-fitting procedure. By convention, most investigators have used variations of the least-squares cosine fitting technique (e.g., Brown & Czeisler, 1992; Nelson, Tong, Lee, & Halberg, 1979) to obtain three measures that describe basic features of the circadian rhythms: (a) the

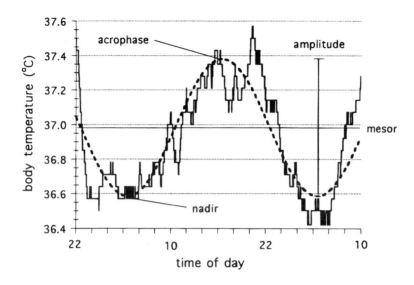

Figure 1. Thirty-six-hour plot of body core temperature, showing smoothed cosine fit and parameters typically employed to describe salient features of the circadian oscillation. *Nadir* and *acrophase* are defined as the minimum and maximum points, respectively, of the fitted curve; *mesor* is the average value of the fitted curve; *amplitude* is defined as the value from peak to trough (or, sometimes, peak to mesor) of the fitted curve.

mesor, or average value of the fitted curve; (b) the *amplitude*, defined as the value from peak to trough of the fitted curve; and (c) the *nadir*, defined as the point on the fitted curve at which the minimum value occurs. Instead of the nadir, some authors choose to report the *acrophase*, which is defined as the point on the fitted curve at which the maximum value occurs. By definition, the nadir and acrophase are 12 hours apart.

The nadir is typically used to designate the phase of the circadian rhythm under investigation. The *phase* of a rhythm describes its occurrence as a function of time, and designation of phase permits one to describe temporal relationships objectively; *phase relationships* are relationships between two or more rhythmic processes or between a circadian rhythm and the 24-hour day. A circadian rhythm is said to be *phase-advanced* when the nadir occurs at an earlier time, relative to a reference point, and it is said to be *phase-delayed* when the nadir occurs at a later time. As I indicate later, this is an important concept in biological rhythms research, because the phase of a rhythm and its temporal relationship to other variables can be altered by various stimuli (e.g., light), and such manipulations often have a significant impact on physiology and behavior.

In addition to the terms just discussed, several additional ones that are employed primarily in studies using the time-free environment (discussed later) should be mentioned. Under these special experimental conditions, in which participants spend days, weeks, or even months in an apartment with no cues to time of day and only limited social contact, their subjective day length is dictated by the endogenous clock. Under these conditions, participants are said to *free-run*, or exhibit *free-running rhythms*. The frequency of the free-running rhythm (i.e., the interval between successive temperature nadirs or some other circadian marker) is referred to as the *free-running period*, or *tau* (t).

Discovery of Circadian Principles

Because of their close link to the solar day, circadian rhythms were long believed to be the product of such environmental cues. The proof that biological rhythms are regulated, instead, by factors inherent to the organism could be derived only from studies of organisms living in the absence of external factors that may provide cues to time of day or, more generally, to the passage of time. The first published study to use this method reported on the daily leaf movements in a plant, *Mimosa pudica* (de Mairan, 1729; cited by Bünning, 1960). Although the plant was kept in total darkness, its leaves continued to exhibit closure and unfolding at times roughly corresponding to dusk and dawn.

The further discovery, a century later, that such leaf movements showed a periodicity close to, but distinctly different from, the natural 24-hour cycle of light and darkness (de Candolle, 1832) provided perhaps the clearest indication that such rhythms are driven by endogenous mechanisms, rather than being the product of environmental stimuli. In the following decades, thousands of investigations established the existence of similar free-running rhythms in species ranging from single-celled organisms to a wide variety of laboratory species. However, another 130 years were to pass before the first attempts were made to study temporal components of human physiology and behavior under analogous experimental conditions.

Human Circadian Rhythms

In the early 1960s, Aschoff and coworkers initiated a series of studies that, over the next 20 years, laid the groundwork for much of what is known today about the human circadian system. (For a comprehensive summary of much of this work, see Aschoff & Wever, 1981; Wever, 1979). All but a few pilot studies were conducted in an underground laboratory consisting of two studio apartments that were free of all environmental cues to time of day. The laboratory was heavily sound-dampened, and the timing and intensity of illumination could be controlled from outside the apartments by the experimenters. In addition, the vast majority of participants were studied in isolation to eliminate possible time cues provided by social contact.

The first experiments conducted in this unique environment (Aschoff, 1965; Aschoff & Wever, 1962) established that adult humans exhibit free-running rhythms of rest and activity averaging slightly longer than 25 hours (see Figure 2). That is, a participant's average "day" continued for about an hour longer than the natural day, although in some people the subjective day continued for a substantially longer period (up to 50 hrs). Participants who thought that they had been in the time-free environment for 3 weeks, for example, were often quite surprised when they were informed that a month or more had elapsed! Further investigations of numerous other systems confirmed that in humans, endogenous daily rhythms tend to free-run at frequencies slightly longer than 24 hours and that all such rhythms typically stay synchronized with one another. (For a complete review, see Moore-Ede, Sulzman, & Fuller, 1982.) This internal organization among rhythms is seen clearly in the usual relationship between the sleep–wake system and the rhythm of body temperature. In the time-free environment, major sleep episodes tend to occur around the low point (nadir) of the temperature rhythm and are terminated several hours after the nadir (see Figure 2). Aschoff and Wever observed remarkable interindividual precision in the period length of the sleep–wake rhythm under these experimental conditions. The average 25-hour rhythms deviated only about 1 half hour between individuals (Wever, 1979).

For any single individual, however, the day-to-day flexibility of the circadian system is both obvious and well documented (Webb & Agnew, 1974). People are not suddenly overcome with sleep at a particular point in their temperature rhythm, and they are not startled awake each morning by a biological alarm clock tied to the temperature

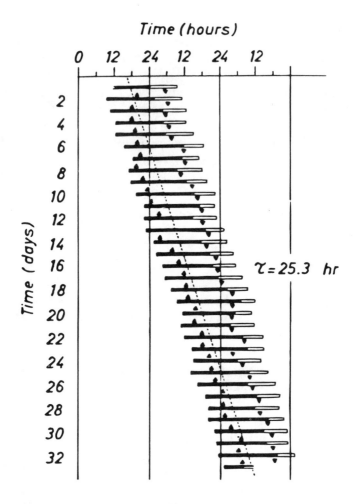

Figure 2. Representation of the free-running rhythms of a 26-year-old male living in a time-free environment for 32 days. Successive circadian periods are shown, one beneath the other, as a function of local time and days in isolation. The free-running period (*t*) in this case was 25.3 hours. Black bars depict activity periods, and open bars represent rest. The maximum (▲) and minimum (▼) of each day's body core temperature are shown as well. From *The Circadian System of Man: Results of Experiments Under Temporal Isolation*, by R. A. Wever, 1979, New York: Springer-Verlag. Reprinted by permission.

cycle. Rather, we routinely shift our bedtimes and wake-up times to accommodate changes in our daily schedules. At the level of individual behavior, therefore, the human circadian system is a "sloppy" system (Campbell, 1984; Campbell & Zulley, 1985, 1989). It is this inherent flexibility in the system that allows our free-running endogenous rhythms to be synchronized, or entrained, by the numerous environmental, behavioral, and social cues that provide the structure of our daily lives.

Napping as a Biological Rhythm

Because most adult humans exhibit a strong propensity to obtain their daily sleep quota in one nightly episode, the human sleep system has traditionally been considered to be monophasic in nature. As illustrated in Figure 2, this assumption seems to be borne out in traditional time-free studies. Although individuals free-run with a period slightly longer than 24 hours, they nevertheless maintain a monophasic sleep–wake organization, with one sleep episode per subjective day. Yet the extent to which such a pattern of sleep and wakefulness is mediated by biology and dictated by societal (or experimental) demands has been questioned (Campbell & Zulley, 1985; Dinges & Broughton, 1989). If the human sleep system is, in fact, monophasic, it would stand as the sole exception to an apparent phylogenetic rule of polyphasic sleep (Campbell & Tobler, 1984). There is now quite convincing evidence, however, that this is not the case. Rather, human sleep is more appropriately viewed as a polyphasic system, with at least two "preferred" phase positions for the occurrence of sleep within the 24-hour day.

In the traditional time-free environment, participants are instructed to lead a "regular" life, that is, to eat three meals in normal sequence and *not* to nap during the subjective day but to sleep only when they are certain that their major sleep period is commencing (e.g., Aschoff, 1965; Weitzman, 1982). In response to such instructions, compliant, well-motivated participants exhibit monophasic, circadian sleep patterns. However, minor changes in experimental instructions result in significant alterations in sleep patterns. Figure 3 shows the frequency of occurrence of sleep episodes taken by a group of study participants living under identical time-free conditions for 72 continuous hours but given the instruction to eat and sleep whenever inclined to do so. Major sleep episodes continue to show a strong propensity to occur in association with the trough of body core temperature, but in addition, under these conditions, there is a marked tendency for a second interval of sleep to occur just before the maximum level of body core temperature is reached. These sleep episodes are differentiated not only by their placement within the 24-hour day but also by their average durations. Sleep periods occurring at about the time of the temperature minimum

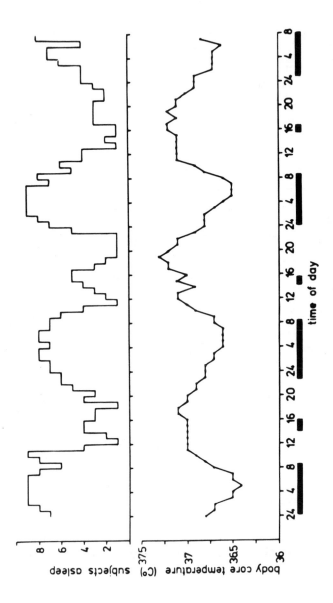

Figure 3. Relationship between sleep episodes and the circadian rhythm of body core temperature recorded in a time-free environment in which individuals were encouraged to eat and sleep whenever inclined to do so. Above the temperature curve (averaged for 9 participants) is a summation histogram of the number of participants asleep during any given hour during the experimental period. Below the temperature curve (black bars) are average onsets and durations of major sleep episodes and naps. From "Ultradian Components of Human Sleep/Wake Patterns During Disentrainment," by S. S. Campbell & J. Zulley, in *Ultradian Rhythms in Physiology and Behavior* (p. 247), ed. by H. Schulz & P. Lavie, 1985, Berlin, Springer-Verlag. Reprinted by permission.

continue for an average of about 8 hours, whereas those initiated at about the maximum are terminated, on average, about 1.5 to 2 hours later. It is clear that under the entrained conditions of normal daily life, the longer sleep episodes correspond to major, nocturnal sleep periods and the shorter sleep episodes correspond to the afternoon sleep periods that we typically refer to as "naps."

The temporal occurrence of sleep and waking episodes is not the only circadian parameter to be influenced by changes in experimental instructions. There is limited evidence to suggest that when individuals are permitted to eat and sleep whenever they wish, rather than asked to follow experimentally circumscribed sleep–wake patterns, the endogenous, free-running period (t) is not 25 hours but, instead, much closer to 24 hours (Campbell, Dawson, & Zulley, 1993; Klerman, Dijk, Czeisler, & Kronauer, 1992). The fact that this fundamental component of circadian rhythmicity is subject to perturbation by behavioral or experimental control serves to emphasize the inherent flexibility of the endogenous circadian timing system. To summarize, both the placement and duration of sleep episodes within the 24-hour day are influenced significantly by the circadian timing system. Although under some circumstances we can sleep at any time, humans exhibit a pronounced tendency to sleep during two specific intervals within the 24-hour day, which are tied to the maximum and minimum levels of body core temperature. How long one is able to maintain a sleep episode depends, in large part, on the phase of the circadian cycle at which the episode is begun. The longest sleep episodes occur in correspondence with the declining portion of the circadian rhythm in body core temperature, and the shortest, with the rising portion. Under normal, entrained conditions, these times correspond to night and day, respectively.

Biological Basis of Circadian Rhythms

At about the time that Aschoff and others were conducting their behavioral studies of human circadian rhythms, Richter (1965) was completing a series of experiments in rats designed to localize the brain areas responsible for circadian rhythm generation. Of the endocrine systems and literally hundreds of brain areas that he experimentally destroyed, only lesions placed in the hypothalamus (see Figure 4) caused alterations in the animals' free-running circadian rhythms (Richter, 1967). Further experiments led to the identification of a more discrete area

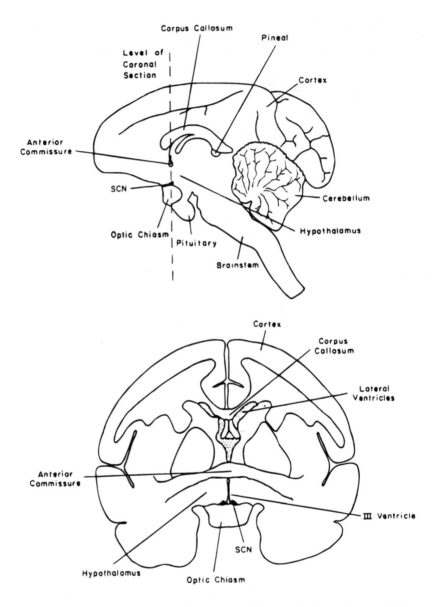

Figure 4. Schematic diagram of the brain of the squirrel monkey: a midline sagittal view (top) and a front view at the plane of the optic chiasm (below). The suprachiasmatic nuclei (SCN) are situated in the hypothalamus directly above the optic chiasm. The SCN are strongly influenced by the environmental light–dark cycle by way of the retinohypothalamic tract and may be influenced by melatonin secretion from the pineal gland. From *The Clocks That Time Us* (p. 156), by M. C. Moore-Ede, F. M. Sulzman, & C. A. Fuller, 1982, Cambridge, MA: Harvard University Press. Reprinted by permission.

within the hypothalamus where ablation caused the total loss of circadian rhythms of feeding, drinking, and activity.

The specific cells involved were subsequently identified by researchers conducting studies to identify neural connections between the visual system and the brain (Moore & Lenn, 1972). On the basis of the knowledge that the daily light–dark cycle is a primary synchronizer of circadian rhythms, Moore and coworkers reasoned that certain retinal projections should terminate in brain areas that control the rhythms. One such projection terminated in the suprachiasmatic nuclei (SCN), and indeed, when these cells were destroyed in laboratory rats, circadian rhythmicity was completely eliminated (Moore & Eichler, 1972; Stephan & Zucker, 1972). Many additional experiments, using numerous techniques (e.g., Inouye & Kawamura, 1979; Lehman et al., 1987; Rusak & Groos, 1982), established in the minds of most scientists that the SCN functions as an endogenously generated circadian pacemaker: a biological clock.

Although it seems certain that the SCN are the locus of a dominant circadian clock, the exact nature and role of the clock remain unclear. A number of studies (e.g., Fuller et al., 1981; Prosser & Satinoff, 1984; Terman & Terman, 1985) have shown that some rhythms actually do persist, often in the ultradian range, following SCN ablation. These findings suggest that there are other brain areas that may have the capacity to function as independent oscillators. For example, rhythmic components of feeding behavior appear to be mediated by areas of the hypothalamus that are separate from the SCN (Mistleberger & Rechtschaffen, 1984; Mistleberger & Rusak, 1989). Similarly, the failure of SCN ablation to affect circadian rhythmicity in visual sensitivity to light in rats (Terman & Terman, 1985) suggests the existence in at least some mammalian species of a retinal pacemaker (Mistleberger & Rusak, 1989).

It has been proposed as well that even the SCN may comprise not one but two or more primary oscillators that are typically joined but may become functionally dissociated under certain conditions. Although a great deal more research is required to clarify the structure and function of the neural mechanisms regulating biological rhythms, the concept of a hierarchy of circadian oscillators, dispersed throughout the brain and possibly other organs (for reviews, see Mistleberger & Rusak, 1989; Moore-Ede et al., 1982), appears to be justified. At least one, and quite possibly several, dominant pacemakers act to synchronize a number of subordinate oscillatory systems to a common frequency. In the absence of influence from the dominant pacemaker or pacemakers, the underlying periodicities of subordinate oscillators may become apparent.

Further research is also required to clarify the role of neuroendocrine systems in circadian regulation; there is a growing body of evidence that various hormones may have a regulatory influence on the timing of circadian rhythms (Mistleberger & Rusak, 1989). Perhaps the most important of these is the system governed by the pineal gland, which serves as the primary locus of melatonin production (for reviews, see Reiter, 1988, 1989). Although the role of melatonin in regulating seasonal reproductive cycles in a number of species has been established, its function in humans remains unclear. Melatonin production is cyclic and is synchronized to the 24-hour environmental light–dark cycle. The recent finding of putative melatonin receptors in the SCN of humans (Reppert, Weaver, Rivkees, & Stopa, 1988) suggests that melatonin may be instrumental in the modulation of entrainment by the light–dark cycle of human circadian rhythms.

Timing of the Circadian System

It was pointed out in a previous section that the human circadian timing system is characterized by a certain degree of lability, or "sloppiness," at least with respect to behavioral expressions of the system (e.g., the timing of sleep and wakefulness). This is by no means a consistent finding across the animal kingdom, however. Rather, the degree of precision with which the timing of circadian rhythms is expressed varies widely across species (Moore-Ede et al., 1982). For example, the hamster exhibits a highly precise circadian rhythm in wheel running, whereas the circadian component of rest–activity in the domestic cat is virtually absent. In addition to differences in precision, there are also species-related variations in free-running period length. A discussion of the complex interactions among species, environmental conditions, physiological state, and other variables that determine period length is beyond the scope of this chapter. However, such differences, as well as those associated with the precision of the timing system, must be considered carefully when inferences are made on the basis of animal studies concerning the nature of human circadian rhythms.

As mentioned earlier, the inherent periodicity of even the most dominant and precise pacemaker becomes apparent only under conditions in which external time cues are completely eliminated, allowing the biological clock to free-run. This is clearly an artificial situation that occurs only under the most stringent laboratory conditions. When circadian rhythms are observed in daily life, out in the real world, they reflect more than the control imposed by a hierarchy of internal pacemakers. They also reveal the powerful influence imposed on the system by factors external to the organism.

Zeitgebers and Entrainment

The term *zeitgeber* (literally, "time giver," in German) was coined by Aschoff (1951) to designate the constellation of external influences that synchronize, or entrain, the endogenous circadian system to an exact frequency. Other terms that are synonymous with zeitgeber include *time cue, synchronizer, entrainer,* and *entraining agent.* Without question, the geophysical cycle of day and night provides the strongest zeitgeber for virtually all organisms. However, other factors, such as ambient temperature, food availability, and physical activity and social cues, have also been demonstrated to entrain endogenous rhythms effectively.

Entrainment does not occur abruptly following the introduction of a zeitgeber. Rather, the circadian system adjusts to new entrainment schedules gradually, with the various overt rhythms (e.g., sleep–wakefulness, body temperature, performance efficiency) often requiring different lengths of time to become fully synchronized to the new time cues. A dramatic yet commonly experienced example of this process of reentrainment is jet lag. Only after about 8 days do the rhythms become resynchronized to one another and entrained to the new zeitgebers (primarily, local time and social cues).

The sleep–wake system, although not one of the measures shown in the figure, is also significantly affected by the shift to newly timed zeitgebers. Because the daily timing of the sleep–wake rhythm is in large part a behavior dictated by social constraints, bedtimes and rising times are often immediately entrained to the new zeitgeber. That is, people choose to time sleep in the new environment to coincide with local time. However, both subjective reports and objective electroencephalographic (EEG) findings indicate that actual sleep time is reduced and sleep quality is drastically compromised during the reentrainment process (Akerstedt, 1985; Dement, Seidel, Cohen, Bliwise, & Carskadon, 1986; Graeber, Dement, Nicholson, Sasaki, & Wegmann, 1986; Graeber, Lauber, Connell, & Gander, 1986; Sasaki, Kurosaki, Mori, & Endo, 1986; Wegmann et al., 1986). As with the other circadian variables discussed, more than a week may be required for sleep to become fully entrained to a shift in the timing of zeitgebers. (For a review, see Winget, DeRoshia, Markley, & Holley, 1984.)

Entrainment by Light and Other External Stimuli

Exposure to environmental light provides one of the strongest natural entraining influences for the human circadian system. Inadequate exposure to light of sufficient intensity has been suggested as a contributing factor in some disorders associated with biological rhythm disturbance, such as seasonal affective disorder. Timed exposure to bright light has been used successfully to treat such disorders (Jacobsen, Wehr, Skwerer, Sack, & Rosenthal, 1987; Lewy, Sack, Miller, & Hoban, 1987; Lewy, Sack, & Singer, 1985; Rosenthal et al., 1984; Sack et al. 1990; Wehr et al., 1986), and timed exposure to light intensities of greater than about 4000 lux has been shown to affect significantly the range of entrainment and phase of circadian rhythms in normal healthy people living in time-free environments (Wever, Polasek, & Wildgruber, 1983). In addition, bright light improves entrainment of the circadian system to non-24-hour schedules in normal people living at home (Eastman & Miescke, 1990), and it is effective in shifting the phase of body core temperature under entrained, laboratory conditions (Czeisler et al., 1989; Dawson & Campbell, 1991; Dijk, Beersma, Daan, & Lewy, 1989) and in the field (Campbell, Dawson, & Anderson, 1993).

This phase-shifting property of bright light exposure has received increasing attention in the past decade as part of an effort to treat sleep–wake disorders thought to involve circadian rhythm abnormalities, such as jet lag, delayed and advanced sleep phase syndrome, and sleep disturbance associated with shift work. By resetting the circadian clock to a more appropriate phase relative to the desired sleep time, improved sleep quality is often achieved.

In many mammals, a pulse of light lasting on the order of minutes is sufficient to induce a circadian phase shift. In humans, however, it appears that substantially longer exposure intervals are required to achieve measurable phase shifts. Likewise, light of considerably higher intensity is required to affect the human circadian system than to induce phase shifts in nonhuman mammals. Primarily because of these differences in the human response to light, the impact of light on the human circadian system was not fully appreciated until 1980, when Lewy and coworkers (Lewy, Wehr, Goodwin, Newsome, & Markey,

1980) demonstrated that light with an intensity of greater than about 2000 lux effectively reduced nighttime melatonin output to daytime levels. Since the publication of this important finding, there has been an explosion in research concerning both basic and clinical aspects of light exposure in humans.

The use of bright light exposure as a therapeutic tool is based on the knowledge that the circadian timing system is differentially sensitive to the influence of light, depending on the phase at which the light stimulus is presented. A light stimulus can cause a phase advance, a phase delay, or no measurable phase shift at all, depending on the time of day the light exposure occurs. This temporally mediated, differential sensitivity to a stimulus can be graphically depicted as a *phase response curve*. Although slight variations exist in the manner in which various species respond to bright light stimuli, general characteristics of the phase response curve are the same for all mammals, including humans.

The Phase Response to Light in Humans

Figure 5 shows a generic phase response curve (PRC) to light. Much of the PRC is composed of an interval during which light exposure causes no perturbation of the circadian clock. That is, light exposure during this interval results in no phase shift. As might be expected, this period corresponds to usual daytime hours, when the likelihood of natural exposure to bright light is high. It clearly would have been maladaptive if our ancestors' endogenous clocks were reset each time they ventured outside their caves during the day. During the first portion of the night, bright light exposure induces phase delays, the magnitude of the shift becoming larger as the night progresses. Then, at a critical point (in humans, corresponding closely to the nadir of body core temperature), light exposure induces not phase delays but, instead, phase advances, the magnitude of the shift becoming *smaller* as the stimulus moves away from this point of inflection. The largest phase delays *and* the largest phase advances are achieved, therefore, when a light stimulus is presented within a relatively narrow time window, centered around the body temperature minimum.

Entrainment by Other Stimuli

Recently, a human phase response curve for melatonin has been established (Lewy, Ahmed, Jackson, & Sack, 1992), which raises the possibility that oral administration of this hormone may also be employed in the

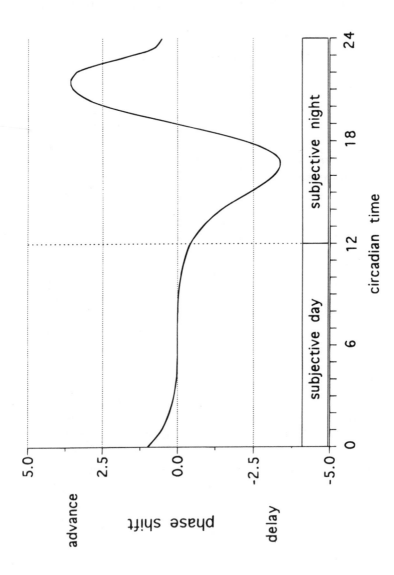

Figure 5. Schematic representation of a phase response curve (PRC) to light. Circadian rhythms may be phase-delayed, phase-advanced, or unaffected by the stimulus, depending on the time of presentation.

treatment of circadian rhythm disturbances. The shape of the PRC for melatonin is essentially a mirror image of that for light, with the largest phase advances being observed following afternoon–evening administration and the largest phase delays occurring after early morning administration. Although the magnitude of the phase shifts obtained with melatonin administration are reduced by a factor of about 10 relative to those achieved with bright light exposure, preliminary studies indicate that timed melatonin administration may promote circadian readjustment in rotating shift workers (Sack, Blood, & Lewy, 1994). Likewise, there is some evidence that melatonin administration may be beneficial in the treatment of jet lag (e.g., Arendt, Aldhous, & Marks, 1986; Arendt & Marks, 1983, 1986).

Other nonphotic zeitgebers include food availability, ambient temperature, physical activity, and social cues. Although these putative entraining agents have been studied extensively in nonhumans, less is known about their influence on the human circadian system. It is surprising that this is the case for social cues, as well. Only one study has specifically examined the strength of social cues as a zeitgeber in humans (Aschoff et al., 1971), and the results of that study are open to alternative interpretations. The finding that some blind individuals living in society continue to exhibit free-running rhythms also raises questions regarding the zeitgeber strength of social cues for the human circadian system.

Conclusion

It needs to be kept in mind that the systematic study of human biological rhythms is a relatively recent endeavor, with virtually all studies having been conducted in the last 30 years. As in any young discipline, there is a strong likelihood that many of the current ideas about how the circadian system functions will undergo revision and reinterpretation, as experimental inquiries become more detailed and investigational tools become more sophisticated. This is likely to be the case with respect to both the way in which the endogenous clock influences physiology and behavior and the manner in which endogenous and external factors influence the clock.

Nevertheless, important strides have been made during the last 3 decades in our understanding of the mechanisms underlying the system of temporal organization that forms the basis of daily life, as well as the impact that this temporal structure has on the regulation of sleep and wakefulness. With regard to sleep, it can be argued that the integration of the study of biological rhythms with sleep research has been as important to the understanding of the nature of sleep as has the development of polysomnography. Whereas EEG permitted detailed examination of sleep's infrastructure, the discovery of a strong circadian contribution to sleep regulation has led to the development of theoretical models that provide a more comprehensive framework within which to view sleep–wake behavior and physiology (Borbely, 1982; Daan, Beersma, & Borbely, 1984).

Moreover, the elucidation of circadian principles of sleep regulation has been indispensable not only to the understanding of many types of sleep disturbance but also to their effective treatment (see chapter 3). For example, the use of timed bright light exposure or melatonin administration to treat some forms of insomnia is the direct result of (a) the identification of related circadian rhythm disturbance in these sleep disorders and (b) the realization that the human circadian system responds to these external stimuli in a phase-response manner. As the understanding of the intimate relationship between the endogenous circadian timing system and sleep–wake regulation continues to grow, more such innovative applications in the treatment of sleep–wake disorders are sure to follow.

REFERENCES

Akerstedt, T. (1985). Shifted sleep hours. *Annals of Clinical Research, 17,* 273–279.

Arendt, J., Aldhous, M., & Marks, V. (1986). Alleviation of jet lag by melatonin: Preliminary results of controlled double blind trial. *British Medical Journal* [Clinical Research], *292,* 476.

Arendt, J., & Marks, V. (1983). Can melatonin alleviate jet lag? [Letter]. *British Medical Journal* [Clinical Research], *287,* 426.

Arendt, J., & Marks, V. (1986). Jet lag and melatonin [Letter]. *Lancet, 2,* 698–699.

Aschoff (1951): Die 24-stunden Periodik der Maus unter konstanten umgebungs bedingungen. ["The 24-hour period of the mouse under constant environmental conditions."] *Naturwissenschaften, 38,* 506–507.

Aschoff, J. (1965). Circadian rhythms in man. *Science, 148,* 1427–1432.

Aschoff, J. (Ed.). (1981). *Biological rhythms.* New York: Plenum Press.

Aschoff, J., Fatranska, M., Giedke, H., Doerr, P., Stamm, D., & Wisser, H. (1971). Human circadian rhythms in continuous darkness: Entrainment by social cues. *Science, 171,* 213–215.

Aschoff, J., & Wever, R. (1962). Spontanperiodik des Menschen bei Ausschluss aller Zeitgeber. ["Spontaneous period of humans in the absence of time cues."] *Naturwissenschaften, 49,* 337–342.

Aschoff, J., & Wever, R. (1981). The circadian system of man. In J. Aschoff (Ed.), *Handbook of behavioral neurobiology* (pp. 311–331). New York: Plenum Press.

Borbely, A. A. (1982). A two process model of sleep regulation. *Human Neurobiology, 1,* 195–204.

Brown, E. N., & Czeisler, C. A. (1992). The statistical analysis of circadian phase and amplitude in constant-routine core-temperature data. *Journal of Biological Rhythms, 7,* 177–202.

Bünning, E. (1960). Opening address: Biological clocks. *Cold Spring Harbor Symposia on Quantitative Biology, 25,* 1–9.

Campbell, S. S. (1984). Duration and placement of sleep in a "disentrained" environment. *Psychophysiology, 21*(1), 106–113.

Campbell, S. S., Dawson, D., & Anderson, M. (1993). Alleviation of sleep maintenance insomnia with timed exposure to bright light. *Journal of the American Geriatric Society, 41,* 829–836.

Campbell, S. S., Dawson, D., & Zulley, J. (1993). When the human circadian system is caught napping: Evidence for endogenous rhythms close to 24 hours. *Sleep, 16,* 638–640.

Campbell, S. S., & Tobler, I. (1984). Animal sleep: A review of sleep duration across phylogeny. *Neuroscience and Biobehavioral Reviews, 8,* 269–300.

Campbell, S. S., & Zulley, J. (1985). Ultradian components of human sleep/wake patterns during disentrainment. In H. Schulz & P. Lavie (Eds.), *Ultradian rhythms in physiology and behavior* (pp. 234–255). Berlin: Springer-Verlag.

Campbell, S. S., & Zulley, J. (1989). Napping in time-free environments. In D. F. Dinges & R. J. Broughton (Eds.), *Sleep and alertness: Chronobiological, behavioral, and medical aspects of napping* (pp. 121–138). New York: Raven Press.

Conroy, R. T., & Mills, J. N. (1970). *Human circadian rhythms.* London: Churchill.

Czeisler, C. A., Kronauer, R. E., Allan, J. S., Duffy, J. F., Jewett, M. E., Brown, E. N., & Ronda, J. M. (1989). Bright light induction of strong (type 0) resetting of the human circadian pacemaker. *Science, 244,* 1328–1333.

Daan, S., Beersma, D. G., & Borbely, A. A. (1984). Timing of human sleep: Recovery process gated by a circadian pacemaker. *American Journal of Physiology, 2,* R161–R183.

Dawson, D., & Campbell, S. (1991). Timed exposure to bright light improves sleep and alertness during simulated night shifts. *Sleep, 14,* 511–516.

de Candolle, A. P. (1832). *Physiologie vegetale.* ["Vegetative Physiology"] Paris: Bechet Jeune.

de Mairan, J. (1729). Observation botanique. *Histoire de L'Academie Royale des Sciences* [Botanical observations], 35–36.

Dement, W. C., Seidel, W. F., Cohen, S. A., Bliwise, N. G., & Carskadon, M. A. (1986). Sleep and wakefulness in aircrew before and after transoceanic flights. *Aviation Space Environmental Medicine, 57*(12), B14–B28.

Dijk, D. J., Beersma, D. G., Daan, S., & Lewy, A. J. (1989). Bright morning light advances the human circadian system without affecting NREM sleep homeostasis. *American Journal of Physiology, 256*, R106–R111.

Dinges, D., F., & Broughton, R. J. (Eds.). (1989). *Sleep and alertness: Chronobiological, behavioral and medical aspects of napping.* New York: Raven Press.

Eastman, C. I., & Miescke, K. J. (1990). Entrainment of circadian rhythms with 26-h bright light and sleep-wake schedules. *American Journal of Physiology, 259*(6 Pt. 2), B1189–B1197.

Fuller, C. A., Lydic, R., Sulzman, F. M., Albers, H. E., Tepper, B., Moore-Ede, M. C. (1981). Circadian rhythm of body temperature persists after suprachiasmatic lesions in the squirrel monkey. *American Journal of Physiology, 241*, 385–391.

Graeber, R. C., Dement, W. C., Nicholson, A. N., Sasaki, M., & Wegmann, H. M. (1986). International cooperative study of aircrew layover sleep: Operational summary. *Aviation Space Environmental Medicine, 57*(12), B10–B13.

Graeber, R. C., Lauber, J. K., Connell, L. J., & Gander, P. H. (1986). International aircrew sleep and wakefulness after multiple time zone flights: A cooperative study. *Aviation Space Environmental Medicine, 57*, B10–B13.

Halberg, F. (1959). Physiologic 24-hour periodicity: General and procedural considerations with reference to the adrenal cycle. *Zeitschrift fuer Vitamin-, Hormon- und Fermentforschung, 10*, 225–296.

Inouye, S. T., & Kawamura, H. (1979). Persistence of circadian rhythmicity in a mammalian hypothalamic "island" containing the suprachiasmatic nucleus. *Proceedings of the National Academy of Science U.S.A., 76*, 5962–5966.

Jacobsen, F. M., Wehr, T. A., Skwerer, R. A., Sack, D. A., & Rosenthal, N. E. (1987). Morning versus midday phototherapy of seasonal affective disorder. *American Journal of Psychiatry, 144*, 1301–1305.

Klerman, E. B., Dijk, D. J., Czeisler, C. A., & Kronauer, R. E. (1992). *Simulations using self-selected light-dark cycles from "free-running" protocols in humans results in an apparent t significantly longer than the intrinsic t.* Paper presented at the 3rd meeting of the Society for Research on Biological Rhythms, Amelia Island, FL.

Lehman, M. N., Silver, R., Gladstone, W. R., Kahn, R. M., Gibson, M., & Bittman, E. L. (1987). Circadian rhythmicity restored by neural transplant: Immunocytochemical characterization of the graft and its integration with the host brain. *Journal of Neuroscience, 7*, 1626–1638.

Lewy, A. J., Ahmed, S., Jackson, J. M., & Sack, R. L. (1992). Melatonin shifts human circadian rhythms according to a phase-response curve. *Chronobiology International, 9*, 380–392.

Lewy, A. J., Sack, R. L., Miller, L. S., & Hoban, T. M. (1987). Antidepressant and circadian phase-shifting effects of light. *Science, 235*, 352–354.

Lewy, A. J., Sack, R. L., & Singer, C. M. (1985). Melatonin, light and chronobiological disorders. *Ciba Foundation Symposium, 117*(1), 231–252.

Lewy, A. J., Wehr, T. A., Goodwin, F. K., Newsome, D. A., & Markey, S. P. (1980). Light suppresses melatonin secretion in humans. *Science, 210*, 1267–1269.

Mistleberger, R. E., & Rechtschaffen, A. (1984). Recovery of anticipatory activity to restricted feeding in rats with ventromedial hypothalamic lesions. *Physiology and Behavior, 33*, 227–235.

Mistleberger, R., & Rusak, B. (1989). Mechanisms and models of the circadian timekeeping system. In M. H. Kryger, T. Roth, & W. Dement (Eds.), *Principles and practice of sleep medicine* (pp. 141–152). Philadelphia: Saunders.

Moore, R. Y., & Eichler, V. B. (1972). Loss of a circadian adrenal corticosterone rhythm following suprachiasmatic lesions in the rat. *Brain Research, 42*(1), 201–206.

Moore, R. Y., & Lenn, N. J. (1972). A retinohypothalamic projection in the rat. *Journal of Comparative Neurology, 146*(1), 1–14.

Moore-Ede, M. C., Sulzman, F. M., & Fuller, C. A. (1982). *The clocks that time us.* Cambridge, MA: Harvard University Press.

Nelson, W., Tong, Y. L., Lee, J. K., & Halberg, F. (1979). Methods for cosinor-rhythmometry. *Chronobiologia, 6,* 305–323.

Prosser, R. A., & Satinoff, E. (1984). Suprachiasmatic leasions alter but do not eliminate circadian body temperature rhythms in rats. *Federation Proceedings, 43,* 906.

Reiter, R. J. (1988). Neuroendocrinology of melatonin. In A. Miles, D. Philbrick, & C. Thompson (Eds.), *Melatonin: Clinical perspectives.* Oxford, England: Oxford University Press.

Reiter, R. J. (1989). The pineal gland. In L. J. De Groot (Eds.), *De Groot's endocrinology.* Philadelphia: Saunders.

Reppert, S., Weaver, D., Rivkees, S., & Stopa, E. (1988). Putative melatonin receptors are located in a human biological clock. *Science, 242,* 78–81.

Richter, C. P. (1965). *Biological clocks in medicine and psychiatry.* Springfield, IL: Charles C. Thomas.

Richter, C. P. (1967). Sleep and activity: Their relation to the 24-hour clock. *Research in Mental Disorders, 45*(8), 8–29.

Rosenthal, N. E., Sack, D. A., Gillin, J. C., Lewy, A. J., Goodwin, F. K., Davenport, Y., Mueller, P. S., Newsome, D. A., & Wehr, T. A. (1984). Seasonal affective disorder: A description of the syndrome and preliminary findings with light therapy. *Archives of General Psychiatry, 41,* 72–80.

Rusak, B., & Groos, G. (1982). Suprachiasmatic stimulation phase shifts rodent circadian rhythms. *Science, 215,* 1407–1409.

Sack, R. L., Blood, M., & Lewy, A. J. (1994). Melatonin administration promotes circadian adaptation to night-shift work. *Sleep Research, 23,* 509.

Sack, R. L., Lewy, A. J., White, D. M., Singer, C. M., Fireman, M. J., & Vandiver, R. (1990). Morning vs. evening light treatment for winter depression. Evidence that the therapeutic effects of light are mediated by circadian phase shifts. *Archives of General Psychiatry, 47,* 343–351.

Sasaki, M., Kurosaki, Y., Mori, A., & Endo, S. (1986). Patterns of sleep–wakefulness before and after transmeridian flight in commercial airline pilots. *Aviation Space Environmental Medicine, 57,* 29–42.

Stephan, F. K., & Zucker, I. (1972). Circadian rhythms in drinking behavior and locomotor activity of rats are eliminated by hypothalamic lesions. *Proceedings of the National Academy of Science U.S.A., 69,* 1583–1586.

Terman, M., & Terman, J. (1985). A circadian pacemaker for visual sensitivity? *Annals of the New York Academy of Science, 453*(1), 147–161.

Webb, W. B., & Agnew, H. W. (1974). Sleep and waking in a time-free environment. *Aeropsace Medicine, 45,* 617–622.

Wegmann, H. M., Gundel, A., Naumann, M., Samel, A., Schwartz, E., & Vejvoda, M. (1986). Sleep, sleepiness, and circadian rhythmicity in aircrews operating on transatlantic routes. *Aviation Space Environmental Medicine, 57,* 53–65.

Wehr, T. A., Jacobsen, F. M., Sack, D. A., Arendt, J., Tamarkin, L., & Rosenthal, N. E. (1986). Phototherapy of seasonal affective disorder: Time of day and suppression of melatonin are not critical for antidepressant effects. *Archives of General Psychiatry, 43,* 870–875.

Weitzman, E. D. (1982). Chronobiology of man: Sleep, temperature and neuroendocrine rhythms. *Human Neurobiology, 1*(3), 173–183.

Wever, R. A. (1979). *The circadian system of man: Results of experiments under temporal isolation.* New York: Springer-Verlag.

Wever, R. A., Polasek, J., & Wildgruber, C. M. (1983). Bright light affects human circadian rhythms. *Pflugers Arch, 396*(1), 85–87.

Winget, C. M., DeRoshia, C. W., Markley, C. L., & Holley, D. C. (1984). A review of human physiological and performance changes associated with desynchronosis of biological rhythms. *Aviation Space Environmental Medicine, 55,* 1085–1096.

Introduction to Sleep Disorders

Saul A. Rothenberg

Disruption of sleep is such a common phenomenon that all the readers of this book are likely to have experienced it at some time in their lives, followed by a return to their regular habits after a few days or weeks. Some readers may have endured sleep disruption for months or years. Estimates of the prevalence of all sleep disorders in the U.S. population vary from 13% to 49% (Bixler, Kales, Soldatos, Kales, & Healey, 1979; Ford & Kamerow, 1989; Shapiro & Dement, 1994). That the state we spend one third of our lives in is so alterable is both remarkable and puzzling, perhaps a reflection of the natural tension between our need for sleep and our need for alertness.

Sleep alterations reflect the impact of many internal and external events in health and sickness. The onset of sleep is sometimes difficult to achieve, requiring a delicate balance among competing needs and changing circumstances. At other times, the urge to sleep is so overwhelming, it is unavoidable. Many changes in sleep pattern are transient and occur in people without significant medical or psychological disorders. Yet some sleep problems go on for years, driven by combinations of aberrant or maladaptive medical and psychological state, environment, and habit. This chapter presents the argument that mental health professionals need to be well versed in recognizing and treating sleep disorders and provides an overview of sleep disorder classification systems. It begins with a description of the many alterations of sleep, brief and protracted, that are troublesome to the sleeper or that are defined as disorders of sleep and that may be addressed with a variety of interventions. Succeeding chapters address in detail the diagnostic interview, laboratory evaluation, specific sleep disorders, and treatment methods.

One of the most interesting and challenging aspects of sleep disorders is their multiplicity of causes. Sleep disorders are often associated with medical conditions, substance use, environmental factors, emotional disorders, or stressful life events (Kryger, Roth, & Dement, 1993). The heart of the evaluation of a sleep complaint is determining the underlying cause of the complaint. The close relation of emotional and mental disorders and daily stress to sleep disorders provides several reasons for mental health professionals, in particular among all health care workers, to understand sleep disorders. The presenting complaint of a patient in a mental health setting may be "difficulty with sleep." Knowing whether a sleep complaint is separate from or related to other disorders is of vital importance. Symptoms of specific sleep disorders may be mistaken for symptoms of diagnosable emotional disorders when the emotional disorders are not present. Excessive daytime sleepiness, for example, may lead a psychologist to inquire about major depression, bipolar disorder, or secondary gains in an adolescent who has trouble waking for school. Yet at least four specific sleep disorders—narcolepsy, obstructive sleep apnea, periodic limb movement disorder, and delayed sleep phase syndrome—may provide a more direct explanation for this symptom. Separating emotional disorders from sleep disorders will help mental health workers provide more appropriately targeted treatments or referrals for their patients.

Sleep disorders may coexist independently with emotional disorders in some people, complicating or decreasing the effectiveness of interventions unless this fact is recognized. Occasionally, sleep disorders exist in a dependent fashion with emotional disorders but are sufficiently severe to warrant separate treatment, as in the case of chronic insomnia related to major depression, generalized anxiety, or adjustment disorders. Mental health professionals may be able to treat the sleep disorder directly or know that the patient needs an appropriate referral whether or not there is a treatable emotional disorder. Parallel interventions for sleep and mood may provide the best therapeutic result for subsets of patients with comorbid disorders. Untreated sleep disturbance may complicate treatment of mental disorders by providing the patient a comfortable diversion that allows them to avoid exploring more painful emotional issues. Emotion-focused treatment may become more effective and time efficient when treatment of sleep disorders either removes self-constructed barriers to progress or gives patients more energy to deal with emotional distress during daytime sessions.

Sleep disorders can persist after the conditions, stress, or emotional conflicts originally generating the sleep disorder are largely resolved. When this occurs, the successful resolution of the original problem may be ambiguous. A clear understanding of conditioned (psychophysiological) insomnia, for example, can help resolve ambiguity and focus treatment methods in effective directions. Left untreated, sleep disorders may be risk factors for development of future emotional disorders (Ford & Kamerow, 1989). A final point for the importance of mental health involvement in sleep medicine is that treatment of many sleep disorders is either primarily cognitive–behavioral, as in the case of insomnia (for which cognitive–behavioral therapy is the preferred long-term intervention), or has a behavioral component, as in weight-loss recommendations or nasal continuous positive airway pressure (CPAP) treatment compliance for obstructive sleep apnea.

When one considers the frequency of sleep complaints in the general population, the variety of underlying causes, and the overlap between the complaints of patients with sleep disorders and the complaints of patients with mental disorders, it is easy to see why several generations of researchers and clinicians have attempted to delineate the characteristics of commonly observed sleep problems. The following section describes similarities and differences in the currently used classification systems for sleep disorders.

Classifications of Sleep Disorders

Since sleep disorders were first classified in the late 19th and early 20th centuries, clinicians and researchers have struggled with organizing sleep disorders into sensible groupings to aid diagnosis and provide a useful framework for understanding etiology. In his seminal work, *Sleep and Wakefulness*, Nathaniel Kleitman (1939) reviewed and analyzed what was known about sleep and sleep disorders. The 15-year period before publication of Kleitman's book was rich with papers describing insomnia and other sleep disorders; debating their causes, similarities, and differences; and coining the terms *dyssomnia* and *parasomnia*, which are used today. Kleitman and his peers of 60 years ago provided insights and directions for classifying sleep disorders that are the basis for several current classification systems. They recognized that sleep disorders may be due to environmental and external factors or internal physiological factors. Furthermore, they observed that internal factors might be related directly to sleep mechanisms or to disease states that are separate from but have a significant impact on sleep. By the early 1930s, Gillespie proposed three major groups: disorders related to amount of sleep (either too much or too little), problems with timing of sleep (now referred to as *circadian disorders*), and various interruptions of sleep (the group Roger named *parasomnias*). Reviews of recent and historical efforts to improve sleep disorders nosologies have been written by Thorpy (1988, 1990).

The first formal sleep disorders nosology was produced by the Association of Sleep Disorders Centers (ASDC) in 1979. The ASDC nosology had four groups of disorders. The first two groups, *disorders of initiating and maintaining sleep* (insomnias) and *disorders of excessive somnolence*, were organized symptomatically because of the greater uncertainty about their etiology than about that of the other two groups—*disorders of the sleep–wake schedule* (circadian rhythm disorders) and *dysfunctions associated with sleep, sleep stages, or partial arousals* (parasomnias)—which were thought to have clearer underlying pathophysiological bases. Although the original ASDC classifications have been modified and revised in the current *International Classification of Sleep Disorders* (ICSD) produced by the American Sleep Disorders Association (1990 and see Appendix A), they were partially incorporated into the North American version of the *International Classification of Diseases, 9th Revision, Clinical Modification* (ICD-9-CM) published by the U.S. Government Printing Office and other publishers (1993 and see Appendix C). The ICD-9-CM is a more specific version of its parent, the *International Classification of Diseases, 9th revision* (ICD-9), originally published by the World Health Organization (1977).

Although different names are sometimes used for the same sleep disorder (see Appendixes A–C), there are three largely overlapping diagnostic schemas available today that use the five-digit number codes of the ICD-9-CM to specify sleep disorders. The ICSD nosology has added a sixth digit for greater specificity. The third nosology, familiar to all mental health workers, is the *Diagnostic and Statistical*

Manual of Mental Disorders (4th ed.; *DSM-IV*), of the American Psychiatric Association (1994 and see Appendix B). Whereas the ICD-9-CM has 2 sections with 19 codes for sleep disorders and the *DSM-IV* has 4 sections with 23 codes, the ICSD has 11 sections with 88 diagnostic codes. However, difference among the three nosologies are not nearly as great as the difference in number of codes implies. For example, the ICSD enumerates sleep disorders associated with mental disorders by listing five categories of mental disorders with multiple examples in each category. The same sleep and mental disorder pairings are covered by two codes in the *DSM-IV* nosology that are called either *insomnia* or *hypersomnia* related to a specific mental disorder. The ICSD and *DSM-IV* labels are slightly different for these categories, but the symptoms and disorders are equivalent.

In fact, the ICSD and *DSM-IV* nosologies are conceptually similar. Both start with the understanding that an individual can sleep too little, too much, or at the wrong time; can manifest behavior during the night that is distressing to the sleeper or to people observing the sleeper; or can have a sleep disorder that is largely attributable to another disorder or external circumstance. The main difference between the ICSD and the *DSM-IV* systems is the greater subdivision of categories and separate disorders in the ICSD.

The *DSM-IV* divides sleep disorders into three main groups. The first group contains *primary sleep disorders* divided into two subgroups, *dyssomnias*, which are alterations in the quality, amount, or timing of sleep, and *parasomnias*, which are behavioral and physiological events occurring during sleep or sleep–wake transitions. The second main group contains *sleep disorders related to another mental disorder*. In this group, although the other mental disorder is considered to be the main problem, an associated sleep disorder is sufficiently severe to warrant separate attention. The third main group contains *other sleep disorders* divided into two subgroups, *sleep disorders related to a medical disorder* and *substance-induced sleep disorders*. Again, the emphasis in this group is on the severity of the sleep complaint that accompanies the other disorder, and the *other disorder* is primary. Hallmarks of the primary sleep disorders are attribution of causality to endogenous sleep–wake or circadian mechanisms and the *absence* of involvement of disorders from the other two groups.

In the ICSD nosology, sleep disorders are also divided into three main groups. Two groups, *dyssomnias* and *parasomnias*, are viewed as relating primarily to sleep, whereas the third group, *sleep disorders associated with medical/psychiatric disorders*, includes disorders that are not primarily sleep disorders but have sleep disturbance as a major feature. The parallel to the *DSM-IV* classification is clear. Dyssomnias include disorders that result in complaints of insomnia or excessive sleepiness, whereas parasomnias are disorders that impinge on or occur during the sleep state and are not primarily insomnia or excessive sleepiness. Dyssomnias are divided into three subcategories: *intrinsic* (internal or endogenous), *extrinsic* (external or exogenous), and *circadian rhythm* sleep disorders. Unlike the earlier ASDC nosology, in this classification the subcategories of dyssomnia are based on the suspected etiology of the sleep disorders and follow the outlines proposed by Kleitman and others. Parasomnias are subdivided into four categories: *arousal disorders, sleep–wake transition disorders, parasomnias usually associated with REM sleep*, and *other parasomnias*. These subcategories are based on a combination of empirical observation and suspected pathophysiology.

The ICD-9-CM is organized differently from the ICSD and the *DSM-IV*. It has two main categories for sleep disorders. One is called *specific disorders of sleep of nonorganic origin* (307.4), whereas the other category, called *sleep disturbances* (780.5), excludes disturbances of nonorganic origin and presumably represents organic sleep disturbances. Many sleep experts are uncomfortable with the organic–nonorganic dichotomy of sleep disorders in the ICD-9-CM because it confuses the emerging understanding of the physiological basis of parasomnias and circadian rhythm disorders. Beyond the attempt to categorize sleep disorders along the broad continuum of organicity, the ICD-9-CM tends to organize sleep disorders according to patient complaint, as in *transient* (304.41) and *persistent* (307.42) *disorder of initiating or maintaining sleep*. Several sleep disorders listed in the ICSD are exceptions and have their own ICD-9-CM codes: *narcolepsy* (347), *altitude insomnia* (298.0), *sleep bruxism* (306.8), and *rhythmic movement disorder* (head banging 307.3). Although the 10th revision of the ICD is modified from the ICD-9-CM, the organic–nonorganic dichotomy is retained.

As knowledge about sleep disorders continues to grow at a rapid rate, it is likely that new information about specific sleep problems will result in an evolving level of sophistication and accuracy of future sleep nosologies with respect to underlying cause. The present classification systems are useful in helping the clinician arrive at a useful differential diagnosis and point the way toward understanding the etiology and pathophysiology of sleep disorders.

Descriptions of Sleep Disorders

Insomnia

Insomnia is a complaint of poor quality, insufficient, or nonrestorative sleep (Buysse & Reynolds, 1990). Most people present with one or more of three forms of insomnia: difficulty falling asleep, difficulty getting back to sleep during the night, or inability to return to sleep, even for a short while, after waking during the night. Insomnia may occur in brief episodes of several days, longer episodes of several weeks, and chronic episodes of months, years, or decades. It can be highly variable in pattern or unremittingly severe. It can be caused by many common and frequently experienced life events. Noisy neighbors, examinations at school, meetings at work, anticipation of important family functions, divorce proceedings, serious health problems, depression, anxiety disorders, chronic illness causing physical discomfort, and conditioned alertness all can be causes of insomnia. Conditioned alertness at bedtime can start with any of the causes of transient or short-term insomnia but can take on a life of its own through repetition, even after the original cause of sleep disruption has resolved. Moreover, any insomnia can be worsened or perpetuated by use of caffeine, nicotine, alcohol, and a variety of over-the-counter and prescribed medications. It is precisely this multifactorial etiology that makes categorizing insomnia so difficult and makes finding its underlying cause so essential and challenging for the health professional who hears this complaint.

The *DSM-IV* nosology describes an insomnia as *primary* when all other mental, medical, and environmental causes have been ruled out. Primary insomnia is closest to psychophysiological (conditioned) insomnia in the ICSD nosology. The best treatment for any complaint of insomnia depends heavily on an accurate assessment of its etiology (Gillin & Byerley, 1990). Hypnotic medication may be useful for short periods of time as an adjunct to nonpharmacological interventions or to help break a vicious cycle of sleeplessness and distress. Behavioral strategies are often more appropriate as long-term solutions (Spielman, Caruso, & Glovinsky, 1987). Many patients with insomnia can benefit from restructuring their bedtime habits and sleep–wake schedules. Restricting time in bed and avoiding excessive time in bed when not sleeping are particularly effective methods for reestablishing healthful sleep patterns. Relaxation training is also a useful intervention for many of these patients. Virtually all insomnias can be reduced to some extent by attention to sleep hygiene rules like keeping regular sleep hours, going to bed only when sleepy, exercising regularly in the late afternoon or early evening, avoiding caffeine within 6 hours of bedtime, avoiding alcohol and nicotine near bedtime, avoiding large meals late at night, and minimizing light, noise, and extremes in temperature in the bedroom.

Restless Legs Syndrome

Restless legs syndrome (RLS) is a disorder with a compelling presentation. Those afflicted with RLS describe it as a creepy, crawly, unpleasant, burning, or itching sensation, usually between the knees and ankles, that sometimes makes it impossible to sit still or lie down for any length of time (Ekbom, 1960). Movement typically relieves the unpleasantness temporarily. One can easily imagine how this disorder would make it difficult for a person to fall asleep or fall back to sleep during the night. RLS is often associated with periodic limb movement disorder, discussed later in conjunction with the hypersomnias. Treatment for RLS is pharmacological (Montplaisir, Lapierre, Warnes, & Pelletier, 1992). Although the mechanism of action is unknown, the dopamine agonists are highly effective at reducing the unpleasant sensations in RLS.

Hypersomnia

Sleep-disordered breathing: Apnea and hypopnea. *Sleep-disordered breathing* is an increasingly recognized medical problem (Young et al., 1993) and the most common reason for an overnight sleep study at a sleep laboratory. As the name implies, this problem occurs only during sleep, with severity varying from mildly disordered to severely disordered sleep (Strollo & Rogers, 1996). At one end of the spectrum is snoring unassociated with breathing disruption. Although simple snoring may pose a relationship problem to a bed partner, it is not a health problem for the snorer without accompanying breathing disruption; however, snoring is often associated with intermittent brief partial to complete cessations of breathing during sleep. When a snorer is sleepy during the day or has symptoms related to cessation of breathing, an evaluation by a physician or sleep specialist is indicated. A partial decrease in airflow for 10 seconds or more is called *hypopnea*. Complete cessation of airflow for 10 seconds or more is called *apnea*. When the

muscles and soft tissue of the throat collapse and partially or completely impede breathing in the face of continued effort to breathe, the
events are called *obstructive*. When partial or complete cessation of airflow occurs in the absence of respiratory effort, the events are called
central.

Obstructive apnea and hypopnea are the most common abnormal
breathing events in affected individuals and may occur several times to
several hundred times during the night. The greater the fragmentation
of sleep caused by the apnea and hypopnea, the greater is the associated daytime sleepiness (Carskadon, Brown, & Dement, 1982).
Excessive daytime sleepiness is one of the hallmarks of severe obstructive sleep apnea (OSA). Central sleep apnea is sometimes associated
with complaints of insomnia, but it may also lead to daytime sleepiness. The treatment of choice for OSA is a nasal CPAP machine, a
device that provides pressurized air that acts like an air splint on the
throat of the sleeping patient. A variety of surgical interventions,
mechanical dental devices, and behavioral strategies may also be useful when tailored to the specific needs of patients with apnea by sleep
professionals.

Periodic limb movement disorder. Another common sleep disorder
is *periodic limb movement disorder* (PLMD), which becomes increasingly
common with age (Ancoli-Israel et al., 1991). In this disorder, contrac-
tions of the muscles of a limb, usually the lower leg, occur at 20- to 40-
second intervals episodically or continually throughout the night. The
etiology of these movements is unknown. Their chief consequence is
disruption of sleep by brief arousals that may or may not follow each
limb movement. As with OSA, when the number of arousals is low,
patients may report difficulty falling asleep or maintaining sleep, but
when the number of arousals is high, leading to significant sleep fragmentation, patients usually complain of excessive daytime sleepiness.
Treatment is pharmacological, with the goal of either raising the
arousal threshold so that limb movements do not awaken the sleeper or
reducing the number of limb movements that occur during the night
(Montplaisir et al., 1992).

Narcolepsy. *Narcolepsy* is a disorder of the neural control mechanisms
that regulate sleep and waking. It has a genetic basis and is inherited in
an autosomal dominant pattern (Aldrich, 1992). The most striking feature of narcolepsy is extreme sleepiness that can overwhelm the person
at any moment, regardless of the number of hours of sleep obtained on
the preceding night. Sleepiness is associated with three other important

symptoms, which collectively are referred to as the *narcoleptic tetrad*. The three are *cataplexy, hypnagogic* or *hypnopompic hallucinations,* and *sleep paralysis*. Each of these symptoms represents a failure of the neural mechanisms that keep the REM sleep state separate from the waking state. Cataplexy is a sudden decrease in muscle tone while awake, often triggered by strong emotion or surprise that can be either positive or negative. The decrease in muscle tone can vary from mild weakness to falling down, unable to move. It is as though the normal loss of muscle tone that accompanies REM sleep at night gets triggered inappropriately during waking. Similarly, hypnagogic or hypnopompic hallucinations, which are vivid visual images or sounds that occur as a person is either falling asleep or waking up from sleep, respectively, appear to be dream imagery starting prematurely, before REM sleep begins, or failing to end promptly after REM sleep. Because the images occur while the narcoleptic patient is awake, they may be misperceived as real and can be frightening. Sleep paralysis occurs as a sleeper is awakening and the normal inhibition of muscle tone during REM sleep fails to end when the sleeper becomes awake. The individual is awake but still cannot move or speak for a brief period of time. Narcolepsy requires a sleep study for proper diagnosis and treatment, in part because single symptoms of the tetrad may occur in the absence of the full syndrome. Treatment of narcolepsy is pharmacological and symptomatic (Mitler, Aldrich, Koob, & Zarcone, 1994).

Circadian Rhythm Disorders

This grouping of sleep and waking disorders originated with the understanding that many behavioral and physiological processes have 24-hour (circadian) patterns that appear to be regulated by a "biological clock" located in the brain. The chief external regulator of the biological clock is light exposure (Dijk et al., 1995). Sleeping, daytime alertness, body temperature, hormonal secretion, and immune system function are synchronized in elegant daily patterns. Sleep disturbances and daytime problems with alertness arise when biological clocks are decoupled from regular sleep–wake schedules or when the body's clock regularly signals readiness for sleep or alertness at socially inconvenient or inappropriate times.

Jet lag. Jet lag arises from an abrupt shift in sleep–wake schedule relative to body clock time that occurs after flying across time zones. Many people experience malaise, fatigue, and disrupted sleep following transoceanic or transcontinental flights, as well as a decrease in those unpleasant consequences occurs as the body clock resynchronizes to the sleep–wake schedule after several days in the new time zone. Jet lag can be minimized by altering the sleep schedule before departure in the direction of the new time zone and by adopting a regular sleep–wake schedule in the new time zone, with exposure to appropriately timed sunlight to help the clock reset: morning sun after flying east and afternoon sun after flying west.

Shift work. There are many variations in how shift workers are asked to change their sleep–wake schedules, differing in the length of time they stay on one schedule and the direction in which their shift is rotated. Each change in work shift represents a circadian challenge similar to the jet lag of a time zone traveler. Alterations in sleep–wake schedules on weekends or on days off may complicate adjustment to evening and night shifts. Difficulty sleeping during the day and maintaining alertness at night are common problems for shift workers. Because of the many variations in shift work patterns in different industries, it is difficult to provide general rules for intervention. For permanent shift workers, keeping the same sleep–wake schedule 7 days a week helps adjustment. Rotating-shift workers may have an easier time adjusting to their shifts if the shifts are rotated from day to evening to night, because the slightly longer than 24-hour biological clock period makes it somewhat easier to delay behaviors than advance them. These workers may also adjust more easily if they alter their sleeping hours by an hour or two in the direction of their next shift a few days before they start the new shift. Recent evidence suggests that taking melatonin, a hormone produced by the pineal gland and released naturally before one's usual bedtime, may help workers shift their biological clocks and adapt to daytime sleep if they take it in the morning before going to sleep (Folkard, Arendt, & Clark, 1993). The difficulty of frequently altering and adopting nontraditional sleep–wake schedules makes it particularly important for a shift worker with sleep–wake complaints to seek help from professionals with circadian rhythm expertise.

Delayed sleep phase syndrome. The fact that human biological clocks have periods slightly longer than 24 hours means that the clock needs to be reset or advanced each day for people to get sleepy at about the same time each night. This is likely accomplished through exposure to light each morning when we awaken. Some people regularly go to sleep late at night and have particular difficulty advancing their bedtimes to earlier hours. They have great difficulty waking for work or school in the morning (Weitzman et al., 1981). Although their presenting complaint might sound like sleep-onset insomnia, it is clearly not the same. When not working or going to school, these individuals can sleep quite well from late at night to late in the morning, if left undisturbed. They appear to have diminished capacity to reset their biological clocks each morning. Treatment may involve delaying sleep around the clock until, after a week or two, it is back to a socially acceptable time. An alternative is to use bright artificial light to help with sleep phase advancing. After they have reset their biological clocks, their adherence to a strict sleep–wake schedule is necessary to keep them from delaying again.

Advanced sleep phase syndrome. The converse circadian problem is also observed. People, usually older, go to sleep early and have a hard time delaying bedtime. As a result, they wake early in the morning, which may be their complaint. However, unlike the early morning awakening that is sometimes a symptom of depression, these individuals have gotten a normal night's sleep that simply began too early. An inability to delay sleep caused by circadian rhythms or an overly sensitive biological clock advancing mechanism may be partly responsible for this disorder. Behavioral adjustment of sleep schedule, bright light exposure late in the day, or evening melatonin administration may help achieve the desired bedtime and sleep hours.

Parasomnia

The group of sleep disorders called *parasomnias* consists of a diverse set of behavioral and physiological events that intrude into sleep, occur during transitions between sleep and waking, or occur during transitions from one sleep stage to another. The *DSM-IV* and ICSD conceptualization and categorization of parasomnias are nearly in complete agreement. The only difference is the greater number of parasomnias listed in the ICSD. Both nosologies make the essential point that most parasomnias involve activation of the central nervous system autonomic, motor, or cognitive processes at inappropriate times during sleep or sleep transitions. ICD-9-CM categories for parasomnias are less coherent in concept, but they cover specific parasomnias as well as broad classes of parasomnias (see Appendix C). An important clinical distinction between dyssomnias and parasomnias is that people with parasomnias most often complain of unusual behaviors during sleep rather than insomnia or excessive sleepiness.

Sleepwalking and sleep terrors. Sleepwalking and sleep terrors are considered disorders of arousal in the ICSD, because these events are thought to represent an incomplete transition to waking from deep sleep. In both disorders, sleep recordings document the presence of brain waves typical of deep sleep, yet the sleepwalker moves as though awake, and the person with sleep terrors appears to be terrified, active, and may vocalize, and often moves (Masand, Popli, & Weilburg, 1995). The amount of activity or terror varies considerably. If left undisturbed, individuals return to sleep and typically have no recollection of the event in the morning. Sleepwalking and sleep terrors are common in young children and decrease in frequency as the child gets older. Occasionally, episodes continue into adulthood. Often the only intervention necessary is ensuring that the sleepwalker does not injure him- or herself by stumbling over or into objects. When the frequency of events is distressing or when risk of injury is significant, consultation with a sleep specialist is recommended. Medication is available that can reduce the likelihood of these events.

REM behavior disorder. Normally, skeletal muscles are paralyzed during REM sleep. In *REM behavior disorder* (RBD), which usually occurs in older individuals, the normal paralysis fails and sleepers may act out their dreams (Schenck, Bundlie, Ettinger, & Mahowald, 1986). When those dreams involve defending oneself from a threat or dangerous situation, the results can be harmful to a bed partner. RBD can be controlled with medication (Schenck & Mahowald, 1990).

Nocturnal seizures. Sometimes unusual behavior at night is related to seizure activity that is not present during the day. Overnight sleep studies or 24-hour EEG studies can evaluate this possibility (Montagna, 1992). If seizure activity is discovered, nocturnal seizures can be treated with the same medications used for daytime seizures.

Bruxism. *Bruxism* consists of grinding one's teeth during sleep. It is a fairly common occurrence that can be treated by having the patient wear a dental appliance at night. Evaluation of the need for such an appliance and construction of the device can be done by a dentist (Attanasio, 1991).

Sleep paralysis and hypnagogic hallucinations. Although these sleep-related events are part of the narcolepsy tetrad (described earlier), each one can occur in isolation in an individual who does not have narcolepsy. They can be frightening experiences in the absence of an explanation of REM sleep physiology and sleep–wake transitions. Fortunately, the events are benign, and a little education about sleep can go a long way toward reducing fears about their meaning.

Conclusion

Disorders of sleep, which may be brief or protracted, are among the most common maladies people suffer. Because of their ubiquity and the ease with which they may be mistaken for symptoms of diverse physical and emotional disorders, it is incumbent on mental health professionals to be familiar with the presentation of frequently encountered sleep symptoms and disorders. When sleep disorders exist as a result of or together with other disorders, parallel treatments may be advantageous. Accurate identification of the sleep problem often leads to more efficacious interventions or referral. Focused treatment, often behavioral, is increasingly available for sleep disorders. Not only can well-informed mental health professionals provide appropriate treatment or referral, but they can also help spread the word that suffering from sleep disorders does not have to be "part of life."

REFERENCES

Aldrich, M. S. (1992). Narcolepsy. *Neurology, 42* (7 Suppl. 6), 34–43.

American Psychiatric Association. (1994). *Diagnostic and statistical manual of mental disorders* (4th ed.). Washington, DC: Author.

American Sleep Disorders Association. (1990). *International classification of sleep disorders: Diagnostic and coding manual.* Rochester, MN: Author.

Ancoli-Israel, S., Kripke, D. F., Klauber, M. R., Mason, W. J, Fell, R., & Kaplan, O. (1991). Periodic limb movements in sleep in community-dwelling elderly. *Sleep, 14,* 496–500.

Association of Sleep Disorders Centers. (1979). Diagnostic classification of sleep and arousal disorders. Prepared by the Sleep Disorders Classification Committee. *Sleep, 2,* 1–137.

Attanasio, R. (1991). Nocturnal bruxism and its clinical management. *Dental Clinics of North America, 35,* 245–252.

Bixler, E. O., Kales, A., Soldatos, C. R., Kales, J. D., & Healey, S. (1979). Prevalence of sleep disorders in the Los Angeles metropolitan area. *American Journal of Psychiatry, 136,* 1257–1262.

Buysse, D. J., & Reynolds. C. F. (1990). Insomnia. In M. J. Thorpy (Ed.), *Handbook of sleep disorders* (pp. 375–433). New York: Marcel Dekker.

Carskadon, M., Brown, E., & Dement, W. (1982). Sleep fragmentation in the elderly: Relationship to daytime sleep tendency. *Neurobiology and Aging, 3,* 321–327.

Dijk, D. J., Boulos, Z., Eastman, C. I., Lewy, A. J., Campbell, S. S., & Terman, M. (1995). Light treatment for sleep disorders: Consensus report. II. Basic properties of circadian physiology and sleep regulation. *Journal of Biological Rhythms, 10*, 113–125.

Ekbom, K. A. (1960). Restless legs syndrome. *Neurology, 10*, 868–873.

Folkard, S., Arendt, J., & Clark, M. (1993). Can melatonin improve shift workers' tolerance of the night shift? Some preliminary findings. *Chronobiology International, 10*, 315–320.

Ford, D., & Kamerow, D. (1989). Epidemiologic study of sleep disturbances and psychiatric disorders: An opportunity for prevention? *Journal of the American Medical Association, 262*, 1479–1484.

Gillin, J., & Byerley, W. (1990). The diagnosis and treatment of insomnia. *New England Journal of Medicine, 322*, 239–348.

International classification of diseases, 9th revision (1977) Geneva: World Health Organization.

International classification of diseases, 9th revision, clinical modification, 4th ed. (1993). Los Angeles: Practice Management Information Corp.

Kleitman, N. (1939). *Sleep and wakefulness.* Chicago: University of Chicago Press.

Kryger, M. H., Roth, T., & Dement, W. C. (Eds.). (1993). *Principles and practice of sleep medicine* (2nd ed.). Philadelphia: Saunders.

Masand, P., Popli, A. P., & Weilburg, J. B. (1995). Sleepwalking. *American Family Physician, 51*, 649–654.

Mitler, M. M., Aldrich, M. S., Koob, G. F., & Zarcone, V. P. (1994). Narcolepsy and its treatment with stimulants: ASDA standards of practice. *Sleep, 17*, 352–371.

Montagna, P. (1992). Nocturnal paroxysmal dystonia and nocturnal wandering. *Neurology, 42* (7 Suppl. 6), 61–67.

Montplaisir, J., Lapierre, O., Warnes, H., & Pelletier, G. (1992). The treatment of the restless leg syndrome with or without periodic leg movements in sleep. *Sleep, 15*, 391–395.

Schenck, C. H., Bundlie, S. R., Ettinger, M. G., & Mahowald, M. W. (1986). Chronic behavioral disorders of human REM sleep: A new category of parasomnia. *Sleep, 9*, 293–308.

Schenck, C. H., & Mahowald, M. W. (1990). Polysomnographic, neurologic, psychiatric, and clinical outcome report on 70 consecutive cases with REM sleep behavior disorder (RBD): Sustained clonazepam efficacy in 89.5% of 57 treated patients. *Cleveland Clinic Journal of Medicine, 57* (Suppl.), S9–S23.

Shapiro, C. M., & Dement, W. C. (1989). ABC of sleep disorders: Impact and epidemiology of sleep disorders. *British Medical Journal, 306*(6892), 1604–1607.

Spielman, A., Caruso, L., & Glovinsky, P. (1987). A behavioral perspective on insomnia treatment. *Psychiatric Clinics of North America, 10*, 541–553.

Strollo, P. J., & Rogers, R. M. (1996). Obstructive sleep apnea. *New England Journal of Medicine, 334*, 99–104.

Thorpy, M. J. (1988). Diagnosis, evaluation, and classification of sleep disorders. In R. L. Williams, I. Karacan, & C. A. Moore (Eds.), *Sleep disorders: Diagnosis and treatment* (2nd ed., pp. 9–25). New York: Wiley.

Thorpy, M. J. (1990). Classification and nomenclature of the sleep disorders. In M. J. Thorpy (Ed.), *Handbook of sleep disorders* (pp. 155–178), New York: Marcel Dekker.

Weitzman, E. D., Czeisler, C. A., Coleman, R. M., Spielman, A. J., Zimmerman, J. C., Dement, W., Richardson, G., & Pollak, C. P. (1981). Delayed sleep phase syndrome: A chronobiologic disorder associated with sleep onset insomnia. *Archives of General Psychiatry, 38,* 737–746.

Young, T., Palta, M., Dempsey, J., Skatrud, J., Weber, S., & Bad, S. (1993). The occurrence of sleep-disordered breathing among middle-aged adults. *New England Journal of Medicine, 328,* 1230–1235.

4

Psychophysiology of Sleep Deprivation and Disruption

James K. Walsh and Scott S. Lindblom

The physiological and psychological effects of sleep deprivation or disruption in humans have been extensively studied over the past 45 years in an attempt to improve understanding of the physiology and function of sleep. Early studies of total sleep deprivation (TSD) were conducted to gain insight into the function of sleep by temporarily eliminating it, much the way early research in localization of brain function relied heavily on neural ablation techniques. Although total sleep loss may not occur as frequently as partial sleep deprivation or sleep disruption in everyday life, there is a practical aspect to this research. The effects of TSD serve as a comparison to improve understanding of the effects of partial sleep loss and sleep disruption. Moreover, there is abundant information that indicates that sleep loss and disruption are epidemic in industrial societies as a result of the relative freedom from the natural light–dark cycle associated with the earth's orbit around the sun. Electric light has led to a 24-hour society, with the availability of shift work, late-night television, all-night grocery stores, and a plethora of other activities for which people sacrifice sleep.

Only recently have researchers become aware of the stunning ramifications of sleep loss (see chapters 4 and 5), the most dramatic of which include incidents such as the Exxon-Valdez oil-spill disaster, the near meltdown of the Three Mile Island nuclear reactor, and the Space Shuttle Challenger explosion. Daily, if not hourly, there are sleep-deprivation-related accidents on our highways and in other modes of transportation. A good portion of school-aged children struggle with algebra, civics, and creative writing under the burden of a sleep debt, with no awareness on the part of educators, parents, or the students themselves. Most researchers believe that *as a nation we have a sleep debt that is every bit as important as the national economic debt.*

The scientific knowledge on which this chapter is based is voluminous and precludes a true critical review. There are nevertheless a number of methodological concerns that are common to virtually all studies of sleep loss or disruption. The reader must be aware of the way in which these factors mediate the data obtained and their interpretation. In particular, the reader should be cautioned about the apparent discrepancy between the effects of sleep deprivation on human performance in the laboratory and the actual impact in society. The inability to conduct blind studies and the Hawthorne effect undoubtedly heighten motivation and performance in all sleep deprivation research. Moreover, practice effects and the scarcity of studies examining higher cognitive functioning are other significant limitations. This body of research should be viewed as characterizing the types of human behaviors most likely to be influenced by sleep loss, rather than as an absolute measure of impairment in real-world situations.

The first section of this chapter reviews factors that modify the response to sleep deprivation. The remaining sections of the chapter review the effects of TSD, partial sleep deprivation (PSD), selective sleep deprivation (SSD), and sleep fragmentation (SF) on human performance and physiology.

Factors Influencing Effects of Sleep Deprivation or Disruption

How an individual responds to sleep loss, whether it is total, partial, selective, or fragmented, is influenced by a variety of factors. The most obvious factor is the magnitude of sleep deprivation or disruption, which is a primary independent variable in most investigations. Other factors that have received attention as mediators of sleep loss effects include circadian rhythms, age, drugs, and motivation. Any study of sleep loss must be interpreted with these factors in mind. Additionally, several specific characteristics of psychomotor tests (i.e., length, pacing, knowledge of results, and difficulty) used to assess human performance after sleep loss can alter research findings, perhaps through motivation changes.

Circadian Rhythms

Marked circadian variation in subjective alertness, physiological sleep tendency, and objective measures of performance has been described (see chapter 2). Regardless of the variable measured, a pronounced decline in alertness and performance occurs between approximately 0200 and 0700 hours, with relatively increased alertness and performance during other times. This circadian influence persists during a period of TSD. Alertness and performance improve (relative to nighttime alertness and performance) during the day after a night without any sleep despite an increase in the time since sleep occurred (Colquhoun, 1971; Kleitman, 1963). In other words, despite an increasing homeostatic drive to sleep, which occurs during sustained wakefulness, the circadian influence results in a temporary improvement in alertness and performance. A subsequent decline occurs during the next circadian trough. There is also evidence that as an individual ages (about the seventh decade) the circadian fluctuations become somewhat blunted, resulting in milder circadian-regulated variation in alertness and performance (see Figure 1; Monk, 1989).

It should be noted that there is not total synchrony among psychological, behavioral, and physiological circadian rhythms. For example, in addition to the major period of increased physiological sleep tendency during the usual sleep time, there is a milder, midafternoon increase, which is followed by a period when sleep is least likely (about 1900–2300 hr). Many behavioral measures show peak performance at the same time that sleep is least likely but do not illustrate a midafternoon dip. On the other hand, subjective ratings of alertness typically peak between 1100 and 1500 hours and show significantly increasing sleepiness just as physiological sleep tendency is decreasing. A discussion of these discrepancies is beyond the scope of this presentation. Nonetheless, the circadian time at which the dependent variable is assessed has the potential to mediate the measured response to sleep loss.

Age

In general, sleep loss or disruption effects in elderly individuals do not differ substantively from those seen in younger individuals. That is, following sleep disruption performance is often impaired, and measures of sleepiness, both subjective and objective, reveal decreased alertness. There is some evidence that older individuals may tolerate

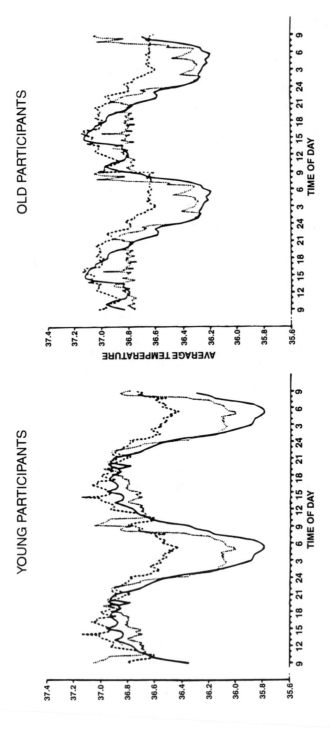

Figure 1. Double-plotted average rectal temperature rhythms under field (——), laboratory (·······), and unmasked (— —) conditions. From "Sleep Disorders in the Elderly: Circadian Rhythm," by T. H. Monk, 1989, *Clinics in Geriatric Medicine, 5,* 335. Reprinted by permission of W. B. Saunders Co.

sleep loss better (i.e., show relatively less impairment) than younger people (Bonnet & Rosa, 1987; Brendel & Reynolds, 1990; Webb, 1985). However, results of these studies may reflect differences in circadian rhythm amplitude or phase, as well as the relatively lower baseline levels in the older adults, which allow for less of a change with sleep disruption or deprivation.

Recovery sleep also exhibits reasonably similar changes in young and older adults following sleep loss or disruption (Bonnet & Arand, 1989). In both groups, total sleep time and sleep efficiency increase, and sleep latency and the amount of Stage 1 sleep decrease. The amount of slow wave sleep (SWS) increases, although more so in young individuals. In fact, with sleep deprivation, sleep of the elderly becomes more similar to the baseline sleep of younger individuals. Rapid eye movement (REM) sleep on the first night following sleep loss does show age differences. REM latency decreases and REM amount remains stable in normal older adults during the first night's recovery sleep, in comparison to the increase in REM latency and decrease in REM amount noted in normal young adults. On the second recovery night, young adults show the REM features that are seen on Night 1 for older adults. The delay in REM "rebound" in younger participants may result from a higher pressure to obtain SWS on the first recovery night (see Table 1; Bonnet, 1994).

Drugs

Stimulants are the drugs most often studied in association with sleep loss, and amphetamine, caffeine, and cocaine have received the most attention. Amphetamine has been shown in a number of trials to improve level of arousal, cognition, and mood during a period of sleep deprivation (Hartmann, Orzack, & Branconnier, 1977; Newhouse et al., 1989). The study by Newhouse and colleagues found a dose-related response but with a varied time course of response among measured parameters. Level of sleepiness, as measured by the Multiple Sleep Latency Test (MSLT), decreased with a 20-mg dose within 1 hour, and the effect persisted for 1–2 hours and then declined steadily to baseline over 7–8 hours. The response to the 10-mg dose was much smaller and disappeared more rapidly. Subjective ratings of sleepiness and fatigue were highly concordant with MSLT data. Cognitive performance tasks also revealed a rapid return to baseline with the 10- and 20-mg doses. However, the 20-mg dose enabled a level of performance to be

Table 1

Effects of Sleep Loss on Recovery Sleep Stages

	Young adults (SD)	Older adults (SD)	Patients with depression	Patients with dementia	Short sleepers	Long sleepers	64-hr older normals	64-hr older insomniacs
Sleep latency	0.38 (0.09)	0.51 (0.11)						
Wake time	0.44 (0.19)	0.59 (0.14)	0.22	0.14	0.13	0.48	0.56	0.52
Stage 1	0.42 (0.12)	0.95 (0.07)	0.61	0.68	0.98	0.60	1.07	1.20
Stage 2	0.87 (0.10)	1.32 (0.25)	1.06	1.08	1.38	0.99	2.36	3.00
Stage 3	0.98	2.06 (0.45)	1.14	1.16				
Stage 4	2.40		1.35	1.12			7.00	5.25
Stage SWS	1.53 (0.11)	1.56 (0.23)	1.23	1.15	1.37	1.52	2.56	3.30
Stage REM	0.89 (0.13)	1.04 (0.09)	0.84	0.78	1.26	1.03	0.26	0.92
Latency to REM	1.01 (0.20)	0.77 (0.20)	2.20	2.00	1.13	1.26	0.35	0.96

Note. Values are the mean percentage of baseline levels of the indicated sleep stages for the indicated groups during the first sleep recovery night after one night of sleep loss, 40 hr or 64 hr (two nights) where indicated. When sufficient studies were available, the standard deviation (*SD*) around the mean percentage is also given. For example, on their recovery night after one night of sleep loss, young adults have a sleep latency that is 38 ± 9% of their baseline sleep latency. SWS = slow wave sleep; REM = rapid eye movement sleep. From "Sleep Deprivation," by M. H. Bonnet, in *Principles and Practice of Sleep Medicine* (p. 62), ed. by M. H. Kryger, T. Roth, and W. C. Dement, 1994, Philadelphia: Saunders. Reprinted by permission of W. B. Saunders Co.

maintained for 12 hours after administration despite an increasing level of sleepiness as measured by the MSLT. The 10-mg dose did not allow this length of performance to be sustained.

Caffeine has been shown to improve task performance between approximately 2300 and 0800 hours, a time that represents mild sleep loss combined with the circadian trough (Borland, Rogers, Nicholson, Pascoe, & Spencer, 1986; Nicholson & Stone, 1980; Walsh et al., 1990). Walsh and colleagues found a significant effect of caffeine ingestion equivalent to approximately 2–4 cups of coffee on two different objective measures of sleepiness–alertness: the MSLT and the Repeated Test of Sustained Wakefulness (RTSW). The MSLT and RTSW were both significantly prolonged after caffeine ingestion, but subjective sleepiness showed little difference between drug and placebo conditions. The effects of caffeine on physiological sleep tendency, ability to sustain wakefulness, and subjective alertness were similar for mild and moderate habitual caffeine users.

Cocaine, like amphetamine and caffeine, has been shown to improve performance following sleep deprivation. A study by Fischman and Schuster (1980) found a reversal in reaction time performance to baseline following administration of 96 mg of inhaled cocaine in sleep-deprived individuals. However, measurements of fatigue and vigor revealed no significant improvement after cocaine administration.

The data from studies of central nervous system stimulants and sleep deprivation are consistent. Provided an adequate dose is used, stimulants allow sleep-deprived individuals to perform at baseline levels for a few hours to as long as 12 hours, often after the objective or subjective evidence of alerting effects has diminished. The question of whether stimulant medication should be used (or in what situations it should be used) to minimize the probability of potentially catastrophic human performance errors when sleep deprivation is unavoidable remains controversial.

Performance Task Characteristics

Human performance following sleep loss or disruption varies with the nature of the task at hand. It appears that the human organism has an amazing capacity to perform reasonably well under the most trying of sleep loss circumstances, provided the affected individual is sufficiently stimulated or motivated and the behavior required is not overly complex (Gulevich, Dement, & Johnson, 1966). This is not to say that sleep loss is benign; most real-world situations provide meager stimulation or motivation to sleep-deprived people when compared with a research environment. The fact that sleep deprivation and disruption experiments cannot be conducted in a blind fashion must not be overlooked. Furthermore, most studies deprive multiple individuals at any given time, allowing interaction among participants. Both of these issues produce high levels of motivation, which tends to reduce impairment from sleep loss. Additionally, because the majority of performance tests used have significant practice effects, repeated testing throughout the period of sleep deprivation reduces the detected performance decrement. Finally, the aspects of human performance that have been studied in sleep deprivation–disruption investigations are largely limited to sustained attention and deductive processing, with few creative or inductive components. To some degree, it is surprising that these experimental limitations have not interfered with the demonstration of any behavioral impairment.

Researchers have identified several characteristics of performance tasks that influence the behavioral effects of sleep loss. These can be categorized to include (a) duration, (b) difficulty, (c) feedback and incentives, (d) pacing (participant- or experimenter-controlled), and (e) type of task (e.g., vigilance, reaction time, memory). Because this research is critical to the understanding of the behavioral effects of total sleep deprivation, a relevant discussion follows.

Total Sleep Deprivation

Behavioral–Psychological Effects

Self-reports of sleepiness–alertness and mood change significantly with TSD. Regardless of the specific dimension or measurement instrument, mood becomes more negative and indices of sleepiness and fatigue increase as TSD persists. In fact, such "subjective" measures are often the first to reveal the negative consequences of sleep deprivation (Johnson, 1982). Other psychological experiences reported by sleep-deprived individuals include visual hallucinations or distortions and feelings of paranoia. At least two nights without sleep are typically needed before visual misperceptions begin, although they may occur earlier if highly visual tasks are performed. Longer periods of TSD are necessary to precipitate paranoid symptoms. Tyler (1955) found that only 2% of 350 participants maintaining wakefulness for 112 hours reported significant symptoms of paranoia. Most investigators agree that the expectations established in the experimental setting and predisposing personality features contribute significantly to an individual's psychological response to sleep loss. It is important to note that mood changes and other psychological symptoms remit when sleep is obtained.

Much of the early published work on human performance in response to sleep loss focused on characteristics of tasks that were sensitive to sleep deprivation or, in contrast, allowed sustained performance for long durations, such as those necessary for military operations. Naitoh and Townsend (1970) reviewed the literature and concluded that the effects of sleep loss on task performance could be minimized if the testing (a) was short in duration, (b) minimized workload, (c) provided knowledge of results, (d) was self-paced, and (e) avoided use of short-term memory. Most research in this area since that time is in agreement with these general conclusions (Bonnet, 1994). Using these five task characteristic categories, we selectively illustrate the well-established behavioral effects of total sleep deprivation.

Duration. An early study by Williams and colleagues revealed that a continuous visual task lasting 2 minutes was significantly affected by sleep deprivation of 70 hours but that the same task extended to 3 minutes was significantly affected by only 50 hours without sleep (Williams, Lubin, & Goodnow, 1959). Another study followed the number of addition problems attempted and the percentage of correct addition problems throughout a period of sleep loss when compared with results obtained at baseline. After one night of TSD, 10 minutes of testing was required to show a significant decline in the number of addition problems attempted and 50 minutes was required to show a significant decrease in percentage of correct problems. After two nights of TSD, only 6 minutes and 10 minutes were required to show a decline in the number attempted and percentage correct, respectively (Donnell, 1969).

Difficulty. The simpler the task, the less it is affected by sleep loss. Simplicity, or workload, can be thought of in terms of the speed of the task as well as the cognitive requirements of the task. By increasing the rate of addition required from one addition problem every 2 seconds to one every 1.25 seconds after two nights of sleep loss, a significant decline in performance was found (Williams & Lubin, 1967), whereas a performance decrement was not apparent when the required rate was one addition problem every 2 seconds. The increased cognitive requirements of a two-step relative to a single-step addition problem also resulted in a significant decline in performance after two nights of sleep loss. Difficulty of a task is, of course, partially determined by the capability or proficiency of the performer. For example, performance decrements were shown to be more extensive in junior surgical house staff than more senior house staff when both were subjected to similar sleep deprivation (Light et al., 1989). Given constancy of other relevant dimensions, such as alertness level and motivation, people perform well-learned tasks better than poorly learned or newly learned tasks.

Feedback and incentives. Wilkinson's early study of serial reaction time found that providing knowledge of results decreased the number of long responses after 30 hours of sleep deprivation when compared with a similar condition in which knowledge of results was not provided (Glenville, Broughton, Wing, & Wilkinson, 1978). This immediate feedback may overcome the effects of sleep loss by increasing the participant's motivation. However, in other studies of reaction time in which participants were required to formulate for themselves how well they were doing, the number of long responses after sleep loss did not decrease (Williams et al., 1959). Performance incentives in the form of financial rewards or fines based on test responses led to a maintenance of baseline performance at 36 hours without sleep. Performance declined over the next 48 hours but remained better than that of the sleep-deprived group without incentives (Horne & Pettitt, 1985). Development of competition by revealing results of testing for the entire test group maintained performance at baseline levels throughout 36 hours of TSD, which was significantly longer than that maintained without announcement of results (Wilkinson, 1961).

Pacing. A self-paced task is more resistant to performance decrements after sleep loss than a task that is experimenter-paced. The lapses in attention, or even "microsleeps," that may occur after sleep deprivation are much less likely to affect performance in a self-paced situation because the timing of task performance is controlled by the individual. Periods of inattention are undetected, and the individual can compensate for these lapses by working faster at other times during the task.

Type of task. Tasks that require passive, sustained attention are most dramatically affected by loss of sleep. To some degree, this effect is determined by task duration, but the characteristics of monotony and sedentary participation are also important. The fact that heightened interest and active participation can enable individuals to forestall the effects of TSD has been demonstrated using performance in "battle games" as the dependent measure and finding no performance decrement even after 50 hours without sleep (Wilkinson, 1964). The short-term memory load of a task is also critical. Early studies of sleep deprivation found that short-term memory was impaired and led investigators to speculate that this was secondary to a decreased ability to encode or an increased inability to rehearse items as they were being presented (Nillson, Backman, & Karlsson, 1989). Some investigators have found no decline in short-term memory performance after sleep loss, but the tests used were usually of a shorter duration than the tests that have shown a decline in performance (Glenville et al., 1978).

Physiological Effects

The majority of the studies that have examined the physiological effects of sleep deprivation have focused on physiological sleepiness; recovery sleep; and neurological, autonomic, and endocrinological variables. In addition, more recent studies have also examined the effects of sleep loss on the immune system, which is the focus of chapter 21. The underlying motivation for examining these effects is similar to that underlying studies of behavioral and psychological consequences: (a) to obtain insight into the function of sleep and (b) to determine potential harmful effects on an individual.

Physiological sleepiness and recovery sleep. The most reliable physiological consequence of sleep deprivation or disruption is physiological sleepiness, or the tendency for an individual to fall asleep in the absence of competing stimuli. In both clinical and experimental settings, the MSLT is widely employed to measure physiological sleepiness. This procedure uses electroencephalographic (EEG) recordings to measure the time it takes for sleep onset to occur on four to six opportunities at 2-hour intervals. The faster sleep onset occurs, the greater the physiological sleepiness. Sleepiness becomes extreme after the loss of a single night of sleep, with most individuals falling asleep within 2 or 3 minutes throughout much of the next day. In fact, available data indicate that there is a direct and predictable relationship between quantity of sleep and physiological sleepiness on the MSLT (Rosenthal, Roehrs, Rosen, & Roth, 1993). Moreover, many authorities believe that the degree of sleepiness, as measured by the MSLT, provides the background capacity for performance. In other words, as sleepiness increases, an individual must increase effort to maintain a stable level of performance. This line of thinking also holds that a person must be very alert to perform optimally.

As studies of sleepiness following TSD would suggest, recovery sleep time increases above baseline. However, a number of studies suggest that the amount of recovery sleep following sleep loss is significantly less than the cumulative debt of lost hours of sleep. A single, 8-hour night of sleep has been shown to allow adequate psychomotor performance after up to 110 hours of continuous wakefulness. Loss of one night of sleep has also been shown to increase total sleep time the following night by approximately 10 to 20% in a 10- to 12-hour recovery sleep period. On the other hand, participants who were allowed a 24-hour period of recovery following either 24 or 48 hours of sleep deprivation recovered 72% and 42% of the total amount of sleep lost, respectively (Rosenthal, Merlotti, & Roehrs, 1991). Thus, although early studies suggested almost trivial increases in sleep time following TSD, methodologically sounder investigations have demonstrated substantial, yet far from 100%, sleep time replacement. Clearly, there is the suggestion of a sleep quality dimension that allows recovery of lost sleep more efficiently.

It is consistent with this hypothesis that examination of the sleep EEG has revealed a number of changes in recovery sleep when compared with baseline sleep. As mentioned previously, in all adults there is an increase in SWS and REM sleep during recovery following sleep loss. If recovery sleep time is limited to about 8 hours, SWS time is increased in the first recovery night, with all other stages and wake time reduced. REM-stage sleep is selectively recovered on the second recovery night. In older adults, who have a less vigorous increase in SWS, Stage 2 sleep amount is preserved or increased during the first recovery night. Other findings in recovery sleep include a decrease in eye-movement density over the second and third REM periods and an increase in spindle activity at the very beginning of sleep (Dijk, Hayes, & Czeisler, 1993; Feinberg & Baker, 1988).

As mentioned earlier, recovery from TSD differs significantly in the young and old. Older adults, who have less efficient baseline sleep than young adults, have increases in sleep efficiency to levels comparable to those of young adults during baseline sleep. Sleep EEG differences include a decrease in REM latency rather than an increase and a diminished SWS increase compared with that of young adults. In addition, sleep-onset REM periods were seen more frequently in older than in younger adults.

Neurological effects. Early studies of extended TSD (at least 8 days) consistently found the development of mild neurological signs, such as nystagmus, myopia, tremor, slurred speech, ptosis, and sluggish corneal reflexes (Kollar, Namerow, Pasnau, & Naitoh, 1968). The findings of nystagmus and myopia led to further studies, which revealed a reduction in convergence for both near and far vision under high visual load, with near vision being more sensitive to progressive sleep deprivation (Horne, 1975). Near point of convergence and stereopsis were found to be maintained (Quant, 1992). Other neurological findings included a hyperactive gag reflex, hyperactive deep tendon reflexes, and an increased sensitivity to pain, all occurring after about 10 days of TSD (Ross, 1965). These neurological changes can be interpreted as a primary central nervous system response or, alternatively, as an effect on the motor neuron. It is important to note that in all cases reversal of the neurological signs occurs after sleep is obtained.

Analysis of the EEG during TSD has revealed a decline in alpha activity while one is awake (Armington & Mitnick, 1959). Alpha activity in the sleep-deprived individual could be increased by an arousing stimulus, which led to the conclusion that the low alpha activity was secondary to drowsiness. It is consistent with this interpretation that delta and theta activity were found to be increased in the waking EEG of sleep-deprived individuals, with no significant change in beta activity (Naitoh, Pasnau, & Kollar, 1971). Often an error in performance occurs during a brief (2–20 sec) period of EEG slowing that has been termed *microsleep* (see Figure 2; Anch, Browman, Mitler, & Walsh, 1988). After about 48 hours without sleep, microsleeps become increasingly more common even when participants are physically active, attesting to the strength of the sleep drive.

More recent spectral analysis of EEG revealed a decrease in interhemispheric correlation between homologous derivations after sleep deprivation. In addition, higher intrahemispheric correlation for all frequency bands and higher absolute power on the faster bands of the spectrum were found. The absolute power of delta was not found to be higher. These results suggest that sleep deprivation produces a loss in interhemispheric coupling and an increase in organization within each hemisphere. These findings are similar to those found in populations with poor cognitive performance (Corsi-Cabrera et al., 1992).

One group of investigators has studied the role of brain catecholamines in the cognitive decline associated with TSD. Participants given alpha-methyl-para-tyrosine (AMPT), a catecholamine synthesis inhibitor, and those who underwent TSD had increased sleepiness without significant decline in the tasks measured. However, participants

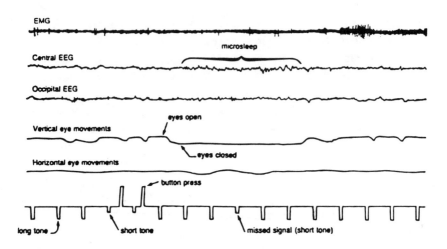

Figure 2. A polysomnographic recording of the electroencephalogram illustrating a microsleep during a vigilant task. EMG = electromyogram; EEG = electroencephalogram. From "The Science of Sleep," by A. M. Anch, C. P. Browman, M. M. Mitler, and J. K. Walsh, in *Sleep: A Scientific Perspective* (p. 16), 1988, Englewood Cliffs, NJ: Prentice-Hall. Reprinted by permission of Prentice-Hall, Inc.

given AMPT who also experienced TSD developed significant decrements in task performance as well as greater sleepiness than those who had one or the other (McCann et al., 1992, 1993). These findings suggest that reduced catecholamine availability may contribute to the sleepiness and performance decline associated with sleep loss.

Of interest is the use of sleep deprivation as a diagnostic or treatment tool in medical disorders. It has long been known that sleep deprivation lowers seizure threshold in susceptible individuals. This phenomenon is used to elicit abnormal EEG events as a conjunct to evaluation of individuals with potential seizure disorders. TSD has also been shown to have an antidepressant effect in approximately half of depressed patients, with endogenous depressives showing the most predictable response (Wu & Bunney, 1990). The mood-altering response usually lasts only until the first sleep occurs, but it has led to numerous investigations in an attempt to determine its etiology. A positive therapeutic response of depression to TSD has been associated with improvement in sleep latency, sleep efficiency, and SWS during recovery sleep. In addition, after TSD, responders have demonstrated a change from increased to decreased blood flow to parts of the limbic system, relative to normals (Ebert, Feistel, & Barocka, 1991), and an increase in blood flow to the left temporal and right parietal cortical regions (Volk et al., 1992). The significance of these findings remains unclear.

Autonomic effects. Changes in body temperature, blood pressure, heart rate, respiratory rate, and skin resistance have been the most frequently studied indices of autonomic nervous system response to TSD. The majority of studies have found a significant but small downward trend in body temperature, with the circadian rhythm of body temperature remaining intact during sleep loss. However, the findings concerning blood pressure, heart rate, and respiratory rate are quite variable, with various authors reporting either no effect or a small increase or decrease (Naitoh, Pasnau, & Kollar, 1971). Of interest is a small study by Horne (1977), who found no change in either mean heart rate or mean respiratory rate but did report increased variability in both measures in response to sleep loss. A lack of standardized procedures and variable degree of sleep loss are likely to have contributed to these inconsistent findings.

A reduction in ventilatory drive to hypoxia and hypercapnia has been shown in sleep-deprived normal people (Schiffman, Trontell, Mazar, & Edelman, 1983). A study of patients with chronic obstructive pulmonary disease (COPD) found a small but significant decrease in forced vital capacity (FVC) and forced expiratory volume in 1 second (FEV1) following one night of sleep loss (Phillips, Cooper, & Burke, 1987). TSD has also been shown to increase the frequency and degree of airway occlusion during sleep in patients who snore (Sullivan, Issa, Berthon-Jones, & Saunders, 1984). The genioglossus muscle, which helps maintain airway patency by pulling the tongue forward during inspiration, has decreased electromyographic (EMG) activity during carbon dioxide rebreathing in awake older adults following sleep loss, suggesting a possible etiology for airway occlusion (Leiter, Knuth, & Bartlett, 1985). Thus, the sleep disruption seen in sleep apnea syndrome may contribute to the underlying pathophysiology of airway collapse during sleep.

The effects of sleep loss on exercise performance are variable, although most studies suggest a reduction in maximal oxygen consumption (VO_2 max) following sleep loss. Blood pH and plasma catecholamine levels have also been reported to be decreased after sleep loss (Chen, 1991). Although the majority of studies agree that maximal exercise performance is decreased after TSD, submaximal exercise does not appear to be affected in all cases (Fiorica, Higgins, Iampietro, Lategola, & Davis, 1968). However, it has been shown that the recovery process may be attenuated by sleep loss even after submaximal exercise (McMurray & Brown, 1984). The attenuated process of recovery from exercise after sleep loss has been postulated to be secondary to a prolonged elevation of the metabolic rate.

TSD has been shown to produce activation of the sympathetic adrenal medullary system and the pituitary adrenal cortical system. However, it has been questioned whether these responses are secondary to the actual sleep loss or to other stressors involved with maintaining an awake state (Naitoh, 1976). A minimal decrease in urinary cortisol, glucose, sodium, and chloride, with a significant increase in urinary urea, has been noted after 72 hours of sleep deprivation, leading to speculation about "shifts in metabolism" as a response to sleep loss (Kant, Genser, Thorne, Pfalser, & Mougey, 1984). No significant changes in plasma cortisol, epinephrine, or norepinephrine levels have been found. The use of positron emission tomography (PET) has revealed no overall change in brain metabolism, but it has shown a decrease in absolute glucose metabolic measurements in the thalamus, basal ganglia, white matter, and cerebellum (Wu et al., 1991).

Endocrinological effects. In addition to serum and urinary levels of cortisol, epinephrine, and norepinephrine, other biochemical indices have been reviewed. Melatonin, which follows a well-established circadian rhythm, is increased in response to TSD (Akerstedt, Froberg, Friberg, & Wetterberg, 1979). However, melatonin levels can be suppressed by exposure to bright light during TSD (Strassman, Qualls, Lisansky, & Peake, 1991a). A majority of studies have suggested no change in levels of adrenocortical or gonadal steroids in response to sleep loss, but one study showed a decrease in 17-OH pregnenolone, 17-OH progesterone, androstenedione, and dihydrotestosterone without a decline in conjugated steroids, follicle-stimulating hormone (FSH), or luteinizing hormone (LH; Akerstedt, Palmblad, de la Torre, Marana, & Gillberg, 1980).

Using a pulse detection program, researchers found LH levels to decline during sleep deprivation independent of melatonin secretion in normal male participants (Strassman, Qualls, Lisansky, & Peake, 1991b). Thyroid hormones and thyroid-stimulating hormone (TSH) were significantly increased after sleep loss (Palmblad, Akerstedt, Froberg, Melander, & von Schenck, 1979). Circadian rhythmicity of growth hormone is lost in response to sleep loss. A field study of 64 healthy males found significant increases in mean serum liver function tests and plasma phosphorous levels. Triglyceride levels and the apoB:apoA ratio decreased, whereas high-density lipoprotein levels increased in the same people (Ilan, Martinowitz, Abramsky, Glazer, & Lavie, 1992). Plasma glucose appears to be unaltered after sleep loss, but some studies have suggested increased insulin resistance with the finding of higher insulin levels in response to an oral glucose tolerance test during TSD with or without exercise (VanHelder, Symons, & Radomski, 1993). The summary of endocrinological findings in response to TSD compiled by Baumgartner and colleagues (1993; see Table 2) reveals the agreement among investigators on the increase in TSH and thyroid hormones (independent of the increase in TSH).

Summary of Effects of TSD

The behavioral and psychological consequences of TSD are widespread and reasonably predictable, although dependent on a wide variety of variables, including duration, difficulty, feedback, pacing, and type of task. It is important to understand these mediating variables when attempting to minimize negative outcomes from unavoidable sleep deprivation. Because large segments of the society are sleep-deprived on a chronic basis, scientists and health professionals must consider the possibility that sleep education could bring about significant reductions in rates of industrial and transportation accidents, mood disorders, educational difficulties, and other societal problems.

A significant number of neurological changes occur following TSD, usually minor in scope and requiring several days without sleep. Furthermore, there appears to be little effect of TSD on the basic measurable parameters of the autonomic system, such as heart rate, respiratory rate, and temperature, independent from a general stress response caused by the experimental setting. However, maximal exercise response appears to be diminished following TSD as measured by VO_2 max, and ventilatory responsiveness to hypercapnia and hypoxia is also blunted by TSD. These findings, as well as the changes in cerebral blood flow, are congruent with the hypothesis of shifts in metabolism or an increase in basal metabolic rate in response to TSD. Although fewer studies are available regarding other endocrinological responses, the decrease in growth hormone and prolactin levels appears quite consistent. Again, these findings may be consistent with a "shift in metabolism" theory, with an increase in the acutely responsive thyroid hormones at the expense of the more chronically active hormones such as growth hormone, prolactin, or LH. Again, it is

Table 2

Neuroendocrine Investigations During Total or Partial Sleep Deprivation in Healthy Participants

Study	n	TSH	T4	T3	fT4	fT3	rT3	Cort	GH	PRL	LH	FSH	E2	T
Baumgartner et al. (1993)	10	←	←	←	←				↑	→	←	↑	←	
Parker et al (1976)	10	←												
Parker et al. (1987)	4	←												
Sack et al. (1988)	8	←												
Brabant et al. (1990)	6	←		←	←	←								
Palmblad et al. (1979)	10	←	←	←	←	←	←							
Gillberg et al. (1981)	12		←											
Weitzman et al. (1983)	6							←						
Saletu et al. (1986)	10							←						
Parker et al. (1969)	5								→					
Parker et al. (1979)	4								→					
Minuto et al. (1981)	3								→					
Calil & Zwicker (1987)	10									→				
Strassman et al. (1987)	11								→	↑				
Sassin et al. (1973)	5									→				
Kapen et al. (1980)	5													
Akerstedt et al. (1980)	12										↑	↑		→
Strassman et al. (1991)	17										↑→			

Note. From "Influence of Partial Sleep Deprivation on the Secretion of Thyrotropin, Thyroid Hormones, Growth Hormone, Prolactin, Luteinizing Hormone, Follicle-Stimulating Hormone, and Estradiol in Healthy Young Women," by A. Baumgartner et al., 1993, *Psychiatry Research, 48,* 155. Adapted by permission of Elsevier Scientific Publishers Ltd.

important to recognize the transient nature of these behavioral, psychological, and physiological changes, which are uniformly reversed when the individual obtains sleep.

Partial Sleep Deprivation

In industrial countries, family, social, and occupational pressures and demands have encouraged lifestyles that deemphasize sleep. Television and other types of entertainment are available on a 24-hour basis. Large segments of the population commute long distances and work long hours, extending the workday and shortening sleep time. School bus schedules start early, and children's activities end late. Moreover, individuals who sleep little are viewed as industrious, whereas those taking time to meet their biological need for sleep are labeled lazy. Many regard sleep as a waste of time or a necessary evil. For these reasons, partial sleep deprivation research has widespread relevance to daily life. PSD is defined as a restriction of total sleep time per 24 hours below the amount required by most individuals. In practice, PSD studies have typically limited sleep to 4 or 6 hours per night for one or more nights. Several studies have attempted to determine the minimal amount of sleep required on an acute or chronic basis before behavioral or physiological decrements are observed.

Behavioral–Psychological Effects

As one might expect from the TSD literature, demonstration of performance deficits as a result of PSD is difficult. Acute sleep restriction studies by Wilkinson found that performance was unaffected by one night of sleep restriction until sleep time was reduced to 2 hours or two nights with sleep reduced to 5 hours (Wilkinson, 1968). Sleep restriction to 5.5 hours per night for 60 days revealed a deficit in vigilance in the last 2 weeks of the study, but other performance measures were unaffected (Webb & Agnew, 1974). A gradual chronic sleep restriction study revealed no decline in performance even at 4.5 hours of sleep (Friedmann et al., 1977). However, examination of mood scales in individuals undergoing chronic sleep deprivation revealed significant differences in fatigue and vigor. Furthermore, the deprived individuals reported poor performance outside of the experimental situation and significant sleepiness when driving or in school.

The occupational effects of acute or chronic sleep restriction recently have received a great deal of attention. Many studies have focused on the performance of resident physicians following a night on call, with sleep usually restricted to less than 5 hours. National attention was directed at this issue following the Libby Zion case, which suggested that inadequate patient care occurred secondary to house staff sleepiness and fatigue. An inclusive review of sleep restriction and house staff performance studies from 1984 to 1991 found that the different methods used in assessing performance resulted in inconsistent findings. However, the authors did note that all studies completed since 1990 revealed significant performance decline following sleep restriction (Leung & Becker, 1992). Although the majority of studies involving surgical house staff have revealed no decline in performance after PSD, these results may be confounded by the inability to separate the acute on-call effects from the chronic sleep deprivation that is likely in the surgical house staff.

Physiological Effects

Sleepiness and recovery sleep. As one might expect, physiological sleepiness increases with the degree of PSD. It is important to note that the effects of PSD on successive nights are cumulative (Carskadon & Dement, 1981). As illustrated in Figure 3, average sleep latency on the MSLT continues to decrease across 7 days of sleep restriction (5 hr per night), indicating that physiological sleepiness continues to rise. Studies over longer periods have not been conducted. Presumably, sleepiness would continue to increase indefinitely provided an individual's sleep need was not met. PSD research has shown that there appear to be substantial interindividual differences in the amount of sleep that constitutes PSD; conversely, the amount of sleep required each night to maintain a high level of alertness during the day (basal sleep need) varies among individuals. In practical terms, PSD occurs whenever the amount of sleep obtained is less than the basal sleep need. Recently, a substantial number of healthy young adults were found to be physiologically sleepy during the day, at a pathological level, despite obtaining 8 hours of sleep at night (Levine, Roehrs, Zorick, & Roth, 1988). Furthermore, these individuals reliably became more alert with 10 hours of sleep per night (Roehrs, Timms, Zwyghuizen-Doorenbos, & Roth, 1989). It appears that even a regular 8 hours of sleep per night constitutes PSD for many individuals.

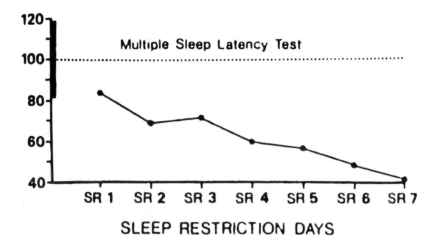

Figure 3. Sleepiness measures for 7 sleep restriction (SR) days are displayed as percentages of 3-day baseline mean scores. Multiple Sleep Latency Test scores were significantly reduced on SR-2 and showed further reduction on each of the sleep restriction days. From "Cumulative Effects of Sleep Restriction on Daytime Sleepiness," by M. A. Carskadon and W. C. Dement, 1981, *Psychophysiology, 18,* Adapted by permission of The Society for Psychophysiological Research, Inc.

SWS retains its predominance in recovery sleep after PSD as it does after TSD. When sleep is restricted for several nights, SWS remains unchanged or is increased after two or more restricted nights, despite continuing PSD. Rapid eye movement (REM) sleep and Stages 1 and 2 are markedly reduced (Webb & Agnew, 1974). When sleep was restricted to the first 4 hours of habitual bedtime for four nights, recovery sleep over two nights revealed a decreased sleep latency, increased total sleep time, and increased REM sleep. SWS was increased only in the first recovery night. Further spectral analysis revealed an increase in the delta band from night to night during sleep restriction, with a decrease in theta–alpha activity after an initial increase (Brunner, Dijk, Tobler, & Borbely, 1990). A study aimed at investigating the hypothesis that SWS serves as a mechanism of energy conservation found that exposure to heat during PSD led to a suppressive effect on the usual SWS increase (Bach et al., 1994). In summary, recovery sleep following PSD is similar to recovery sleep after TSD, with initial SWS recovery and secondary REM sleep recovery. The reason for the predominant slow wave recovery remains speculative, but the suppressive effect of heat on SWS recovery argues for the theory that it may serve a function in energy conservation.

Other physiological effects. The effects of sleep restriction on neurological, autonomic, and endocrinological systems presumably are similar, although of a lesser magnitude, to the findings with TSD. The response of patients with depression or the diagnosis of patients with seizure disorders has been the focus of most studies regarding the neurological effects of PSD; PSD appears to be as efficacious as TSD in the diagnosis of seizure disorders and in determining a response to depression (Schilgen & Tolle, 1980). One would suspect a diminished respiratory drive in response to hypoxia and hypercapnia with minimal changes in blood pressure, heart rate, or temperature regulation after sleep restriction, as is the case with TSD. However, no well-designed studies have investigated these autonomic parameters after sleep restriction. A small study involving 4 patients with mild to moderate obstructed sleep apnea (OSA) found a significant increase in the number of respiratory events when sleep was limited to 4 hours a day (Stoohs & Dement, 1993). This result parallels the findings in TSD. PSD has also been found to increase the number of respiratory events in healthy full-term infants (Canet, Gaultier, D'Allest, & Dehan, 1989).

The effects of PSD on subsequent exercise performance has been examined. Gross motor performance such as treadmill running, sprint swimming, and muscular strength and power are maintained under conditions of PSD. However, submaximal performance, as measured by different weight-lifting tasks, declined after three successive nights of 3 hours of sleep (Reilly & Piercy, 1994). A single night of 3 hours of sleep has been shown to decrease maximum oxygen consumption and significantly increase heart rate and ventilation at submaximal exercise (Mougin et al., 1991). Met-enkephalin, β-endorphin, and cortisol levels are not affected by submaximal exercise after sleep restriction, but lactate levels are increased (Mougin et al., 1992).

Studies investigating the endocrinological effects of sleep restriction have found an increase in TSH, thyroid hormones, estradiol, and LH, a decrease in prolactin, and no change in growth hormone or FSH (see Table 2; Baumgartner et al., 1993). The reason for the increase in LH in response to PSD (LH decreases in response to TSD) is unclear.

Summary of Effects of PSD

Performance decrements have been documented in response to acute PSD if the sleep restriction is sufficient (≤ 2 hr per night or ≤ 5 hr in 2 nights). It is surprising, that relatively minor performance impairment has accompanied up to 8 weeks of experimental PSD. However, the studies not only suffer from the methodological shortcomings of all sleep deprivation research but also involve very small samples of non-randomly selected individuals. Perhaps only those with a relatively short daily biological sleep need would volunteer for participation. On the other hand, humans may be able gradually to adapt to shortened daily sleep amounts. Horne (1988) proposed the concept of "core sleep," suggesting that beyond about 5 hours per night, sleep becomes optional, that is, has relatively little restorative value. In the following section, we review studies of physiological sleep tendency that do not support the concept of optional sleep. Clearly more research is needed in this area to provide insight and guidance with respect to sleep quantity and human performance, health, and safety.

The physiological changes in the neurological, autonomic, and endocrinological systems in response to PSD are reasonably consistent with the changes found in response to TSD. However, the physiological effects of weeks, months, or years of PSD in humans remain uncharted, despite the fact that large segments of society adhere to lifestyles that result in PSD of significant durations. Although the animal literature is not the focus of this chapter, the seminal work of Rechtschaffen and colleagues must be mentioned here briefly. In a series of experiments, these researchers have demonstrated that rats deprived of 80% or more of their baseline sleep died within 10 to 30 days, whereas control animals deprived of about 25–30% of baseline sleep survived without any of the physiological deterioration seen in the more severely deprived rats (Rechtschaffen, Bergmann, Everson, Kushida, & Gilliland, 1989). It seems likely, therefore, that prolonged or severe PSD has marked physiological effects in humans. Whether or not this critical degree of PSD ever occurs in the real world must be determined.

Selective Sleep Deprivation

Selective sleep deprivation (SSD) refers to the elimination of a specific stage of sleep, usually by arousals after the stage has been identified, throughout one or more complete nights of sleep. These experiments have been carried out in an attempt to determine the function of the different stages of sleep. For practical reasons, only Stage 4, slow wave sleep (Stages 3 and 4), and REM deprivation investigations have been performed. Attempts to deprive individuals of either Stage 1 or Stage 2 would result in near total sleep deprivation, at least on the first night or two, because these stages appear to be biological antecedents of other stages. The majority of studies eliminated or minimized time spent in a specific stage of sleep by awakening the participant when the physiological recording showed signs of that stage. For example, REM sleep deprivation is performed by awakening the individual when the onset of REM sleep is identified. Because the person must spend some time (at least a few seconds) in REM sleep for identification to occur, REM deprivation is never complete. Additionally, studies of non-REM (NREM) deprivation involve a significant reduction in the amount of REM because in most cases development of REM occurs after a period of NREM. One additional methodological limitation of SSD studies is the confounding influence of sleep fragmentation, which results from the large number (often 50 to 100) of experimental awakenings required to prevent any sleep stage.

REM sleep deprivation has received the most attention of all the SSD manipulations, in large part because of the strong relationship between REM and dreaming. Because of the popularity of Freud and other psychoanalytic writers, who emphasized dreams and the unconscious, in the 1950s and 1960s there was profound interest in the potential psychological consequences of preventing dreams. Initial studies of REM deprivation found that participants who were awakened each time they attempted to go into REM sleep had an increased frequency of attempts at engaging in REM sleep (Agnew, Webb, & Williams, 1967). These findings led to the conclusion that there was a need, or biological pressure, for REM sleep or its psychological dimension, dreaming. A large number of studies followed, examining the behavioral, performance, and physiological effects of REM deprivation in an attempt to understand the "need" for REM sleep. Studies of SWS or Stage 4 deprivation are fewer in number and generally focus on the issue of the differential restorative capacity of various sleep stages.

Behavioral–Psychological Effects

Early studies of REM deprivation reported resultant anxiety, irritability, and difficulty concentrating. However, subsequent studies using reliable psychological testing found no significant changes specific to REM deprivation (Agnew, Webb, & Williams, 1967; Lubin, Moses,

Johnson, & Naitoh, 1974). That is, irritability or other mild symptoms were also seen with sleep disruption that approximated the disruption of the REM deprivation technique but allowed normal amounts of REM. These studies have shown no basis for the early hypothesis that REM sleep is necessary for maintaining sanity. Subsequent theories regarding the role of REM sleep have been proposed, with the drive-facilitation and the information processing theories receiving the most attention. The drive-facilitation theory suggests that REM deprivation creates a state of heightened drive tension. Many animal studies found that REM deprivation resulted in an increase in sexual behavior, aggressiveness, and hunger. However, when applied to humans, these findings have not been convincingly reproduced.

Animal studies also led to the information processing theory of REM sleep. This theory suggests that REM deprivation impairs memory and the processing of information required to make adaptive changes. REM-deprived rats revealed impaired memory for tasks learned before REM sleep loss, but these findings—an apparent increased rate of forgetting in response to REM deprivation—have not been successfully duplicated in humans. However, a cleverly designed study that measured improvement rather than decrements in performance found that the selective disruption of REM sleep resulted in no improvement in the performance of a basic visual discrimination task for which improvement was shown after a normal night's sleep and after non-REM disruption. The authors concluded from this study that the "process of human memory consolidation is strongly dependent on REM sleep" (Karni, Tanne, Rubenstein, Askenasy, & Sagi, 1994, p. 681). Although REM sleep does not appear necessary for maintaining performance of tasks already learned (i.e., there was no effect on proficiency), REM sleep deprivation appears to result in an inability to improve performance of a new task.

The predominance of slow-wave sleep in the recovery sleep of sleep-deprived individuals suggests an important role of SWS in human performance, physiology, or both. However, the few studies examining the effects of SWS deprivation have found either no significant decrement or a very small decrement in performance (Agnew et al., 1967; Johnson, Naitoh, Moses, & Lubin, 1974). Contrary to these findings, the study discussed earlier in which REM deprivation led to an inability to improve performance of a newly learned task also found that SWS deprivation resulted in a small but significant decline in performance on a previously learned task.

Physiological Effects

Sleepiness and recovery sleep. One study investigated whether SWS is more important than other sleep stages for determining sleepiness or alertness the following day. Participants were deprived of SWS by awakenings, underwent controlled awakenings during Stages 1 and 2, and slept undisturbed in a third condition. MSLT scores revealed significant reductions in alertness during the SWS deprivation and control disruption conditions, relative to undisturbed sleep, but no difference between those two groups (Walsh, Hartman, & Schweitzer, 1994). These data support the suggestion that total sleep time is more important than the sleep stage composition of sleep. Recently, the MSLT has been used to assess sleepiness–alertness following REM deprivation when compared with a control sleep disruption condition (Rosenthal et al., 1994). In this study, REM-deprived participants showed no increase in physiological sleep tendency, even though total sleep time on deprivation nights was reduced by over 2 hours when compared with baseline. The control disruption, on the other hand, resulted in reduced alertness comparable to that expected with reduced total sleep time. These data can be interpreted to suggest that REM deprivation may have an alerting effect, perhaps consistent with the antidepressant effect reported with REM deprivation. Other investigators have found equivalent levels of sleepiness as measured by the MSLT in individuals deprived of REM sleep or Stage 2 sleep (Glovinsky, Spielman, Carroll, Weinstein, & Ellman, 1990).

The most remarkable findings concerning SSD are the effects on sleep stages during deprivation and recovery nights. REM deprivation leads to an increase in the number of awakenings necessary to deprive individuals of REM. Furthermore, the amount of REM sleep is elevated on recovery nights, without a significant change in SWS (Dement, 1960). These observations have led to use of the term "REM pressure," because the organism appears to have a biological need for REM.

Stage 4 deprivation leads to recovery sleep similar to that seen with TSD: an increase in Stage 4 sleep on the first recovery night and a subsequent increase in REM sleep on the second and third recovery nights (Agnew et al., 1967). Similar to the results concerning REM sleep, it was found that individuals deprived of Stage 4 sleep make increasing efforts to enter Stage 4 and have increased Stage 4 sleep when sleep is undisturbed. A comparison of Stage 4 and REM sleep deprivation found that participants required a greater number of arousals to deprive them of Stage 4 than REM sleep. These arousals were earlier in the sleep episode in contrast to those for REM sleep deprivation, in which the arousals were more frequent later in the sleep episode (Agnew, Webb, & Williams, 1964).

Other physiological effects. The physiological effects of SSD have not been well studied. There have been only a few selective studies examining the effects of SSD on the neurological and autonomic systems and no studies on exercise performance or endocrinological changes. The neurological studies focused on the response to depression; similar to TSD and PSD, REM deprivation was found to be effective in obtaining a response in endogenous depression (Vogel et al., 1975). In fact, the majority of antidepressant medications available today suppress REM sleep. These findings suggest a role of REM sleep or related processes in depression. No studies have been performed that examine the short- or long-term neurological consequences of REM or NREM deprivation.

REM and NREM deprivation and their effects on ventilation have been studied. Neither type of SSD demonstrated the blunted response to hypercapnia and hypoxia seen in the majority of TSD studies. No change in waking ventilation was found, but an increased frequency of breaths, in which ventilation was reduced below the range for tonic REM, was found during recovery sleep following both REM and NREM deprivation. The authors speculated that disruption of REM and NREM sleep may lead to perpetuation of apnea episodes and arousals found in the sleep apnea syndrome (Neilly, Kribbs, Maislin, & Pack, 1992).

Summary of Effects of SSD

The demonstration in early SSD investigations that there is a pressure for both SWS and REM led to a great deal of research directed at the consequences of SSD, with the rationale that there must be negative outcomes from SSD if an organism so strongly attempts to enter the state. Nevertheless, the yield from these studies has to date been rather meager. No physiological or psychological consequences, save one, have been identified, other than those that occur with sleep disruption or deprivation of any sort. Recent REM-deprivation studies have indicated that memory consolidation may be one possible function of REM.

Sleep Fragmentation

Sleep fragmentation (SF) refers to the occurrence of multiple brief arousals from sleep, typically without awareness or recollection on the part of the sleeper. Recognition of the significance of SF emanates from investigations of sleep apnea syndrome, periodic limb movement disorder, and the sleep of the elderly, which have demonstrated that when brief (2–20 sec) arousals are frequent, individuals become physiologically sleepy during the day despite obtaining what appears to be adequate sleep at night. Conversely, if patients with sleep apnea have periods of undisturbed sleep during the night, the degree of sleepiness during the day is mild (Bonnet, Downey, Wilms, & Dexter, 1986). These observations prompted experimental studies of the relationship between SF and the restorative property of sleep, as indexed by performance, mood, and physiological sleep tendency during waking hours.

Behavioral–Psychological Effects

A number of experimental studies have shown that restorative sleep must be continuous. Normal sleepers who were aroused for a few seconds with auditory stimuli after every minute of sleep for two consecutive nights had performance decrements and subjective sleepiness equal to those found after TSD for 40–64 hours (Bonnet, 1985). These changes occurred despite the fact that the participants averaged about 6 hours of sleep between arousals. Another experimental study compared three SF conditions: (a) an arousal every minute, (b) an arousal every 10 minutes, and (c) an arousal at each sleep onset following 2.5 hours of undisturbed sleep. Performance decrements were less in the 10-minute condition and the least in the 2.5-hour condition compared with the every-minute condition (Downey & Bonnet, 1987). In an attempt to determine the significance of different indices of arousal, Bonnet (1987) disturbed the sleep of normal individuals every 2 minutes of sleep on two consecutive nights in three different weeks. The experimental definition of *induced arousal* varied among weeks; the different types of arousal were (a) a verbal response to the stimulus, (b) a change in body position in response to the disturbance, and (c) an increase in EEG frequency in response to the stimulus. Significant differences in performance decrements were not found among the conditions, but all conditions resulted in a decline in morning vigilance performance and an increase in objective morning sleepiness when compared with baseline. Thus, arousals need not produce movement or behavior to produce daytime impairment. It is interesting that only the condition that required conscious arousal resulted in a change in the mood scale, with these participants reporting an increase in subjective sleepiness (Bonnet, 1987).

A single study suggested that older individuals are less sensitive to the effects of experimental SF than young adults (Bonnet, 1989), although circadian rhythm or other differences might also account for the observed differences between age groups. In summary, performance decrements from SF are dependent on the frequency of the arousals (or periods of consolidated sleep) and, perhaps, the age of the individual. Only an EEG change is needed to disrupt significantly the restorative process of sleep. The negative consequences of SF seem to be relatively independent of the amount of sleep obtained at the various sleep stages.

Arousal thresholds also differ between young and old adults. In a study in which young and old participants had their sleep fragmented by a series of ascending tones from an audiometer, the young adults were found to have significantly higher arousal thresholds (Bonnet, 1989). The arousal threshold increased rapidly early in the night on both nights of sleep disturbance in the young adults, but it increased in the older adults only during the second night of sleep disruption (Figure 4). In the study by Downey and Bonnet described earlier, in which three different conditions of fragmentation were used in young adults, arousal thresholds increased significantly across Night 1 but not Night 2 in the every-minute condition. The 10-minute condition did not result in an increase in arousal thresholds until the middle of the second night, and the 2.5-hour condition did not result in an increase until the last third of both nights of disturbed sleep.

Physiological Effects

Sleepiness and recovery sleep. It is consistent with the performance decrements seen following SF that physiological sleepiness increases as well (Stepanski, Lamphere, Badia, Zorick, & Roth, 1984). When a nap was fragmented experimentally, subsequent physiological sleepiness was strongly related to the frequency of induced arousals (Levine, Roehrs, Stepanski, Zorick, & Roth, 1987). Elderly individuals have more arousals from sleep than do young adults and are sleepier during the day. Furthermore, there is a significant correlation between arousal

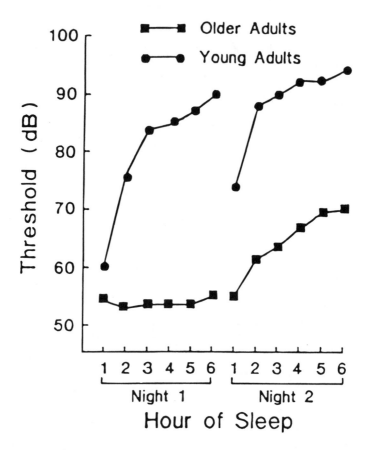

Figure 4. Auditory arousal threshold by hour and disruption night in young and older participants. Young adult thresholds were significantly higher at all test points except the first. Significant increases were seen in the young adults at Hours 2 and 3 on the first night and at Hour 2 in the second night in the older group. From "The Effect of Sleep Fragmentation on Sleep and Performance in Younger and Older People," by M. H. Bonnet, 1989, *Neurobiology of Aging, 10,* 22. Reprinted by permission of Pergamon Press.

frequency and the degree of physiological sleepiness during the daytime in older people (Carskadon, Brown, & Dement, 1982).

The effect of fragmented sleep on recovery sleep is similar to that of TSD or PSD. When allowed to sleep without disturbance, individuals who have had their sleep significantly fragmented demonstrate rebounds in SWS and REM sleep. The amount and placement of each may vary and is likely dependent on the SF condition. For instance, when sleep is disrupted every minute, SWS and REM sleep are essentially eliminated. This leads to an SWS rebound on the first recovery night and an REM rebound on the second recovery night, comparable to the effects of TSD. However, when sleep is disturbed every 10 minutes, only 50% of SWS and 25% of REM sleep are eliminated. The 2.5-hour condition described earlier resulted in a 25% reduction in SWS and a 65% reduction in REM sleep. The 10-minute and 2.5-hour conditions resulted in only moderate rebounds in SWS on the first recovery night and, therefore, a tendency toward increased REM sleep in the first and second recovery nights (Downey & Bonnet, 1987).

Other physiological effects. Controlled studies of the physiological effects of SF are rare. Bonnet, Berry, and Arand (1991) found that metabolism was increased by measuring oxygen consumption and carbon dioxide production when sleep was experimentally disturbed in normal people. Another controlled study found that two nights of SF did not result in an impairment in the ventilatory response to hypercapnia (Espinoza, Thornton, Sharp, Antic, & McEvoy, 1991). This result is comparable to the findings with NREM and REM deprivation but differs from the findings of decreased ventilatory responsiveness to hypercapnia and hypoxia after TSD.

Transient arousals from sleep, as seen in SF, result in elevations in blood pressure by an average of 25%. Additionally, arousals are associated with cardioacceleration and increased sympathetic neural activity (Shepard, 1992). The link between arousals and the development of ventricular arrhythmias is tenuous, but cases of sudden death and life-threatening arrhythmias have been reported in otherwise healthy individuals (Wellens, Vermeulen, & Durrer, 1972).

Summary of Effects of SF

Sleep fragmentation, if frequent enough and independent of the level of arousal, can result in performance decrements and physiological sleepiness comparable to the effects of total sleep deprivation. Recovery sleep following sleep fragmentation also shows strong similarities to that following TSD or SSD, depending on the fragmentation rate. If the fragmentation rate is sufficiently high to greatly reduce the amount of SWS or REM, these stages rebound in a fashion similar to that after TSD or SSD. The physiological consequences of SF, other than sleepiness, are largely unstudied; however, one investigation of metabolism during SF suggested further similarity between SF and sleep deprivation.

Conclusion

Sleep deprivation, in its complete or incomplete form, has been used for decades as a research strategy to understand the function of human sleep and its components. Unfortunately, the function or functions of sleep remain for future science to explain. Much more recently, scientists and health care providers have recognized the widespread health and safety effects of sleep deprivation in modern society. A review of experimental studies reveals consistent, but relatively unimpressive, physiological and behavioral consequences of sleep deprivation and disruption in the controlled laboratory environment, with the exception of marked increases in physiological sleep tendency. Interpretation of these results, especially those dealing with human performance, must be made with caution because there are methodological flaws and shortcomings that limit the generalizability of these research findings to the real-world situation. The significance of sleepiness has not been accurately and fully delineated in experimental settings. However, there is substantial evidence from studies of night-shift workers, students, sleep apnea patients, and other individuals exhibiting significant sleepiness that sleep deprivation and disruption have profound effects on the lives of millions. Investigators must now look at sleep deprivation research not only as helping to understand the function of sleep but also as fundamental to improving the health and safety of humans in modern society.

REFERENCES

Agnew, H. W., Webb, W. B., & Williams, R. L. (1964). The effects of stage four sleep deprivation. *Electroencephalography and Clinical Neurophysiology, 17,* 68–70.

Agnew, H. W., Webb, W. B., & Williams, R. L. (1967). Comparison of stage four and 1-REM sleep deprivation. *Perceptual and Motor Skills, 24,* 851–858.

Akerstedt, T., Froberg, J. E., Friberg, Y., & Wetterberg, L. (1979). Melatonin excretion, body temperature, and subjective arousal during 64 hours of sleep deprivation. *Psychoneuroendocrinology, 4,* 219–225.

Akerstedt, T., Palmblad, J., de la Torre, B., Marana, R., & Gillberg, M. (1980). Adrenocortical and gonadal steroids during sleep deprivation. *Sleep, 3,* 23–30.

Anch, A. M., Browman, C. P., Mitler, M. M., & Walsh, J. K. (1988). The science of sleep. In Anch, A. M., Browman, C. P., Mitler, M. M., & Walsh, O. K.

(Eds.), *Sleep: A scientific perspective* (pp. 1–21). Englewood Cliffs, NJ: Prentice-Hall.

Armington, J. C., & Mitnick, L. L. (1959). Electroencephalogram and sleep deprivation. *Journal of Applied Physiology, 14,* 247–250.

Bach, V., Maingourd, Y., Libert, J. P., Oudart, H., Muzet, A., Lenzi, P., & Johnson, L. C. (1994). Effect of continuous heat exposure on sleep during partial sleep deprivation. *Sleep, 17,* 1–10.

Baumgartner, A., Dietzel, M., Saletu, B., Wolf, R., Campos-Barros, A., Graf, K. J., Kurten, I., & Mannsmann, U. (1993). Influence of partial sleep deprivation on the secretion of thyrotropin, thyroid hormones, growth hormone, prolactin, luteinizing hormone, follicle stimulating hormone, and estradiol in healthy young women. *Psychiatry Research, 48,* 153–178.

Bonnet, M. H. (1985). Effect of sleep disruption on sleep, performance, and mood. *Sleep, 8,* 11–19.

Bonnet, M. H. (1987). Sleep restoration as a function of periodic awakening, movement, or electroencephalographic change. *Sleep, 10,* 364–373.

Bonnet, M. H. (1989). The effect of sleep fragmentation on sleep and performance in younger and older people. *Neurobiology of Aging, 10,* 21–25.

Bonnet, M. H. (1994). Sleep deprivation. In M. H. Kryger, T. Roth, & W. C. Dement (Eds.), *Principles and practice of sleep medicine* (pp. 50–67). Philadelphia: Saunders.

Bonnet, M. H., & Arand, D. L. (1989). Sleep loss in aging. *Clinics in Geriatric Medicine, 5,* 405–420.

Bonnet, M. H., Berry, R. B., & Arand, D. L. (1991). Metabolism during normal, fragmented, and recovery sleep. *Journal of Applied Physiology, 71,* 1112–1118.

Bonnet, M. H., Downey, R., Wilms, D., & Dexter, J. (1986). Sleep continuity theory as a predictor of EDS in sleep apneics. *Sleep Research, 15,* 105.

Bonnet, M. H., & Rosa, R. R. (1987). Sleep and performance in young adults and older insomniacs and normals during acute sleep loss and recovery. *Biological Psychology, 25,* 153–172.

Borland, R. G., Rogers, A. S., Nicholson, A. N., Pascoe, P. A., & Spencer, M. B. (1986). Performance overnight in shiftworkers operating a day-night schedule. *Aviation, Space, and Environmental Medicine, 57,* 241–249.

Brendel, D. H., & Reynolds, C. F. (1990). Sleep stage physiology, mood, and vigilance responses to total sleep deprivation in healthy 80-year-olds and 20-year-olds. *Psychophysiology, 27,* 677–685.

Brunner, D. P., Dijk, D. J., Tobler, I., & Borbely, A. A. (1990). Effect of partial sleep deprivation on sleep stages and EEG power spectra: Evidence for non-REM and REM sleep homeostasis. *Electroencephalography and Clinical Neurophysiology, 75,* 492–499.

Canet, E., Gaultier, C., D'Allest, A. M., & Dehan, M. (1989). Effects of sleep deprivation on respiratory events during sleep in healthy infants. *Journal of Applied Physiology, 66,* 1158–1163.

Carskadon, M. A., Brown, E. D., & Dement, W. C. (1982). Sleep fragmentation in the elderly: Relationship to daytime sleep tendency. *Neurobiology of Aging, 3,* 321–327.

Carskadon, M. A., & Dement, W. C. (1981). Cumulative effects of sleep restriction on daytime sleepiness. *Psychophysiology, 18,* 107–113.

Chen, H. (1991). Effects of 30-h sleep loss on cardiorespiratory functions at rest and in exercise. *Medicine and Science in Sports and Exercise, 23,* 193–198.

Colquhoun, W. P. (1971). Circadian variations in mental efficiency. In W. P. Colquhoun (Ed.), *Biological rhythms and human performance* (pp. 39–107). London: Academic Press.

Corsi-Cabrera, M., Ramos, J., Arce, C., Guevara, M. A., Ponce-deLeon, M., & Lorenzo, I. (1992). Changes in the waking EEG as a consequence of sleep and sleep deprivation. *Sleep, 15,* 550–555.

Dement, W. (1960). The effect of dream deprivation. *Science, 131,* 1705–1711.

Dijk, D., Hayes, B., & Czeisler, C. A. (1993). Dynamics of electroencephalographic sleep spindles and slow wave activity in men: Effect of sleep deprivation. *Brain Research, 626,* 190–199.

Donnell, J. M. (1969). Performance decrement as a function of total sleep loss and task duration. *Perceptual and Motor Skills, 29,* 711–714.

Downey, R., & Bonnet, M. H. (1987). Performance during frequent sleep disruption. *Sleep, 10,* 354–363.

Ebert, D., Feistel, H., & Barocka, A. (1991). Effects of sleep deprivation on the limbic system and the frontal lobes in affective disorders: A study with Tc-99m-HMPAO SPECT. *Psychiatry Research, 40,* 247–251.

Espinoza, H., Thornton, A. T., Sharp, D., Antic, R., & McEvoy, R. D. (1991). Sleep fragmentation and ventilatory responsiveness to hypercapnia. *American Review of Respiratory Disease, 144,* 1121–1124.

Feinberg, I., & Baker. T. (1988). Response of delta (0–3 Hz) EEG and eye movement density to a night with 100 minutes sleep. *Sleep, 11,* 473–487.

Fiorica, V., Higgins, E. A., Iampietro, P. F., Lategola, M. T., & Davis, A. W. (1968). Physiological responses of men during sleep deprivation. *Journal of Applied Physiology, 24,* 167–176.

Fischman, M. W., & Schuster, C. R. (1980). Cocaine effects in sleep-deprived humans. *Psychopharmacology, 72,* 1–8.

Friedmann, J., Globus, G., Huntley, A., Mullaney, D., Naitoh, P., & Johnson, L. (1977). Performance and mood during and after gradual sleep reduction. *Psychophysiology, 14,* 245–250.

Glenville, M., Broughton, R., Wing, A. M., & Wilkinson, R. T. (1978). Effects of sleep deprivation on short duration performance measures compared to the Wilkinson auditory vigilance task. *Sleep, 1,* 169–176.

Glovinsky, P. B., Spielman, A. J., Carroll, P., Weinstein, L., & Ellman, S. J. (1990). Sleepiness and REM sleep recurrence: The effects of stage 2 and REM sleep awakenings. *Psychophysiology, 27,* 552–559.

Gulevich, G., Dement, W., & Johnson, L. (1966). Psychiatric and EEG observations on a case of prolonged (264) wakefulness. *Archives of General Psychiatry, 15,* 29–38.

Hartmann, E., Orzack, M. H., & Branconnier, R. (1977). Sleep deprivation deficits and their reversal by *d*- and *l*-amphetamine. *Psychopharmacology, 53,* 185–189.

Horne, J. A. (1975). Binocular convergence in man during total sleep deprivation. *Biological Psychology, 3,* 309–319.

Horne, J. A. (1977). The effect of sleep deprivation upon variations in heart rate and respiration rate. *Experientia, 33,* 1175–1176.

Horne, J. A. (1988). Core and optional sleep. In J. A. Horne (Ed.), *Why we sleep* (pp. 180–217). London: Oxford University Press.

Horne, J. A., & Pettitt, A. N. (1985). High incentive effects on vigilance performance during 72 hours of total sleep deprivation. *Acta Psychologica, 58,* 123–139.

Ilan, Y., Martinowitz, G., Abramsky, O., Glazer, G., & Lavie, P. (1992). Prolonged sleep-deprivation induced disturbed liver functions, serum lipid levels, and hyperphosphatemia. *European Journal of Clinical Investigation, 22,* 740–743.

Johnson, L. C. (1982). Sleep deprivation and performance. In W. B. Webb (Ed.), *Biological rhythms, sleep, and performance* (pp. 111–142). New York: Wiley.

Johnson, L. C., Naitoh, P., Moses, J. M., & Lubin, A. (1974). Interaction of REM deprivation and stage 4 deprivation with total sleep loss: Experiment 2. *Psychophysiology, 11,* 147–159.

Kant, G. J., Genser, S. G., Thorne, D. R., Pfalser, J. L., & Mougey, E. H. (1984). Effects of 72 hours sleep deprivation on urinary cortisol and indices of metabolism. *Sleep, 7,* 142–146.

Karni, A., Tanne, D., Rubenstein, B. S., Askenasy, J. J. M., & Sagi, D. (1994). Dependence on REM sleep of overnight improvement of a perceptual skill. *Science, 265,* 679–682.

Kleitman, N. (1963). *Sleep and wakefulness,* Chicago: University of Chicago Press.

Kollar, E. J., Namerow, N., Pasnau, R. O., & Naitoh, P. (1968). Neurologic findings during prolonged sleep deprivation. *Neurology, 18,* 836–840.

Leiter, J. C., Knuth, S. L., & Bartlett, D. (1985). The effect of sleep deprivation on activity of the genioglossus muscle. *American Review of Respiratory Disease, 132,* 1242–1245.

Leung, L., & Becker, C. E. (1992). Sleep deprivation and house staff performance: Update 1984–1991. *Journal of Medicine, 34,* 1153–1159.

Levine, B., Roehrs, T., Stepanski, E., Zorick, F., & Roth, T. (1987). Fragmenting sleep diminishes its recuperative value. *Sleep, 10,* 590–599.

Levine, B., Roehrs, T., Zorick, F., & Roth, T. (1988). Daytime sleepiness in young adults. *Sleep, 11,* 39–46.

Light, A. I., Sun, J. H., McCool, C., Thompson, L., Heaton, S., & Bartle, E. J. (1989). The effects of acute sleep deprivation on level of resident training. *Current Surgery, 46,* 29–30.

Lubin, A., Moses, J. M., Johnson, L. C., & Naitoh, P. (1974). The recuperative effects of REM sleep and stage 4 sleep on human performance after complete sleep loss: Experiment I. *Psychophysiology, 11,* 133–146.

McCann, V. D., Penetar, D. M., Shaham, Y., Thorne, D. R., Gillin, J. C., Sing, T. C., Thomas, M. A. & Belenky, G. (1992). Sleep deprivation and impaired cognition. Possible role of brain catecholamines. *Biological Psychiatry, 31,* 1082–1097.

McCann, V. D., Penetar, D. M., Shaham, Y., Thorne, D. R., Sing, H. C., Thomas, M. L., Gillin, J. C., & Belenky, G. (1993). Effects of catecholamine depletion on alertness and mood in rested and sleep deprived normal volunteers. *Neuropsychopharmacology, 8,* 345–356.

McMurray, R. G., & Brown, C. F. (1984). The effect of sleep loss on high intensity exercise and recovery. *Aviation, Space, and Environmental Medicine, 55,* 1031–1035.

Monk, T. H. (1989). Sleep disorders in the elderly: Circadian rhythm. *Clinics in Geriatric Medicine, 5,* 331–345.

Mougin, F., Simon-Rigaud, M. L., Davenne, D., Renaud, A., Garnier, A., Kantelip, J. P., & Magnin, P. (1991). Effects of sleep disturbances on subsequent physical performance. *European Journal of Applied Physiology, 63,* 77–82.

Mougin, F., Simon-Rigaud, M. L., Mougin, C., Bourdin, H., Jacquier, M. C., Henriet, M. T., Davenne, D., Kantelip, J. P., Magnin, P., & Gaillard, R. C. (1992). Met-enkephalin, β-endorphin and cortisol responses to sub-maximal exercise after sleep disturbances. *European Journal of Applied Physiology, 64,* 371–376.

Naitoh, P. (1976). Sleep deprivation in human subjects: A reappraisal. *Waking and Sleeping, 1,* 53–60.

Naitoh, P., Pasnau, R. O., & Kollar, E. J. (1971). Psychophysiological changes after prolonged deprivation of sleep. *Biological Psychiatry, 3,* 309–320.

Naitoh, P., & Townsend, R. E. (1970). The role of sleep deprivation research in human factors. *Human Factors, 12,* 575–585.

Neilly, J. B., Kribbs, N. B., Maislin, G., & Pack, A. I. (1992). Effects of selective sleep deprivation on ventilation during recovery sleep in normal humans. *Journal of Applied Physiology, 72,* 100–109.

Newhouse, P. A., Belenky, G., Thomas, M., Thorne, D., Sing, H. C., & Fertig, J. (1989). The effects of *d*-amphetamine on arousal, cognition, and mood after prolonged total sleep deprivation. *Neuropsychopharmacology, 2,* 153–164.

Nicholson, A. N., & Stone, B. M. (1980). Heterocyclic amphetamine derivatives and caffeine on sleep in man. *British Journal of Clinical Pharmacology, 9,* 195–203.

Nillson, L. G., Backman, L., & Karlsson, T. (1989). Priming and cued recall in elderly, alcohol intoxicated and sleep deprived subjects: A case of functionally similar memory deficits. *Psychological Medicine, 19,* 423–433.

Palmblad, J., Akerstedt, T., Froberg, J., Melander, A., & von Schenck, H. (1979). Thyroid and adrenomedullary reactions during sleep deprivation. *Acta Endocrinologica, 90,* 233–239.

Phillips, B. A., Cooper, K. R., & Burke, T. V. (1987). The effect of sleep loss on breathing in chronic obstructive pulmonary disease. *Chest, 91,* 29–32.

Quant, J. P. (1992). The effect of sleep deprivation and sustained military operations on near visual performance. *Aviation, Space, and Environmental Medicine, 63,* 172–176.

Rechtschaffen, A., Bergmann, B. M., Everson, C. A., Kushida, C. A., & Gilliland, M. A. (1989). Sleep deprivation in the rat: X. Integration and discussion of the findings. *Sleep, 12,* 68–87.

Reilly, T., & Piercy, M. (1994). The effect of partial sleep deprivation on weightlifting performance. *Ergonomics, 37,* 107–115.

Roehrs, T., Timms, V., Zwyghuizen-Doorenbos, A., & Roth, T. (1989). Sleep extension in sleepy and alert normals. *Sleep, 12,* 449–457.

Rosenthal, L., Folkerts, M., Fortier, J., Sicklesteel, J., Roehrs, T. A., & Roth, T. (1994). The effects of selective REM deprivation on daytime sleepiness. *Sleep Research, 23*, 422.

Rosenthal, L., Merlotti, L., & Roehrs, T. A. (1991). Enforced 24-hour recovery following sleep deprivation. *Sleep, 14*, 448–453.

Rosenthal, L., Roehrs, T. A., Rosen, A., & Roth, T. (1993). Level of sleepiness and total sleep time following various time in bed conditions. *Sleep, 16*, 226–232.

Ross, J. J. (1965). Neurologic findings after prolonged sleep deprivation. *Archives of Neurology, 12*, 399–403.

Schiffman, P. L., Trontell, M. C., Mazar, M. F., & Edelman, N. H. (1983). Sleep deprivation decreases ventilatory response to CO_2 but not load compensation. *Chest, 84*, 695–698.

Schilgen, B., & Tolle, R. (1980). Partial sleep deprivation as therapy for depression. *Archives of General Psychiatry, 37*, 267–271.

Shepard, J. W., Jr. (1992). Hypertension, cardiac arrhythmias, myocardial infarction, and stroke in relation to obstructive sleep apnea. *Clinics in Chest Medicine, 13*, 437–458.

Stepanski, E., Lamphere, J., Badia, P., Zorick, F., & Roth, T. (1984). Sleep fragmentation and daytime sleepiness. *Sleep, 7*, 18–26.

Stoohs, R. A., & Dement, W. C. (1993). Snoring and sleep-related breathing abnormality during partial sleep deprivation. *New England Journal of Medicine, 328*, 1279.

Strassman, R. J., Qualls, C. R., Lisansky, E. J., & Peake, G. T. (1991a). Elevated rectal temperature produced by all-night bright light is reversed by melatonin infusion in men. *Journal of Applied Physiology, 71*, 2178–2182.

Strassman, R. J., Qualls, C. R., Lisansky, E. J., & Peake, G. T. (1991b). Sleep deprivation reduces LH secretion in men independently of melatonin. *Acta Endocrinologica, 124*, 646–651.

Sullivan, C. E., Issa, F. G., Berthon-Jones, M., & Saunders, N. A. (1984). Pathophysiology of sleep apnea. In N. A. Saunders & C. E. Sullivan (Eds.), *Sleep and breathing* (pp. 299–364). New York: Marcal Dekker.

Tyler, D. B. (1955). Psychological changes during experimental sleep deprivation. *Diseases of the Nervous System, 16*, 293–304.

VanHelder, T., Symons, J. D., & Radomski, M. W. (1993). Effects of sleep deprivation and exercise on glucose tolerance. *Aviation, Space, and Environmental Medicine, 64*, 487–492.

Vogel, G. W., Thurmond, A., Gibbons, P., Sloan, K., Boyd, M., & Walker, M. (1975). REM sleep reduction effects on depression syndromes. *Archives of General Psychiatry, 32*, 765–777.

Volk, S., Kaendler, S. H., Weber, R., Georgi, K., Maul, F., Hertel, A., Pflug, B., & Hor, G. (1992). Evaluation of the effects of total sleep deprivation on cerebral blood flow using single photon emission computerized tomography. *Acta Psychiatry Scandinavia, 86*, 478–483.

Walsh, J. K., Hartman, P. G., & Schweitzer, P. K. (1994). Slow-wave sleep deprivation and waking function. *Journal of Sleep Research, 3*, 16–25.

Walsh, J. K., Muehlbach, M. J., Humm, T. M., Dickins, Q. S., Sugerman, J. L., & Schweitzer, P. K. (1990). Effect of caffeine on physiological sleep tendency and ability to sustain wakefulness at night. *Psychopharmacology, 101,* 271–273.

Webb, W. B. (1985). A further analysis of age and sleep deprivation effects. *Psychophysiology, 22,* 156–161.

Webb, W. B., & Agnew, H. W., Jr. (1974). The effects of a chronic limitation of sleep length. *Psychophysiology, 11,* 265–274.

Wellens, H. J. J., Vermeulen, A., & Durrer, D. (1972). Ventricular fibrillation occurring on arousal from sleep by auditory stimuli. *Circulation, 46,* 661–665.

Wilkinson, R. T. (1961). Interaction of lack of sleep with knowledge of results, repeated testing, and individual differences. *Journal of Experimental Psychology, 62,* 263–271.

Wilkinson, R. T. (1964). Effects of up to 60 hours sleep deprivation on different types of work. *Ergonomics, 7,* 175–186.

Wilkinson, R. T. (1968). Performance tests for partial and selective sleep deprivation. *Progress in Clinical Psychology, 8,* 28–43.

Williams, H. L., & Lubin, A. (1967). Speeded addition and sleep loss. *Journal of Experimental Psychology, 73,* 313–317.

Williams, H. L., Lubin, A., & Goodnow, J. J. (1959). Impaired performance with acute sleep loss. *Psychology Monographs, 73,* 1–26.

Wu, J. C., Bunney, W. E. (1990). The biological basis of an antidepressant response to sleep deprivation and relapse: Review and hypothesis. *American Journal of Psychiatry, 147,* 14–21.

Wu, J. C., Gillin, J. C., Buchsbaum, M. S., Hershey, T., Hazlett, E., Sicotte, N., & Bunney, W. E. (1991). The effect of sleep deprivation on cerebral glucose metabolic rate in normal humans assessed with positron emission tomography. *Sleep, 14,* 155–162.

Public Policy and Sleep Disorders

Mary A. Carskadon and Jennifer F. Taylor

The fields of sleep research and sleep disorders medicine have made significant progress in many areas over the last 40 years, yet the impact of sleep problems on society remains great. This chapter reviews the development of sleep disorders medicine in the United States and assesses the present situation vis-à-vis sleep and society as established through the efforts of the National Commission on Sleep Disorders Research, highlighting a number of areas needing additional attention. Sleep disorders affect millions of patients and their families directly, and the consequences of sleep disorders and insufficient sleep drain societal resources as well.

Historical Perspective on Sleep Disorders Medicine

The discovery of REM sleep and its relationship to dreaming ushered in the modern era of sleep research in the early 1950s (Aserinsky & Kleitman, 1953). Psychiatrists were first to pursue the study of this nocturnal phenomenon, inspired by the potential of REM sleep to provide a window on the unconscious. In short order, sleep phenomena became the focus of investigation for a variety of North American scientists, who organized the Association for the Psychophysiological Study of Sleep (APSS) in the early 1960s. The APSS began with a solid cadre of young psychiatrists, psychologists, and physiologists, of whom a dozen convened in 1967 to hammer out the standard criteria for evaluating human sleep (Rechtschaffen & Kales, 1968).

The early 1960s also marked the first significant advances toward an understanding of sleep disorders. For example, U.S. and Japanese investigators unlocked part of the mystery of narcolepsy in 1963, when they independently described the relationship of the unusual symptoms of this disorder—cataplexy, sleep paralysis, hypnagogic hallucinations—with the early appearance of REM sleep at sleep onset (Rechtschaffen, Wolpert, Dement, Mitchell, & Fisher, 1963; Takahashi & Jimbo, 1963). Meanwhile, in Europe, the sleep apnea syndrome—a disorder destined to become a driving force behind the second great expansion of interest in sleep disorders—was described (Jung & Kuhlo, 1965; Gastaut, Tassinari, & Duron, 1965).

In 1970, William C. Dement of Stanford University established the first sleep disorders clinic in the United States with the goal of providing a specialist's attention to patients with sleep disorders. In 1975, the first handful of sleep clinicians met in Chicago and founded an alliance aimed at establishing guidelines for evaluating and treating sleep disorders and for certifying the skills of clinicians in this field. Prominent among this early group were psychologists and physicians trained in psychiatry and neurology. In 1979, the Association of Sleep Disorders Centers (ASDC) published the first comprehensive classification system for sleep disorders (Association of Sleep Disorders Centers, 1979). Sleep apnea was by this time clearly identified as a major sleep disorder with significant consequences for waking function. The careful assessment of daytime sleepiness became a focus of research in the late 1970s and early 1980s, largely spurred by close clinical investigation of the two major disorders of excessive sleepiness: narcolepsy and sleep apnea.

The 1980s saw an exponential expansion in the number of sleep disorders centers and clinicians specializing in sleep disorders. The report of a successful treatment for obstructive sleep apnea—nasal continuous positive airway pressure—propelled this expansion (Sullivan, Issa, Berthon-Jones, & Eves, 1981). The availability of an effective nonsurgical treatment for this disorder served to amplify the interest in sleep disorders, particularly on the part of pulmonary physicians. The description of another new disorder in 1986—one with a vivid and characteristic presentation—was a significant landmark (Schenck, Bundlie, Ettinger, & Mahowald, 1986); that the REM sleep behavior disorder had heretofore been overlooked signaled for many the depth of the gulf separating clinical observation from illnesses of the night.

The decade of the 1980s was capped by the publication of the first comprehensive textbook of sleep medicine (Kryger, Roth, & Dement, 1989), which has since gone into a second edition (Kryger, Roth, & Dement, 1994), and a pediatrics volume has been written (Kryger & Ferber, 1995). The sleep disorders nosology was reconfigured and expanded in an international diagnostic system for sleep disorders (International Classification of Sleep Disorders, 1990) under the auspices of the American Sleep Disorders Association (ASDA), the revamped version of the ASDC. The present U.S. membership of the ASDA includes approximately 2,360 individuals and 236 sleep disorders centers (American Sleep Disorders Association, 1994).

The National Commission on Sleep Disorders Research

In the midst of this growing interest in sleep disorders, there arose a concern that these disorders have a significant impact on society but were poorly understood and little known beyond the sleep disorders cognoscenti. This concern was met in 1988 by the U.S. Congressional establishment of the National Commission on Sleep Disorders Research (NCSDR). Commission members were appointed, and the first meeting was held on March 28, 1990. William C. Dement of Stanford University was elected chair, and Joseph A. Piscopo, vice-chair. Administrative responsibility for the commission was assumed by the National Institute on Aging, whose representative to the commission, Andrew A. Monjan, served as executive secretary. The appointed and *ex officio* members of the NCSDR included a broad representation of interested people: sleep and circadian rhythms scientists, clinicians, patients, patient advocates, and representatives of several government agencies, most prominently the National Institutes of Health (NIH), as well as the Uniformed Services, Veterans Administration, and Centers for Disease Control.

The charge by Congress to the NCSDR was threefold:

1. To conduct a comprehensive study of the present state of knowledge of the incidence, prevalence, morbidity, and mortality resulting from sleep disorders and of the social and economic impact of such disorders.
2. To evaluate the public and private facilities and resources (including trained personnel and research activities) available for the diagnosis, prevention, and treatment of as well as research into such disorders.

3. To identify programs (including biological, physiological, behavioral, environmental, and social programs) by which improvement in the management and research into sleep disorders can be accomplished.

The process adopted by the NCSDR to accomplish these tasks included public hearings and the initiation of a set of working groups to gather information and prepare position papers. Eight public hearings were held over the course of approximately 15 months. Testimony was presented by a wide variety of individuals: patients and their family members, sleep disorders experts, basic scientists in the areas of sleep research and circadian rhythms, educators, and representatives from industry, the military, and regulatory agencies. Working groups were formed around several cross-cutting issues, such as basic sciences research, cardiopulmonary disorders, narcolepsy and neurological disorders, mental health, life span (early development, aging, and women's issues), shift work and transportation, insomnia, and several others. Commission members worked with experts from these fields to compile position papers. Along with the data gathered in the course of the hearings, the position papers served as the information base for the NCSDR deliberations, which culminated in the submission of the executive report to Congress in January of 1993 (National Commission on Sleep Disorders Research, 1993).

Report of the National Commission

The major findings of the NCSDR are summarized in Exhibit 1; several are discussed in this chapter. The scope of the problem is quite large: On the basis of extrapolations from extant epidemiological data, the NCSDR concluded that chronic primary sleep disorders affect about 40 million U.S. residents and that about half again as many experience sleep disorders on an intermittent or recurrent basis. Obstructive sleep apnea syndrome (SAS) and insomnia were singled out by the NCSDR as the most prevalent chronic sleep disorders, affecting nearly 20 million and 16.25 million adults, respectively. Approximately one-quarter million Americans have narcolepsy, one of the most thoroughly studied chronic sleep disorders. Other sleep disorders have an unknown prevalence; however, the NCSDR report raised an important issue: the strong association of sleep disturbance with mental and substance abuse disorders. For example, insomnia is a predictor for the subsequent occurrence

Exhibit 1

Findings of the NCSDR

- Millions of Americans are affected by sleep disorders.
- Sleep disorders affect all age groups.
- The problem will grow.
- Too little research has been conducted in women.
- Minorities and the poor have too little access to sleep medicine.
- Americans are seriously sleep-deprived with disastrous consequences.
- The cost is high in dollars, lives, and human suffering.
- There is a pervasive failure of knowledge transfer.
- There are serious gaps in research.
- Alarmingly few young investigators are in "the pipeline".

Note. NCSDR = National Commission on Sleep Disorders Research.

of depression (Ford & Kamerow, 1989). Several clear messages emerged from the commission's estimates of the prevalence of sleep disorders. First, improved epidemiological data are needed to provide better estimates of the prevalence of sleep disorders. Second, given the commission's estimates and the known availability of clinical resources, the numbers of persons with undiagnosed and untreated sleep disorders were thought to be exceedingly high. Third, present resources are inadequate to meet the clinical needs.

The NCSDR report also emphasized that sleep disorders affect persons of all ages, although specific prevalence rates are available for only a few disorders (e.g., sleep apnea, insomnia, narcolepsy) and certain age groups. In the very young, sudden infant death syndrome (SIDS) is thought to be a sleep-related disorder of unknown etiology affecting 8–10,000 infants each year. In some infants, congenital malformations of the face and jaw may lead to sleep apnea, and as many as 1 in 4 children under 5 years may experience some kind of sleep disturbance. Particularly for infants and young children, a sleep disorder may affect the entire family. The prevalence of major sleep disorders in adolescence is unknown, although adolescents may have heightened susceptibility to certain problems, perhaps circadian rhythm disorders in particular (Dahl & Carskadon, 1995). The prevalence of many sleep disorders, most particularly sleep-disordered breathing and periodic limb movement disorder, increases across adulthood and into old age. Sleep disorders associated with multiple drug use and dementia may also be prominent in the elderly.

The NCSDR report cited evidence that the problem of sleep disorders in the United States is destined to worsen in tandem with the aging of the U.S. population. Many of the major sleep disorders have age as a primary risk factor, hence escalating the problems over the next several decades. The NCSDR report projected that by the year 2010, sleeping problems will affect 79 million, and excessive sleepiness, 40 million Americans.

As with many medical conditions, sleep disorders in women have not been studied nearly to the same extent as in men. As meager as the data are for women, the effects of race and ethnicity on sleep disorders are even less well studied. These gaps in knowledge may seriously compromise professionals' ability to generalize from assumptions regarding sleep disorders and their impact.

One of the most striking findings of the commission was the "pervasive failure of knowledge transfer" (National Commission on Sleep Disorders Research, 1993, p. 24) regarding sleep. This deficit was found to affect virtually every level of training and education. Despite the major advances in diagnosis and treatment of sleep disorders in the last 3 decades, little of this knowledge has become part of educational curricula. One of the activities sponsored by the NCSDR was a survey of "Deans of Education, Directors of Undergraduate Education and Course Directors in Medicine, Physiology, Neural Science, Behavioral Science, Psychiatry, Neurology, Family Practice and Pediatrics at 126 accredited medical schools in the United States" (Rosen, Rosekind, Rosevear, Cole, & Dement, 1993, p. 250). This survey found that sleep and sleep disorders medicine received an average of less than 2 hours of total teaching time, and 37 of the schools responding reported no teaching time allocated to sleep disorders. A separate study of pediatrics training found a similarly limited amount of teaching about sleep disorders (Mindell, Moline, Zendell, Brown, & Fry, 1994). The extent of training in sleep disorders that occurs in clinical psychology, nursing, and other clinical programs has not been formally surveyed; however, informal testimony to the commission revealed a lack of such training across the board. The commission hearings also revealed that curricular training in sleep physiology, sleep hygiene, and sleep disorders is not available throughout the normal educational span, including grammar school, junior and senior high school, college, and graduate training.

The educational gap spans business and management schools as well, even though future business managers of businesses will one day be supervising workers and dealing with issues of shift work, sleep deprivation, and sleep-related performance impairment.

The impact of this pervasive ignorance is felt most poignantly at the level of the individual patient. Time after time, patients speaking at the NCSDR hearings noted not just the delay in adequate diagnostic assessment but also the difficulties faced by themselves or family members owing to the lack of understanding on the part of members of the community: teachers, employers, and friends. The testimony of one mother is illustrative:

> My son has narcolepsy. . . . He has been branded by the local education system as lazy, day dreaming, incompetent, lacking imagination and motivation. . . . It's time the medical and educational system woke up to the fact that this is a medical disorder. The ridicule, humiliation, and labeling must be stopped and replaced by knowledge. (National Commission on Sleep Disorders Research, 1993, p. 19)

The costs of sleep disorders to society were estimated by the NCSDR at billions of dollars per year. Work commissioned by the NCSDR based on 1990 statistics led to the conclusion that the direct societal costs of sleep disorders (as well as sleep deprivation and circadian factors) amount to $15.9 billion annually. Direct costs include costs of such items as hospitalization, treatment, and provider fees. The NCSDR estimated that the total societal costs—including such indirect economic costs as loss of productivity resulting from disability or premature demise— might be 10-fold greater, approximately $150 billion. A recent publication (Leger, 1994) provided detailed calculations of the total costs of accidents owing to sleepiness on the basis of 1988 statistics. Leger's conclusion was that the economic impact of sleepiness-related accidents in the United States during 1988 was between $43.15 and $56.02 billion.

In addition to the economic price of sleep disorders to society, the price paid by individuals is disturbingly high. Years of suffering resulting from the failure to receive adequate diagnosis and treatment can rob individuals of educational opportunities, economic advancement, and life itself. Patients and family members testifying at NCSDR hearings provided evidence in heart-wrenching detail:

- *Sleep apnea.* My undetected sleep disorder robbed me of the chance to continue the educational process. . . . Individual potentials . . .

withered and remained undeveloped within me, and at 46 years of age, I struggle to convince myself that I am fortunate to have a job, a mainstream job, that pays all of $15,000 a year. . . . (National Commission on Sleep Disorders Research, 1993, p. 24)

- *Sudden infant death syndrome.* It was a few days past Christmas two years ago. . . . She endeared herself to everyone with her flirting and her laughter. She was my perfect little angel. . . . Karen put her down for a nap at 4:30 pm and found her dead at ten minutes till five. . . . In a matter of a few moments her life of promise was gone, and our road of grief was only beginning. (National Commission on Sleep Disorders Research, 1993, p. 15)

- *Insomnia.* I had a major breakdown due to insomnia, work overload and other emotional problems. I had to take time off my job to try to recover, but recovery eluded me, and the job I loved drifted daily ever further out of my reach. . . . The sleepless nights continued along with the horror-filled days. . . . The insomnia had worn me down to the point where I couldn't care for myself. . . . I was really scared that I'd never be able to pick up the pieces of my life, and would have to sit an emotional, sleepless cripple for the rest of my life. (National Commission on Sleep Disorders Research, 1993, p. 16)

- *Narcolepsy.* I have lived with the symptoms of narcolepsy for at least 45 years. . . . Prior to diagnosis, I was directly responsible for several near-fatal automobile accidents. I received diagnosis only because of a 3-paragraph article in the San Francisco Chronicle. . . . The simple joys and pleasures everyone takes for granted . . . would, for the most part, be denied me. I would literally sleep the rest of my life away. (National Commission on Sleep Disorders Research, 1993, p. 16)

One area wherein the cost of sleep disorders has been neither well described nor well recognized is regarding the elderly. The incidence of many sleep disorders increases with age. For example, the prevalence of sleep apnea in middle-aged adults is estimated to be 4% in women and 9% in men (Young et al., 1993); in the elderly, however, the estimated prevalence of sleep-disordered breathing ranges from 28% to 62% (Ancoli-Israel & Coy, 1994). Similarly, the prevalence of sleep-related periodic limb movements in the elderly is estimated to be 45% (Ancoli-Israel et al., 1991). These high prevalence rates have led some to suggest that such sleep-related phenomena are a part of the natural aging process and of no consequence. Ancoli-Israel and Coy (1994) argued eloquently that the older patient must be assessed as is the younger:

> Elderly should be treated just like other age groups, that is, if they present with sleepiness, it is important to determine whether that sleepiness is caused by medications, circadian rhythm changes, periodic

limb movements in sleep or SAS. Excessive daytime sleepiness in any age group is not normal behavior. (p. 81)

Societal stereotypes must be replaced by knowledge about sleep disorders.

The recommendations of the NCSDR are outlined in Exhibit 2. The first of these has already come to pass. As part of the 1993 National Institutes of Health (NIH) Revitalization Act, the National Heart, Lung, and Blood Institute was authorized to establish the National Center on Sleep Disorders Research. The National Center advisory board has recently been established, and that body is working on the priorities for the center. Funding for the center is unfortunately not at a level that will support the goals set by the NCSDR. In fact, the funding is approximately 10% of the NCSDR recommendation. Nevertheless, the center

---

Exhibit 2

Recommendations of the NCSDR

1. Establish a national center within an existing institute of the NIH ($16.4 million).
2. Strengthen ongoing programs of the NIH (including ADAMHA) and other agencies (with an immediate increase of $55.8 million above existing levels for research in sleep and sleep disorders).
3. Establish accountability in all federal agencies concerned with sleep and sleep disorders following a study by the Office of Science Technology Policy to establish feasibility of a coordinating body ($1.1 million).
4. Increase levels of federal support for sleep and sleep disorder research, training, and career development ($2.5 million).
5. Ask congress to encourage education and awareness of sleep disorders to the full range of health care professionals, particularly those in primary care ($4 million).
6. Urge federal government to undertake a major public awareness– education campaign about sleep disorders to educate American public ($3.25 million).

Note.   NCSDR = National Commission on Sleep Disorders Research; NIH = National Institutes of Health; ADAMHA = Alcohol, Drug, and Mental Health Administration.

is poised to assist in the coordination of efforts within the federal government and in cooperation with nongovernmental groups (e.g., the National Sleep Foundation and the ASDA).

The NCSDR endorsed the efforts of the NIH and the Alcohol, Drug, and Mental Health Administration (ADAMHA) and urged them to continue to expand their research efforts. The center was not conceived by the commission as a mechanism to replace, but rather as a way to augment and support, the efforts of these agencies. The NCSDR prepared a blueprint that detailed areas and mechanisms in need of new research funding. Current fiscal realities limit the likelihood that these recommended initiatives will receive adequate attention in the short term. Nevertheless, the NCSDR has provided a clear assessment of the major gaps. One of the other recommendations—the establishment of federal accountability—was intended to help identify a mechanism that would span the entire federal purview to include not just NIH and ADAMHA but any agencies whose functions involve issues raised by sleep disorders.

The remaining recommendations of the NCSDR pointed to initiatives that were considered urgent and central to many of the major problems identified in the course of the commission's proceedings. Specific funds were recommended to support research training and career development in sleep and sleep disorders. The NCSDR recommended that Congress encourage and support dissemination of information about sleep disorders to all health care professional training programs. The final recommendation urged the development of a campaign to educate the public about sleep and sleep disorders.

Conclusion

The National Commission on Sleep Disorders Research served the purpose defined for it in the Congressional initiative. Steps taken since the commission was founded and since its report was filed point to its lasting impact on the nation. Implementation of its full menu of recommendations is unlikely, yet the gains in terms of the establishment of the National Center for Sleep Disorders Research and in highlighting the scope of the problems have provided incremental progress for the field. As always, grass roots interest will be the key to sustaining and augmenting the gains made by the NCSDR. Patient groups, as well as scientists and clinicians with a grasp of the issues, will need to bolster the efforts of the National Center and of the various institutes and federal agencies involved in pushing back the rivers of ignorance.

The scope of the problems presented by sleep disorders is vast and includes not only the individual patient but also the health and well-being of all Americans. A variety of roles exist for psychology and behavioral medicine in the efforts to identify, treat, and understand sleep disorders, as well as in the efforts to provide education to people in many levels of society. Clearly, many if not most sleep disorders benefit from behavioral treatment approaches. Significant inroads have already been made in the treatment of insomnia (Morin, 1993; Spielman, Saskin, & Thorpy, 1987). More work needs to be done for patients in other diagnostic categories of sleep disorders. Of particular importance are the opportunities to educate patients of all ages about healthy approaches to sleep behavior. Psychologists and other behavioral scientists are well positioned to pursue the initiatives identified by the NCSDR and to push forward the knowledge transfer that is so urgently needed.

REFERENCES

American Sleep Disorders Association. (1994, November). A glance at the continuing growth of the ASDA membership. *ASDA Update,* p. 5.

Ancoli-Israel, S., & Coy, T. (1994). Are breathing disturbances in elderly equivalent to sleep apnea syndrome? *Sleep, 17,* 77–83.

Ancoli-Israel, S., Kripke, D. F., Klauber, M. R., Mason, W. J., Fell, R., & Kaplan, O. (1991). Periodic limb movements in sleep in community-dwelling elderly. *Sleep, 14,* 496–500.

Aserinsky, E., & Kleitman, N. (1953). Regularly occurring periods of eye motility, and concomitant phenomena, during sleep. *Science, 118,* 273–274.

Association of Sleep Disorders Centers (ASDC), Sleep Disorders Classification Committee. (1979). Diagnostic classification of sleep and arousal disorders. *Sleep, 2,* 1–137.

Dahl, R. E., & Carskadon, M. A. (1995). Sleep and its disorders in adolescence. In M. H. Kryger & R. Ferber (Eds.), *Principles and practice of sleep medicine in the child,* (pp. 19–27). Philadelphia: Saunders.

Ford, D. E., & Kamerow, D. B. (1989). Epidemiological study of sleep disturbances and psychiatric disorders. An opportunity for prevention? *Journal of the American Medical Association, 262,* 1479–1484.

Gastaut, H., Tassinari, C., & Duron, B. (1965). Etude polygraphique des manifestations episodiques (hypniques et respiratoire) diurnes et nocturnes du syndom de Pickwick. [Polygraphic study of the diurnal and nocturnal episodic manifestations (sleep and breathing) of the Pickwick syndrome]. *Reviews of Neurology, 112,* 568–579.

International Classification of Sleep Disorders. (1990). *Diagnostic and coding manual.* Rochester, MN: American Sleep Disorders Association.

Jung, R., & Kuhlo, W. (1965). Neurophysiological studies of abnormal night sleep and the Pickwickian syndrome. In K. Akert, C. Bally, & J. P. Schadé (Eds.), *Sleep mechanisms: Progress in brain research* (Vol. 18, pp. 141–159). Amsterdam: Elsevier.

Kryger, M. H., & Ferber, R. (Eds.). (1995). *Principles and practice of sleep medicine in the child.* Philadelphia: Saunders.

Kryger, M. H., Roth, T., & Dement, W. C. (Eds.). (1989). *Principles and practice of sleep medicine.* Philadelphia: Saunders.

Kryger, M. H., Roth, T., & Dement, W. C. (Eds.). (1994). *Principles and practice of sleep medicine* (2nd ed.). Philadelphia: Saunders.

Leger, D. (1994). The cost of sleep-related accidents: A report for the national commission on sleep disorders research. *Sleep, 17,* 84–93.

Mindell, J. A., Moline, M. L., Zendell, S. M., Brown, L. W., & Fry, J. M. (1994). Pediatricians and sleep disorders: Training and practice. *Pediatrics, 94*(2, Pt. 1), 194–200.

Morin, C. M. (1993). *Insomnia: Psychological assessment and management.* New York: Guilford Press.

National Commission on Sleep Disorders Research. (1993). *Wake up America: A national sleep alert* (Vol. 1). Executive summary and executive report. Washington, DC: Author.

Rechtschaffen, A., & Kales, A. (Eds.). (1968). Berger, R. J., Dement, W. C., Jacobson, A., Johnson, L. C., Jouvet, M., Monroe, L. J., Oswald, I., Roffwarg, H. P., Roth, B., & Walter, R. D. *A manual of standardized terminology, techniques and scoring system for sleep stages of human subjects.* Los Angeles: UCLA Brain Information Service/Brain Research Institute.

Rechtschaffen, A., Wolpert, E., Dement, W. C., Mitchell, S., & Fisher, C. (1963). Nocturnal sleep of narcoleptics. *Electroencephalography and Clinical Neurophysiology, 15,* 599–609.

Rosen, R. C., Rosekind, M., Rosevear, C., Cole, W. E., & Dement, W. C. (1993). Physician education in sleep and sleep disorders: A national survey of U.S. medical schools. *Sleep, 16,* 249–254.

Schenck, C. H., Bundlie, S. R., Ettinger, M. G., & Mahowald, M. W. (1986). Chronic behavioral disorders of human REM sleep: A new category of parasomnia. *Sleep, 9,* 293–308.

Spielman, A. J., Saskin, P., & Thorpy, M. J. (1987). Treatment of chronic insomnia by restriction of time in bed. *Sleep, 10,* 45–56.

Sullivan, C. E., Issa, F. G., Berthon-Jones, M., & Eves, L. (1981). Reversal of obstructive sleep apnea by continuous positive airway pressure applied through the nares. *Lancet, 1,* 862–865.

Takahashi, Y., & Jimbo, M. (1963). Polygraphic study of narcolepsy with special reference to hypnagogic hallucination and cataplexy. *Folia Psychiatrica Neurologica Japonica, 7*(Suppl.), 343–347.

Young, T., Palta, M., Dempsey, J., Skatrud, J., Weber, S., & Badr, S. (1993). The occurrence of sleep-disordered breathing among middle-aged adults. *New England Journal of Medicine, 328,* 1230–1235.

II

Diagnostic Methods and Tools for the Evaluation of Sleep Disorders

6

The Diagnostic Interview and Differential Diagnosis for Complaints of Insomnia

Arthur J. Spielman and Paul B. Glovinsky

Trouble sleeping is one of the most common health complaints in the general population and is especially prevalent in patients with psychological problems (Gallup Organization, 1991; Mellinger, Balter, & Uhlenhuth, 1985). The American Psychological Association estimated that each year approximately 600,000 visits to psychologists are due to insomnia complaints (see National Commission on Sleep Disorders Research, 1992); therefore, insomnia is too ubiquitous to be left solely to the sleep specialist. Although difficult cases should be referred to experts at sleep disorders centers, the psychologist's expertise in the evaluation of multidetermined problems and the administration of nondrug treatments makes psychological referral appropriate for the majority of patients with insomnia. Furthermore, patients prefer the behavioral approaches that psychologists offer (Morin, Gaulier, Barry, & Kowatch, 1992).

When the patient's history is suggestive of an underlying physiological disorder such as a sleep-related respiratory disturbance or periodic leg movements, referral to a sleep disorders center is advisable. Evaluation in these cases should include overnight polysomnography. In other cases, the insomnia is readily understood as secondary to a medical disorder such as arthritis or chronic bladder infection. In these cases, the psychologist may consult with the treating physician regarding containment of secondary sleep disruption. In still other instances, insomnia is the central complaint but the clinical picture is

125

complicated by long-term reliance on sleeping pills. In these cases, the psychologist is positioned to collaborate with the physician, introducing behavioral and other nondrug therapies as medication is tapered.

When faced with a patient complaining of insomnia that does not appear secondary to a situational disturbance or medical condition, the clinician may be tempted to respond reflexively, suggesting a line of treatment out of familiarity and confidence in the treatment rather than out of regard for the intricacies behind the symptom. These therapeutic avenues include psychotherapy, referral to a physician for hypnotic or psychotropic medication, minimization of the problem, and general prescriptions for stress reduction, lifestyle changes, and sleep hygiene. Any of these may in fact constitute an appropriate clinical response. However, it is our contention that the choice of treatment could be more specifically based on the patient's presenting history if clinicians knew what questions to ask regarding sleep and sleep disturbance. The task becomes one of delineating the particular and often idiosyncratic factors that led to the initial complaint to achieve diagnostic specificity and administer a focused, effective treatment. The assessment approach we recommend requires the patient and the clinician to shift attitudes in line with the nature of insomnia and use a daily sleep diary in conjunction with a comprehensive history (Spielman & Glovinsky, 1991).

In this chapter, we begin with a discussion of how a focused clinical assessment informs the choice of treatment for complaints of insomnia. The nature of the complaint itself provides a fruitful starting point, but it is important to broaden the scope of inquiry to include the entire course of the sleep disturbance, including factors that predisposed the patient towards developing insomnia, factors that precipitated the acute disturbance, and factors that perpetuate the condition. The multiple determinants of insomnia are stressed, necessitating a review of general psychological functioning, medical factors, possible disturbances within sleep itself, the contribution of lifestyle choices and pressures, and habits relating specifically to bedtime and sleeping. The use of a simple sleep log in depicting and delineating these various determinants is presented. The chapter closes with a series of short clinical vignettes illustrating how the sleep log can play a critical role in organizing the complex determinants leading to the complaint of insomnia.

The Assessment

The History

Complaint. The clinician's inquiry, with the help of survey questionnaires, provides the fundamental historical view of the patient's sleep disturbance. The patient's description of the complaint may be key to understanding it and providing effective treatment. The complaint points to the part of the night that is most problematic (e.g., trouble falling asleep, staying asleep, or getting back to sleep in the morning; inability to sleep at the desired time).

Identifying which part of the night is disturbed is important in understanding the problem as well as selecting and customizing treatment. Sleep-onset difficulty that is characteristic of delayed sleep phase syndrome (Weitzman et al., 1981), for example, is responsive to bright light exposure in the morning, whereas nighttime exposure would exacerbate the problem (Rosenthal et al., 1990). In other insomnia conditions, knowing what part of the night is most disturbed is also useful in devising a rational sleep schedule. A common initial intervention is prescribing less time in bed. This is the essential feature of sleep-restriction therapy (Spielman, Saskin, & Thorpy, 1987), but it is also common practice as a part of multicomponent treatments (Hoelscher & Edinger, 1988; Morin, 1993; Morin, Kowatch, Barry, & Walton, 1993). In general, to reduce time in bed when the patient's sleep disturbance is at the beginning of the night, the prescribed time of retiring is set later. Conversely, in cases with early-morning awakenings, the time of arising is set earlier to produce a more compact sleeping period. These therapeutic maneuvers allow the treatment to start by minimizing the initial loss of sleep that restricted time in bed imposes.

Another value of the complaint is that it guides inquiry to the relevant domain. A patient's report of inadequate amount or quality of sleep, for example, requires the clinician to determine whether the daytime consequences are attributable to a sleep disturbance or, alternatively, reflect aspects of psychological problems. Fatigue and irritability, for example, are common features of both insomnia and dysthymic disorder.

Course. The age of onset of the complaint may generate specific hypotheses to be tested while the history is taken. Stage of development, typical challenges at different stages of life, and the expected level of functioning at different ages are all areas of fruitful inquiry that place the problem in a larger context.

Unraveling the chain of factors that contribute to a case of insomnia requires a focus on the course of the disorder (see Exhibit 1). The historical formulation weaves the connections among the premorbid picture of sleep, the initial insomnia, changes over time, and the current sleep disturbance. An appreciation of the blend of predisposing, precipitating, and perpetuating factors often helps the clinician to select a set of interventions that address different components of the problem.

As we have discussed previously (Spielman, 1986; Spielman, Caruso, & Glovinsky, 1987; Spielman & Glovinsky, 1991), understanding the time course and additive nature of three historical factors is helpful (see Figure 1). On top of the relatively constant predisposing factors, the precipitating factors appear at the onset of the insomnia and, in general, diminish with time. The perpetuating factors increase as the sleep disturbance becomes chronic.

Predisposing factors. *Predisposing factors* are conditions that set the stage for insomnia and may determine whether the problem becomes chronic. An emotionally reactive individual will have sleep problems when worries mount. A "night person," who dreads the morning and comes alive at night, is inclined to sleep onset problems. An individual without sleep disturbance but chronically taking steroids has a lowered threshold to development of nocturnal arousal.

Exhibit 1

Issues of Importance in the Course of Insomnia

Predisposing, precipitating, and perpetuating factors (see Figure 1)
Duration of the problem (transient, short-term, chronic)
Changes over time:

- Stable versus getting worse or better
- Duration and circumstances of asymptomatic periods
- Seasonal variation
- Severity covaries with other problems (e.g., medical, psychiatric, stress-related) or changes in sleep habits and hygiene that may perpetuate the problem (see Exhibit 2)

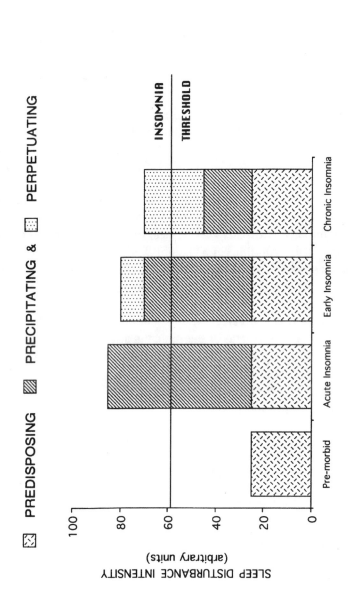

Figure 1. The contributions to insomnia change with time. From "A Behavioral Perspective on Insomnia Treatment," by A. J. Spielman, L. S. Caruso, & P. B. Glovinsky, 1987, *Psychiatric Clinics of North America, 10,* 541–553. Adapted with permission of W. B. Saunders Co.

Long-term psychological disorders and physiologically based hyperarousal are key elements in models of chronic insomnia (Hauri & Fisher, 1986; Kales, Caldwell, Preston, Healey, & Kales, 1976; Spielman & Glovinsky, 1991). The internalization of psychological conflicts may burden the individual with ruminative worry or anxious anticipation. Somatization of conflicts or constitutionally high physiological arousal are obstacles to sleep that present long-term challenges for some individuals.

Precipitating factors. The importance of precipitating factors is intuitively obvious, whereas appreciation of the other two factors is more easily overlooked (Spielman, 1986). Whether the insomnia began gradually or suddenly, both patient and clinician typically focus on concurrent conditions to figure out what precipitated the problem. Understanding the trigger often provides enough information to formulate an initial treatment. For instance, one can change the timing and dosage of theophylline in a patient being treated for asthma. A problem may cease after the resolution of a depressive reaction produced by a job loss. A patient can be advised not to indulge in espresso after work.

Perpetuating factors. Perpetuating factors develop after insomnia begins. They may be a result of the patient's attempt to cope with the sleep disturbance. In many cases, the original cause of the sleep problem has long subsided, but the perpetuating factors are sufficient to maintain the sleep disturbance (see Exhibit 2). Sleeping late in the morning after a bad night, for example, may be a reasonable way to

---

Exhibit 2

Factors That Commonly Perpetuate Insomnia

Too much time in bed
Variable retiring and arising times
Unpredictability of sleep
Concern about daytime deficits
Napping, dozing, and nodding
Fragmentation of sleep
Maladaptive conditioning
Caffeine consumption
Hypnotic and alcohol ingestion

limit the deleterious effects of sleep loss. Although it may improve mood, performance, and alertness the next day, the irregularity of the sleep schedule that oversleeping produces may make it difficult to fall asleep the following night. Thus, the sleep problem is sustained.

Insomniacs who worry about the detrimental effect of too little sleep on their health may remain in bed for long periods "resting to keep the immune system strong." The repeated experience of being awake resting in bed during the night establishes a habit that does not promote the bed as a cue for sleep (Bootzin & Nicassio, 1978). This maladaptive conditioning interferes with sleep.

Although it is clear that napping during the day may reduce the propensity for sleep at night, some insomniacs are caught in a vicious cycle. Daytime napping may alleviate the deficits of sleep loss, however, it leads to inadequate nocturnal sleep. Less well recognized is the effect of very brief dozing or "spacing out" in front of the TV in the evening. When it is time to retire, the individual may become activated (e.g., through bathroom rituals or setting the alarm), and the window of opportunity for sleep is closed.

For effective long-term treatment, the patient should understand the developmental chain of factors that can contribute to the problem. The clinician may make a statement like either of the following:

> There's more to your insomnia now than when it first began. In addition to the psychological blow caused by the end of your marriage, your response to the sleep disturbance may be compounding the problem. In other words, the way you have coped with the insomnia may now be making things worse. You have been napping and drinking more coffee to help restore your alertness and vitality. While this has helped you maintain your functioning, nighttime sleep may be suffering as a consequence.
>
> Your sleep problem may have less to do with the end of your marriage and more to do with your having learned that your bed is a place for agitation, not repose. You now regularly toss and turn in bed for hours before you finally get to sleep. The bed may have become a cue that triggers worries about sleep; it's become a place to toss and turn. As the hour of sleep approaches and the bed beckons, you have learned to worry about the upcoming trials and tribulations. This worry itself is interfering with your ability to fall asleep.

Multiple determinants of insomnia. A comprehensive evaluation places the complaint in a historical perspective and surveys psychological issues, medical status, lifestyle, sleep habits, and the response to trial treatments. In addition, the possible role of physiological abnormalities during sleep should be considered. Patients may first visit the doctor with great certainty about the cause of their problem. One individual is convinced that the sleep disturbance is due to a biological abnormality of the brain; another person is sure that emotional difficulties are at the root of the condition; and a third sees the problem as a result of external stress. Because the patient is often at least in part correct, and to help foster rapport, it is important to start where the patient indicates the problem resides. However, it is equally important to cast a wide net, encouraging the patient to explore all the influences on sleep posed by psychological adaptation, organic factors, lifestyle, and sleep hygiene. Even if one factor predominates, it is beneficial to uncover a set of supporting factors. In fact, these relatively minor contributions to the problem may be the easiest to remedy. Addressing these factors will likely produce a modest initial improvement, helping motivate the patient to tackle more central but entrenched causes of insomnia.

Many patients are baffled by their sleep disturbance and report that the only problems in their life are the worry about sleeplessness and the fatigue, irritability, and other daytime consequences of insomnia. In these cases, we also emphasize that we will need to undertake a comprehensive review to root out the cause of the problem. In addition, we acknowledge that insomnia itself imposes stress and worry and that we can deal directly with this vicious cycle: insomnia → sleep worries and daytime deficits → arousal → insomnia, and so on (Kales et al., 1976).

The clinician's response should be measured because the outward presentations of insomnia are deceptively uniform; although few presenting complaints exist, there are endless combinations of factors that result in sleep disturbance. This underlying complexity does yield to a systematic inquiry. A comprehensive approach informs the patient that there are many ways of attacking the problem. For example, a patient may emphasize that the stress of performing on the job has become an intrusive presleep preoccupation and that going to sleep early maximizes the sleep eventually obtained. This patient must learn that this practice is counterproductive over the long run and relatively easy to correct. In another case, although it may be self-evident that sleep disturbance is produced by the disruptions attendant on divorce, the connection is less apparent when the bedroom environment has become conditioned to elicit disturbing memories of the former partner. Reestablishing the bedroom as a comfortable haven, by moving furniture, redecorating, and removing the cues associated with the former partner, may be the appropriate first step in treating the sleep problem. Any improvement may render the patient more amenable to further adjustments, initiating a lengthier process of adaptation to a new status as a single person. In summary, any step in the right direction, toward sleep, builds momentum and the motivation to deal with more central issues. Toward this end the practitioner may say the following:

> I see how you understand the problem. We are also going to look for anything else that may be adding to the situation. It is important for you to try to identify all the contributions to the sleep disturbance. We will be systematically looking at your psychological well-being, medical status, possible physiological problems during sleep, lifestyle, and sleep habits for clues to what's wrong and how to help you. For example, I have seen patients who understand that stress on the job triggered the problem; however, they often do not appreciate that the habit of bringing projects home from the office and working late into the evening interferes with sleep. Let's come up with a list of contributing factors to address in your treatment.

Psychological functioning. Just as night follows day, so does sleep disturbance follow psychological distress. Arousal from the ruminations and anxieties of psychological concerns may postpone or interrupt sleep. As thinking and feeling depart from the neutral zone, sleep suffers. Worrying about potential danger and the excited anticipation of reward both can undo sleep. Similarly, affective arousal such as anxiety and depression are common disturbers of sleep. The use of insomnia as a diagnostic criterion in a number of psychiatric disturbances is evidence that sleep may be seen as a bellwether of psychic struggles (see Table 1). In addition, insomnia problems are coded independently of mental disorders as *primary insomnia, breathing-related sleep disorder, circadian rhythm sleep disorder*, and *sleep disorder due to a general medical condition* (American Psychiatric Association, 1994).

The common role that psychiatric disorders and psychological functioning play in insomnia requires a focus on mental life in the interview and suggests the use of psychological tests such as the Minnesota Multiphasic Personality Inventory (MMPI; Hathaway & McKinley, 1983) or various depression and anxiety scales. In a series of studies, one group demonstrated that a substantial proportion of insomniacs are characterized by a few MMPI profiles (Kales & Kales, 1984). The authors of these correlational studies concluded that an inhibitory

Table 1

Psychiatric Disorders That Have Insomnia as a Diagnostic Criterion

Disorder	DSM-IV code
Major depressive episode	327
Dysthymic disorder	300.4
Generalized anxiety disorder	300.02
Acute stress disorder	308.3
Posttraumatic stress disorder	309.81
Separation anxiety disorder	309.21
Insomnia related to another mental disorder	307.42
Substance-related disorders	
Substance-induced sleep disorder	various
Alcohol withdrawal	291.8
Caffeine intoxication	305.90
Amphetamine withdrawal	292.0
Cocaine withdrawal	292.0
Nicotine withdrawal	292.0
Opioid withdrawal	292.0
Sedative, hypnotic, or anxiolytic withdrawal	292.0

Note. DSM-IV = *Diagnostic and Statistical Manual of Mental Disorders* (4th ed.). From *Diagnostic and Statistical Manual of Mental Disorders* (4th ed.), by the American Psychiatric Association, 1994, Washington, DC: Author. Adapted with permission of the American Psychiatric Association.

personality style is typical of insomniacs. They reasoned that when psychological conflicts are internalized, the result is physiological arousal, which is at odds with sleep.

Investigation of the patient's inner world often leads to an understanding that illuminates the causes of the sleep problem and directs the clinician to useful interventions. We also recommend the careful assessment of (a) the capacity of intrusive ideation and worry to prevent sleep, (b) the patient's beliefs and attitudes about sleep, and (c) the patient's expectations of treatment. These areas may provide possibilities for intervention to correct self-defeating thoughts.

Medical factors. Insomnia is common secondary to the pain and discomfort associated with a variety of somatic disorders. Physicians often assume that their treatment of organic disorders and associated pain and discomfort will be sufficient eventually to resolve the accompanying insomnia. Although we are not aware of systematic data that bear on this assumption, clinical experience is replete with examples of cases of insomnia that did not resolve following successful treatment of a medical condition. In our experience, for example, substantial numbers of patients were given sleeping pills following surgery or other interventions, and this drug use continued because the sleep disturbance was not resolved. Similarly, patients attempt to cope with certain physical problems by going to sleep early, sleeping in, resting in bed during the day, and taking naps to keep their "immune system healthy." In some cases, these coping strategies lead to long-term sleep problems. The continuation of sleep problems may be due to the development of drug dependency (Gillin, Spinweber, & Johnson, 1989), the weakening of the association of the bed with sleep (Bootzin & Nicassio, 1978), or the desynchronization of circadian processes (Moore-Ede, Czeisler, & Richardson, 1983).

Another type of problem is the insomnia that is produced directly by pharmacological treatment. It is well known, for example, that prednisone and some drugs for asthma, high blood pressure, and depression may produce insomnia (Walsh, Hartman, & Kowall, 1994). A number of strategies, including changing the time of drug administration, using drugs with a different side effect profile, or adding a sedating drug to the regimen, are available to ameliorate this problem. Therefore, a comprehensive drug history is an essential part of the evaluation for insomnia.

Intrasleep abnormalities. To assess the presence of some primary sleep disorders, the clinician needs to make specific inquiries. All patients should be asked about a feeling of restlessness in their legs (nonarticular discomfort) before bedtime. The patient's description of restless legs syndrome (see American Sleep Disorders Association [ASDA], 1990) may include a feeling of tightness or a drawing in the calf or thigh. These feelings usually occur at night while the patient is sedentary. Temporary relief is obtained by walking or moving the legs.

Although patients are usually unaware of breathing irregularities during sleep, they may have been told that they snore loudly, stop breathing, grunt, or snort while asleep. These descriptions by the patient or bed partner suggest a sleep-related respiratory disturbance such as obstructive sleep apnea syndrome (see ASDA, 1990). The observation of pauses in breathing without snoring suggests other types of sleep-related respiratory disturbances such as central alveolar hypoventilation (see ASDA, 1990).

Another problem that the patient is usually unaware of is brief, recurrent limb (most frequently, foot) movements during sleep. Difficult to elicit by interview, periodic limb movement disorder (see ASDA, 1990) is not rare and is associated with complaints of difficulty staying asleep, early-morning awakenings, or nonrefreshing sleep.

A definitive evaluation of insomnia includes the nocturnal monitoring of multiple physiological variables, a procedure called *nocturnal polysomnography*, and in the morning, obtaining the patient's subjective report of the sleep experience. A nocturnal polysomnographic recording may be the best or only way to detect abnormalities of sleep that produce insomnia, such as periodic limb movements, alpha intrusion in sleep, and sleep-disordered breathing (see ASDA, 1990). However, a nocturnal polysomnogram is not necessary in the assessment of the vast majority of cases of insomnia, and we refer readers to the recent Standards of Practice Committee report (1995) issued by the ASDA on this subject.

General domains to survey in assessment. The patient's spontaneous narrative often leaves out important features that should be investigated for more complete understanding. Table 2 lists features of the history that should be elicited from the patient to help depict the nature of the insomnia. Understanding and, in some cases, modifying the patient's expectations and attitudes are crucial to success (Morin, 1993). Many patients are looking for an immediate solution. They have tolerated their insomnia long enough, and now that they are seeking professional help, they expect the solution to come overnight. It is helpful if the clinician can shift the focus from a short-term solution to the long view.

Insomnia generally takes weeks or months to improve under the best of conditions. If the clinician's initial approach raises the patient's expectations and focuses them onto a single night or two, this increased attention can itself lead to arousal and be counterproductive. To help both the clinician and the patient learn to step back and take a longer view of the problem, a regular schedule of office visits or telephone contact should be established. Depending on the case, contact once per week to once every 3 weeks is optimal.

Insomnia is often the product of a confluence of factors, and its treatment requires a tailored mix of interventions (Hauri, 1993). Some people respond to rigid constraints on sleep, others to learning new associations

Table 2

Insomnia: General Domains and Specific Issues to Survey

General domains	Specific issues
Circumstances surrounding the onset	Age of onset, precipitating events, sudden or gradual onset
Severity and frequency	Every night, episodic, specific nights, situationally specific
Daytime consequences	Fatigue, sleepiness, napping, cognition, performance, and mood
Past treatments	Adequacy of trial, efficacy
Factors that ameliorate	Sleep in nonhabitual environments, sleep prior to a day with no commitments
Factors that exacerbate	Sleep on Sunday nights, anxiety when seeing the clock at night
Specific areas of importance	
Medical	Pain, discomfort, and treatments that interfere with sleep
Pharmacological	Activating drugs, sedating drugs that break down the regularity of the sleep–wake cycle, side effects
Psychiatric	Depression, anxiety
Work	Stress, work schedule
Family	Childhood habit of staying up late with a parent who was a "night owl" or waiting for a parent to return from late night drinking

between bedtime cues and sleep. Some people need a time set aside for worry before going to bed; others need to unwind. The variability of sleep hinders the quick assessment of any intervention, so that oftentimes treatments are best presented in phases, with modifications and new interventions made every few weeks.

This approach results in a treatment that is not determined from the outset but rather is altered in the light of the patient's reports. The detached, observational stance encouraged for the patient does more than reduce expectations and buffer the patient against nightly fluctuations in sleep. It puts the patient in a position to give more accurate and complete information about treatment response, enlists the patient as a collaborator over the long haul, and prevents discouragement before the treatments finally take hold.

To engender the long view, the practitioner may say the following:

> I understand your distress, but you have had this sleeping problem for years. There are three reasons not to try to fix the problem overnight. First, the kind of treatments that could help you get adequate sleep within a few days will not necessarily address the underlying problems that are causing your sleeping difficulty. Therefore, these quick solutions are often not effective over the long term. Second, we need some time to see what the problem is in detail. This close look will yield the understanding of what is wrong and how to treat it. Third, in my experience it takes more than days or a few weeks for this type of sleep disturbance to resolve. So, put up with the problem for another month or so, and we will figure it out. I am aiming for a treatment that will make your sleep robust for the long haul.

Sleep habits and lifestyle. The use of a daily diary is invaluable in the assessment of insomnia and response to treatment (Monk et al., 1994). The sleep log focuses the patient on day-to-day details as opposed to a retrospective history, which tends to collapse this information. It also underscores the importance of looking at patterns over time. If possible, the sleep log should be filled out for 1 week or more before the initial office visit to document the problem with a level of detail that can suggest areas for fruitful inquiry and treatment. If the log is sent home with the patient after the first visit, it can be customized to represent better the factors identified during the evaluation as salient. The information generated by the diary (see Exhibit 3) allows a detailed analysis of the nature of the problem, including (a) sleep pattern; (b) the effect of sleep habits (e.g., variable sleep schedule, tossing and turning for long periods of time in bed); (c) the effectiveness of the patient's coping strategies (e.g., extra time in bed to get extra sleep, napping, increased caffeine consumption, and "sleeping in" on weekends); (d) the effect of practices of everyday living on sleep (e.g., exercise, alcohol, cigarettes). Related areas that are not elicited from the sleep log should be covered in the interview, including (a) activities during the wind-down period right before bedtime (e.g., working, socializing, talking on the phone); (b) activities that take place in bed (e.g., eating, playing board games, and in general making the bed the hub of evening activities); and (c) aspects of the sleeping environment (e.g., snoring bed partner, intrusive pet, noise).

Exhibit 3

The Sleep Log: 24-Hour Perspective

Sleep: Timing, duration, and pattern
          Sleep schedule (bedtime, uptime)
          Sleep-onset latency
          Awakenings
          Sleep amount
          Sleep on weekends compared with weekdays
          Dozing and napping
          Subjective rating—adequacy of sleep
Wake: Type, amount, and time of ingestion
          Alcohol
          Caffeine
          Medication
          Nicotine
          Other drugs
      Time and duration
          Outdoor light exposure
          Vigorous exercise
      Subjective rating
          Alertness–sleepiness
          Fatigue
          Cognition
          Performance
          Mood

The Sleep Log

We suggest that practitioners who do not have sleep expertise use a simple sleep diary; although it sacrifices some information, it is user-friendly from the perspective of both the patient and clinician (see Figure 2). The graph format, with successive 24-hour periods depicted by stacked horizontal grids, enables the clinician's eye to synthesize dozens of details readily. The patient is instructed to use four symbols on the 24-hour grid to depict aspects of the sleep pattern and caffeine use. A darkened dot representing "lights out" is placed at the time the patient begins trying to sleep. An open dot represents "lights on." This indicates when the patient ends the night by getting out of bed. Sleep is shown by a horizontal line bounded by verticals that mark sleep onset and sleep offset. Awakenings are therefore identified by the gaps between the sleep marks. The final symbol is a C, which indicates the time of

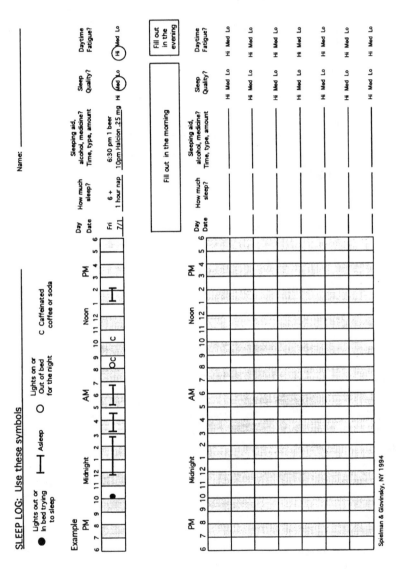

Figure 2. A sample of a user-friendly sleep log.

consumption of caffeine-containing drinks. These four symbols are easy to use and interpret. As is illustrated later, additional symbols should be used to customize the sleep log to enable the patient to indicate the timing of other events or symptoms of potential importance.

Next to each 24-hour grid is a set of questions about sleep that night and fatigue the next day. Following the date, the patient is asked to add up all the sleep obtained that night and to indicate how much sleep occurred during napping. A space is provided for the time, type, and amount of any sleeping aid, alcohol, or medicine the patient may have taken. Sleep quality and daytime fatigue are then rated as *hi, med,* or *lo.*

The most reliable information is obtained if the patient fills out the 24-hour grid and answers all questions (except concerning daytime fatigue) in the morning shortly after getting up. At the end of the day, the rating of daytime fatigue is the final entry. An example is provided in Figure 2 to illustrate the proper completion of the sleep log. Once completed, the clinician should ascertain whether the log indeed reflects the patient's complaint. Occasionally, extraordinary events such as vacations, recent jet travel across time zones, or the accommodation of a house guest may lead to a false picture.

Case Illustrations

In this section, we illustrate the usefulness of the daily sleep log in understanding typical cases of chronic insomnia. We also discuss other kinds of information that are helpful in evaluation and in outlining treatment strategies. The format of each vignette includes background information and daily sleep logs to encourage professionals to develop hypotheses and questions about the case. The reader can then see how we understood the problem from the sleep diary and compare his or her formulation to ours.

Because our purpose is to demonstrate the role of the sleep log in the assessment of insomnia, we have limited the types of cases in these vignettes. There are no cases of insomnia produced by such common causes as pain, concurrent medical problems, medications, periodic limb movements during sleep, and sleep-disordered breathing. These and other conditions unfold from the history or require specialized assessment techniques such as polysomnographic recordings. Our purpose is to help the clinician to deal with the common types of insomnia treated in the office setting. In some of the cases to follow, the sleep log has been customized to yield extra information. The sleep log we use (see Figure 2) includes a number of items that we have deleted from the case illustrations for the sake of simplicity.

Case 1

A 23-year-old male medical student complains of "trouble getting to sleep as far back as I can remember." Because he needs to attend 9:00 a.m. classes, the long sleep latencies during the week result in short sleep duration and daytime weariness. Although he makes it to class on time, he is so groggy he doesn't get much out of the first few classes each day.
   Sleep log analysis (see Figure 3).

- The sleep problem is limited to difficulty falling asleep; there is no trouble staying asleep.
- The patient attempts to compensate for morning grogginess with coffee.
- The problem resolves on the weekend, when he is released from the constraints of a sleep schedule.

   Formulation. This may be a case of a mismatch between the patient's internal timing for sleep and the demands of school scheduling. This "night owl" is going to bed early during the week and trying to sleep at a time when his circadian clock is still set for waking activities. The sleep-onset difficulty is absent on weekends, when the patient chooses to go to sleep later and is able to catch up by sleeping late into the day. Diagnosis: delayed sleep phase syndrome (Weitzman et al., 1981; also see ASDA, 1990). Some patients with similar patterns may be experiencing school anxiety, with the result that falling asleep proves difficult on school nights. Diagnosis: adjustment sleep disorder (see ASDA, 1990).
   Treatment options. A daily regimen of bright light exposure is recommended, using either outdoor light or indoor artificial light of greater than 2500 lux (Lewy, Wehr, Goodwin, Newsome, & Markey, 1980; Rosenthal et al., 1990) for a half hour to 2 hours starting right after waking in the morning. The patient will begin to get drowsy earlier and fall asleep earlier in the evening. He will be able to accumulate more sleep before his alarm clock rings. Waking at the same time 7 days a week also is necessary. Sleeping late shifts the patient's internal clock, so that falling asleep at the desired time becomes a problem again. Once the patient's sleep is shifted earlier, morning bright light exposure should be tapered and discontinued.

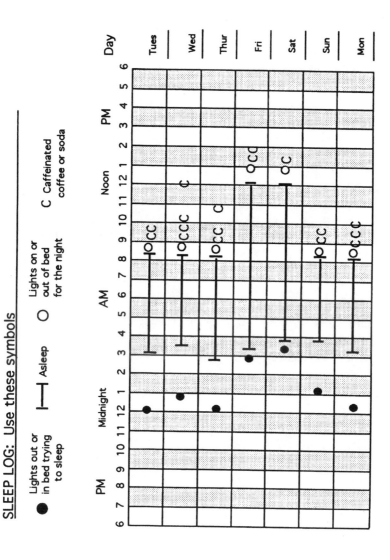

Figure 3.   Case 1: "trouble getting to sleep" and groggy in the morning.

A second method of realigning internal circadian rhythms with external schedule demands is chronotherapy (Weitzman et al., 1981). It can exploit this patient's tendency to have an easier time staying awake longer than going to sleep earlier. Chronotherapy involves a progressive 3-hour delay in bedtime and time of arising. Of course, as chronotherapy involves nearly a week of acute mismatch between prescribed bedtimes and typical social or vocational obligations, in practice it is often deferred until a vacation or temporary leave is scheduled.

Case 2

A 40-year-old public relations executive complains of long sleep latencies, frequent awakenings, early morning awakenings, and daytime fatigue. These problems began 2 years ago following a miscarriage.

Sleep log analysis (see Figure 4).

- The complaint of difficulty both falling and staying asleep is confirmed.
- Time of retiring and arising are regular.
- The patient is spending too much time in bed: approximately 9.5 hours per night.

Formulation. The patient may be experiencing ruminative and intrusive thoughts that are directly or symbolically related to the miscarriage. Questions regarding the impact and meaning of the precipitating event need to be explored, along with an evaluation for depression. Diagnosis: dysthymic disorder or major depressive disorder (American Psychiatric Association, 1994).

In many cases of chronic insomnia, the impact of the precipitating factor has long since dissipated, and the sleep disturbance has taken on a life of its own (Spielman, 1986). This patient has regular retiring and arising times, but she is spending too much time in bed. This produces a shallow, fragmented, overextended sleep. Diagnosis: inadequate sleep hygiene (see ASDA, 1990). Although it is not present in this case, insomnia also may be perpetuated by napping, irregular time of retiring and arising, use of caffeine or alcohol, unpredictability of sleep, or worry over daytime deficits.

Treatment options. Psychotherapy to explore the impact of the miscarriage and any continuing repercussions is recommended, as well as an evaluation for antidepressant medication.

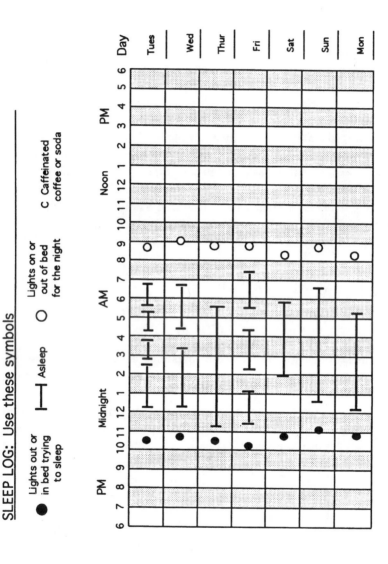

Figure 4.   Case 2: a mix of sleep-onset and maintenance difficulties and daytime lethargy following a miscarriage.

Sleep-restriction therapy limits the amount of time spent in bed and is an effective means of consolidating sleep, reducing night-to-night variability, and shortening the time it takes to fall asleep (Glovinsky & Spielman, 1991; Spielman, Saskin, & Thorpy, 1987). Because this patient estimates that she is sleeping about $5\frac{1}{2}$ hours per night, she would be assigned a restricted time in bed of $5\frac{1}{2}$ hours. Gradually extending her time in bed by 15–30 minutes per week will ensure that sleep will remain consolidated until an optimal sleep schedule is established.

Case 3

A 65-year-old male psychoanalyst complains, "I am waking too early in the morning and get fatigued during the day, especially in the evening. I have no trouble falling asleep. I believe I have a masked depression." This problem has been relatively constant for the past 4 years; no precipitating event is apparent. To cope with the hours alone in the morning, he takes an hour-long walk on awakening.

Sleep log analysis (see Figure 5).

- Prominent sleepiness and napping exclusively in the evening
- Early retiring time, 9:00 to 10:30 p.m.
- Very rapid sleep onset
- Early morning awakening
- Time in bed limited to about 7 hours

Formulation. Although some of these features certainly raise the possibility of a depressive disorder, this pattern of early evening drowsiness and 7 hours spent in bed is more characteristic of a phase shift of the sleep–wake cycle. The timing of sleep has been shifted (advanced) to an earlier than desired clock time. This phase shift is a common part of the aging process. Diagnosis: advanced sleep phase syndrome (see ASDA, 1990) associated with aging.

This patient's morning walk may be contributing to the early-morning awakening problem. Retinal exposure to outdoor light in the early morning produces a shift in circadian rhythms. The direction of this shift is to advance the cycle, so that the time he goes to sleep and the time he wakes up will tend to occur at an earlier clock hour. On further inquiry, the patient reported that his problem was exacerbated in the spring and summer. Diagnosis: advanced sleep phase syndrome, morning bright light stimulation producing a phase advance of the endogenous circadian oscillator (see ASDA, 1990).

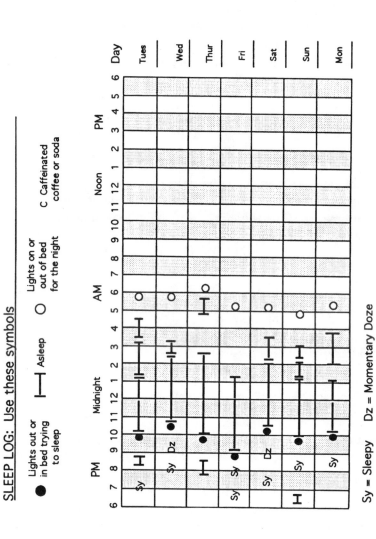

Figure 5. Case 3: early-morning awakenings that terminate sleep.

When early-morning awakening is cited as a chief complaint, depression is often an underlying factor. Sleep laboratory studies of depression have shown that the internal structure of sleep is altered in a number of other ways, including earlier appearance of the first REM sleep of the night, frequent eye movements in the first REM period, and reduced amounts of deep slow wave sleep (Reynolds & Kupfer, 1987). In addition, a diurnal mood variation—feeling worse in the morning—may also be present. Diagnosis: major depressive disorder (American Psychiatric Association, 1994).

Treatment options. Antidepressant medications are indicated if the sleep problem is part of a major depressive disorder. Prescribing bright light exposure for an hour or two in the evening and limiting early-morning exposure will produce a phase-delay shift to correct the early-morning awakening (Campbell, Dawson, & Anderson, 1993). Depending on one's latitude on the earth, outdoor light at dusk occurs late enough to be effective for only about 8–12 weeks at about the time of the summer solstice. Therefore, artificial indoor light of sufficient intensity (>2500 lux) may need to be used at other times of the year (contact the Society for Bright Light Therapy, New York, NY).

Case 4

A 30-year-old female freelance writer complains, "I can't depend on my sleep, and I have to nap to compensate."
   Sleep log analysis (see Figure 6).

- Irregular bedtimes
- Napping at different times of the day
- Too much time in bed

Formulation. This patient forfeited the benefits of regular bedtimes and thus weakened or desynchronized her underlying circadian rhythm organization. She has less propensity to sleep at night and an increase in daytime sleepiness. Her subjective experience is that she lacks the ability to sleep adequately and remain alert all day. Such patients may have a self-image that includes extraordinary sensitivity to sleep loss or unique sleep requirements. This patient may feel she needs to make special allowances in her lifestyle to accumulate whatever sleep she can. This may be one aspect of a more global personal vulnerability. Diagnoses: irregular sleep–wake pattern, inadequate sleep hygiene (see ASDA, 1990), personality disorder (American Psychiatric Association, 1994).

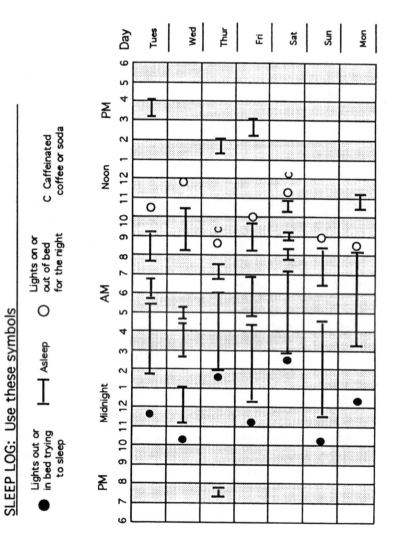

Figure 6.   Case 4: loss of confidence in the ability to sleep.

Treatment options. This type of case often requires the combination of general psychotherapeutic and specific sleep therapy approaches. Gains resulting from sleep restriction and improved sleep hygiene can be quickly lost unless some psychological resiliency is established. A strong therapeutic alliance will help to get the patient through early stages of treatment when she will not be able to fall back on naps, extra time in bed, and lying down and resting. Addressing the patient's misconceptions about her sleep requirement may help her cope with the demands that treatment will impose (Lacks & Morin, 1992). Sanctioning the occasional use of a hypnotic is often helpful in this type of patient. This limits cumulative sleep loss and reduces the patient's excessive worry about sleeplessness.

Case 5

A 52-year-old female teacher complains, "Since my teens, I've had trouble falling asleep. Once every month or so, before an important event, it's even worse. I guess I just can't stop my mind from racing."

Sleep log analysis (see Figure 7).

- A sleep-onset problem that varies in severity is confirmed.
- On Saturday night, the patient goes to sleep later, 12:30 a.m., and still takes an hour to fall asleep.
- The patient is spending too much time lying in bed, awake, in the evening and perhaps too much time trying to sleep: about 8 1/2 hours.

Formulation. When the condition is exclusively sleep-onset insomnia, one needs to know if the patient is "just getting going" at night (a "night-owl's" pattern) and if the problem remits when she can set her own schedule. On inquiry, she reports being most alert in the morning and fatigued at night; on weekends and vacations, she goes to sleep later but still has difficulty falling asleep. Therefore, delayed sleep phase syndrome presenting as sleep-onset insomnia (see Case 1) is not likely.

The patient spends her evenings in bed talking on the phone, snacking, watching TV, and correcting papers. Engaging in nonsleep activities in bed may have weakened the association (maladaptive conditioning) between the bed and sleep (Bootzin & Nicassio, 1978). Worrying whether the upcoming night will be "typically bad or horrible," she dreads going to sleep. Entertaining a psychiatric diagnosis

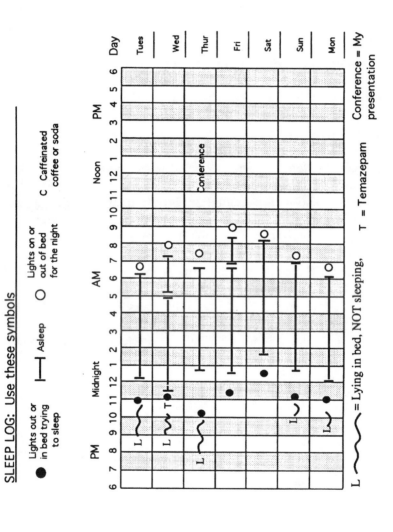

Figure 7.   Case 5: ruminations while trying to sleep.

such as generalized anxiety disorder, the practitioner performed a focused psychological inquiry but did not find significant anxiety, depression, or generalized ruminative state to qualify for such a diagnosis. Her worrying is limited to the sleep problem and its consequences. The issues that appear to be contributing to the sleep-onset difficulties include maladaptive conditioning, too much time in bed, and anticipatory anxiety regarding sleep. Diagnoses: psychophysiological insomnia and inadequate sleep hygiene (see ASDA, 1990).

Treatment options. Stimulus control instructions (Bootzin & Nicassio, 1978) designed to address the maladaptive conditioning include the following: (a) Use the bed only for sleep (and sex); (b) if not asleep within about 15 or 20 minutes, get out of bed; (c) go back to bed again when sleepy, and repeat (b) if necessary; (d) get up at the same time every day; and (e) eliminate napping.

A stress-reduction program may help this patient regulate the flood of ideas and her reactivity to upcoming events. In addition, relaxation, paradoxical intention, and guided imagery training (Hauri, 1991; see the review in Espie, 1991) may help to relieve muscle tension and focus the mind on nonworrisome ideation. These presleep tasks create a ritual transition buffer period between active waking and relaxed readiness for sleep. The cares and concerns of the day are put aside and nighttime rituals are engaged in that help relax the body and quiet the mind. Additional help getting drowsy in the evening can be provided by bright light exposure in the morning. The use of a benzodiazepine hypnotic medication on the nights before especially significant events appears appropriate.

Case 6

A 35-year-old man complains, "I have no trouble falling asleep, but I can't stay asleep. I usually can fall back to sleep in the morning and get my best sleep." Half of the time, during the morning awakening, the patient stays in bed trying to sleep, and the other half, he gets up and reads or has breakfast. Before he goes back to sleep, he turns off his alarm.

Sleep log analysis (see Figure 8).

- No set time to wake up in the morning
- Usually awake between 5:00 and 7:00 a.m. and usually asleep between 7:30 and 9:00 a.m.

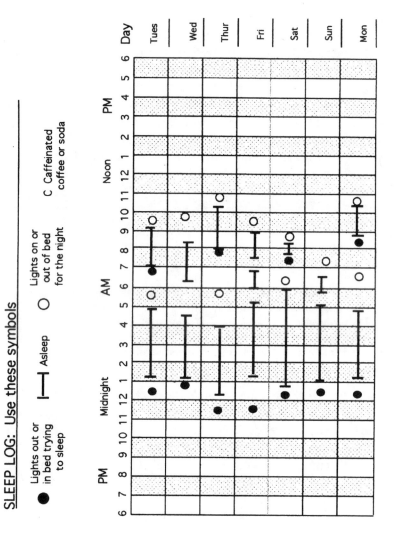

Figure 8.   Case 6: long awakening in the morning followed by a return to sleep.

Formulation. The split sleep pattern—long morning awakening followed by a substantial amount of sleep—may have become a habit. To get as much sleep as possible, the patient sets no limits on his time in bed. This may have allowed the two sleep fragments to drift apart (Wehr, 1991).

Treatment options. Setting a strict wake-up time that curtails time in bed (as in sleep-restriction therapy) will begin the process of eliminating the habitual pattern. Initially, this produces mild sleep deprivation because the patient is not able to take his *ad libitum* nap in the morning. As treatment proceeds, nocturnal wakefulness will be minimized and longer sleep obtained. Bright light exposure first thing in the morning may facilitate the consolidation of the two sleep fragments. Alternatively, the short-term use of a benzodiazepine hypnotic in conjunction with strict limits to the time allowed for sleep may be effective.

Case 7

A 45-year-old businessman complains, "I don't get enough sleep."
Sleep log analysis (see Figure 9).

- Regular and short sleep schedule on weekdays yields short sleep durations of 5 hours or fewer.
- On weekends, he sleeps in and, compared with weekdays, gets over 45% more sleep.
- He drinks about five cups of coffee per day during the week.
- He has mild difficulty both falling and staying asleep

Formulation. Although the patient's sleep schedule is fairly regular, there is a consistent and large difference in the amount he sleeps on weekdays versus weekends. This strategy of catching up on sleep on weekends is not without benefit, but it may be perpetuating the sleep problems. Sleeping more and later on weekends may be setting the stage for difficulty falling asleep on Sunday, Monday, and other nights. Diagnosis: inadequate sleep hygiene (see ASDA, 1990).

This pattern may be associated with the worries and demands of the patient's work schedule and, possibly, caffeine consumption. If he is constantly under time pressure, he may be working late or rushing to do chores in the morning. Achieving and staying asleep is not easy under these conditions. Diagnosis: generalized anxiety disorder (American Psychiatric Association, 1994).

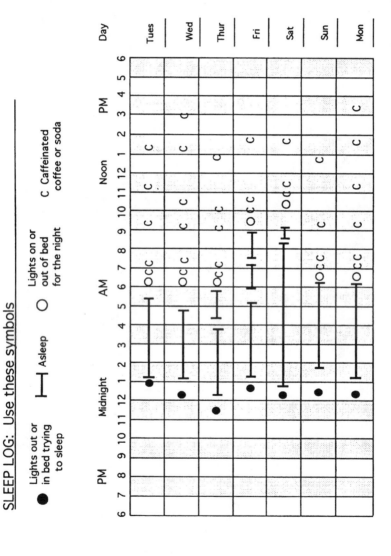

Figure 9. Case 7: insufficient sleep.

Table 3
Case Illustrations

Case	Clinical features–differential diagnosis	Treatment options	Diagnoses
1	Sleep-onset problems only Problem resolves when there is no wake-up schedule (e.g., weekends, vacations)	Bright light exposure on awakening in the morning No sleeping late Chronotherapy	Delayed sleep phase syndrome Adjustment sleep disorder Psychophysiological insomnia
2	Difficulty falling and staying asleep Onset after miscarriage Regular retiring and arising times Too much time in bed	Psychotherapy Sleep-restriction therapy Relaxation and imagery training Antidepressants	Dysthymic disorder Inadequate sleep hygiene Major depressive disorder
3	Early-morning awakening Sleepiness in the evening Early retiring time Bright light exposure in the morning	Restrict light exposure in the morning (Artificial) bright light exposure in the evening Antidepressants	Advanced sleep phase disorder Major depressive disorder

	Symptoms	Interventions	Diagnoses
4	Irregular bedtimes Napping at different times of the day Peremptory need to sleep whenever possible Psychopathology	Sleep-hygiene instructions Sleep-restriction therapy Address sleep myths Psychotherapy Intermittent hypnotic medication	Irregular sleep–wake pattern Inadequate sleep hygiene Personality disorder
5	Chronic sleep-onset problems Worsens with anticipatory anxiety and rumination Trouble falling asleep present on weekends and vacations Hours of talking, eating, working in bed Too much time in bed	Stimulus control instructions Relaxation and guided imagery training Stress reduction Bright light exposure in the morning Occasional hypnotic medication	Psychophysiological insomnia Inadequate sleep hygiene Generalized anxiety disorder
6	Early-morning awakening Long awakenings Habitual return to sleep in the morning No set wake-up time in the morning	Sleep-restriction therapy Bright light exposure in the morning Short-term hypnotic medication	Irregular sleep–wake pattern
7	Short sleep duration during the week Long sleep duration on weekends Difficulty falling and staying asleep Five cups of coffee per day	Regular bedtimes on weekdays and weekends to equalize sleep time Stress reduction Cut caffeine consumption	Inadequate sleep hygiene Generalized anxiety disorder

Treatment options. Consistent sleep from night to night needs to be established. Strictly enforced retiring and arising times should be set. The habitual arising time necessary on weekdays to meet the patient's work schedule should be set as the out-of-bed time 7 days per week. The patient should cut coffee intake by half, with no consumption allowed after noon, and institute a wind-down period in the evening with no business-related work allowed and no stimulating phone calls. A stress-reduction program might also be considered.

Conclusion

As illustrated by this series of cases, the symptom of insomnia is produced by a range of conditions (see Table 3). The clinician is in the best position to help if the evaluation process casts a wide net to capture the multiple contributions to the problem. The sleep log is invaluable in snaring patterns of activities and practices that play a role in the sleep disturbance. The clinician is no longer limited to offering symptomatic relief with the administration of sedative hypnotics. Advances in understanding as well as the development of new nonpharmacological treatments allow the selection of interventions that address specific problems.

REFERENCES

American Psychiatric Association. (1994). *Diagnostic and statistical manual of mental disorders* (4th ed.). Washington, DC: Author.

American Sleep Disorders Association. (1990). *The international classification of sleep disorders. Diagnostic and coding manual.* Lawrence, KS: Allen Press.

Bootzin, R. R., & Nicassio, P. M. (1978). Behavioral treatments for insomnia. In M. Hersen, R. E. Eisler, & P. M. Miller (Eds.), *Progress in behavior modification* (Vol. 6, pp. 1–45). New York: Academic Press.

Campbell, S. S., Dawson, D., & Anderson, M. W. (1993). Alleviation of sleep maintenance insomnia with timed exposure to bright light. *Journal of the American Geriatric Society, 41,* 829–836.

Espie, C. A. (1991). *The psychological treatment of insomnia.* New York: Wiley.

Gallup Organization. (1991). *Sleep in America.* Princeton, NJ: Author.

Gillin, J. C., Spinweber, C. L., & Johnson, L. C. (1989). Rebound insomnia: A critical review. *Journal of Clinical Psychopharmacology, 9,* 161–172.

Glovinsky, P. B., & Spielman, A. J. (1991). Sleep restriction therapy. In P. Hauri (Ed.), *Case studies in insomnia* (pp. 49–63). New York: Plenum Press.

Hathaway, S. R., & McKinley, J. C. (1983). *The Minnesota Multiphasic Personality Inventory*. Minneapolis: University of Minnesota Press.

Hauri, P. J. (Ed.). (1991). *Case studies in insomnia*. New York: Plenum Press.

Hauri, P. J. (1993). Consulting about insomnia: A method and some preliminary data. *Sleep, 16*, 344–350.

Hauri, P. J., & Fisher, J. (1986). Persistent psychophysiological (learned) insomnia. *Sleep, 2*, 38–53.

Hoelscher, T. J., & Edinger, J. D. (1988). Treatment of sleep-maintenance insomnia in older adults: Sleep period reduction, sleep education, and modified stimulus control. *Psychology and Aging, 3*, 258–263.

Kales, A., Caldwell, A. B., Preston, T. A., Healey, S., & Kales, J. D. (1976). Personality patterns in insomnia. *Archives of General Psychiatry, 33*, 1128–1134.

Kales, A., & Kales, J. D. (1984). *Evaluation and treatment of insomnia*. New York: Oxford University Press.

Lacks, P., & Morin, C. M. (1992). Recent advances in the assessment and treatment of insomnia. *Journal of Consulting and Clinical Psychology, 60*, 586–594.

Lewy, A. J., Wehr, T. A., Goodwin, F. K., Newsome, D. A., & Markey, S. P. (1980). Light suppresses melatonin secretion in humans. *Science, 210*, 1267–1269.

Mellinger, G. D., Balter, M. B., & Uhlenhuth, E. H. (1985). Insomnia and its treatment: Prevalence and correlates. *Archives of General Psychiatry, 42*, 225–232.

Monk, T. H., Reynolds, C. F., III, Kupfer, D. J., Buysse, D. J., Coble, P. A., Hayes, A. J., Machen, M. A., Petrie, S. R., & Ritenour, A. M. (1994). The Pittsburgh sleep diary. *Journal of Sleep Research, 3*, 111–120.

Moore-Ede, M. C., Czeisler, C. A., & Richardson, G. S. (1983). Circadian timekeeping in health and disease: Part 2. Clinical implications of circadian rhythmicity. *New England Journal of Medicine, 309*, 530–536.

Morin, C. M. (1993). *Insomnia: Psychological assessment and management*. New York: Guilford Press.

Morin, C. M., Gaulier, B., Barry, T., & Kowatch, R. A. (1992). Patients' acceptance of psychological and pharmacological therapies for insomnia. *Sleep, 15*, 302–305.

Morin, C. M., Kowatch, R. A., Barry, T., & Walton, E. (1993). Cognitive-behavior therapy for late-life insomnia. *Journal of Consulting and Clinical and Psychology, 61*, 137–146.

National Commission on Sleep Disorders Research. (1992). *Wake up America: A national sleep alert*. Washington, DC: Department of Health and Human Services.

Reynolds, C. F., & Kupfer, D. J. (1987). Sleep research in affective illness: State of the art. *Sleep, 10*, 199–215.

Rosenthal, N. E., Joseph-Vanderpool, J. R., Levendosky, A. A., Johnston, S. H., Allen, R., Kelly, K. A., Soutre, E., Schultz, P. M., & Starz, K. E. (1990). *Sleep, 13*, 354–361.

Spielman, A. J. (1986). Assessment of insomnia. *Clinical Psychology Reviews, 6,* 11–25.

Spielman, A. J., Caruso, L. S., & Glovinsky, P. B. (1987). A behavioral perspective on insomnia treatment. *Psychiatric Clinics of North America, 10,* 541–553.

Spielman, A. J., & Glovinsky, P. B. (1991). The varied nature of insomnia. In P. Hauri (Ed.), *Case studies in insomnia* (pp. 1–15). New York: Plenum Press.

Spielman, A. J., Saskin, P., & Thorpy, M. J. (1987). Treatment of chronic insomnia by restriction of time spent in bed. *Sleep, 10,* 45–56.

Standards of Practice Committee, American Sleep Disorders Association. (1995). Practice parameters for the use of polysomnography in the evaluation of insomnia. *Sleep, 18,* 55–57.

Walsh, J. K., Hartman, P. G., & Kowall, J. P. (1994). Insomnia. In S. Chokroverty (Ed.), *Sleep disorders medicine* (pp. 219–239). Boston: Butterworth-Heinemanna.

Wehr, T. (1991). The durations of human melatonin secretion and sleep respond to changes in daylength (photoperiod). *Journal of Clinical Endocronology and Metabolism, 73,* 1276–1280.

Weitzman, E. D., Czeisler, C., Coleman, R., Spielman, A. J., Zimmerman, J., Dement, W. C., Richardson, G., & Pollak, C. P. (1981). Delayed sleep phase syndrome: A chronobiological disorder with sleep onset insomnia. *Archives of General Psychiatry, 38,* 737–746.

Chapter

7

The Diagnostic Interview and Differential Diagnosis for Complaints of Excessive Daytime Sleepiness

Jeanine L. White and Merrill M. Mitler

Excessive daytime sleepiness, once considered a benign complaint, is now known to have serious individual and societal consequences. Occupational and social functioning is severely affected by the inability to stay alert or awake. Excessive sleepiness increases the probability of automobile fatalities (Findley, Weiss, & Jabour, 1991) and compromises public safety (Mitler, 1991). When the effects of excessive sleepiness are severe, the ability for complex performance deteriorates (Dement, Carskadon, & Richardson, 1978). As a result, excessively sleepy individuals are frequently perceived as unmotivated or uninterested in their responsibilities, which in turn may lead to decreased employability and self-esteem. Depression may develop because of these secondary effects of sleepiness. Excessive daytime sleepiness is the most common sleep-related reason for a person to seek professional help. This chapter discusses the clinical factors related to a complaint of excessive daytime sleepiness and outlines a diagnostic interview strategy.

If left unrecognized and untreated, chronic sleep loss or sleep disorders can have far-reaching effects on society. For example, adolescents are an important subpopulation prone to developing excessive daytime sleepiness. Carskadon et al. (1980) found that during puberty there is an increased physiological need for sleep. However, environmental influences, such as less parental supervision of bedtimes, demands of part-time jobs, and earlier start of morning classes in high school can limit the opportunity for adequate sleep. Because of disrupted or shortened sleep and the resulting daytime sleepiness, cognitive development can be compromised (Guilleminault, Eldridge, Simmons, & Dement, 1976). Chronic sleep deprivation may also explain in part the irritability, apathy, and heightened emotional sensitivity often seen during adolescence. In a 5-day sleep deprivation study, adolescents whose sleep time was progressively shortened endorsed frequently more negative mood state items than those who were allowed to sleep full nights (Carskadon, 1990).

Factors Related to Daytime Sleepiness

The complaint of excessive daytime sleepiness involves three interrelated factors: (a) the quantity of sleep one receives, (b) the quality of sleep, and (c) time-of-day (i.e., circadian rhythm) factors.

Sleep Quantity

The importance of obtaining adequate sleep is often disregarded or denied and, as a result, sleep may be sacrificed for social or occupational reasons. Sleepiness promotes sleep-seeking behavior and heightens the ability to fall asleep (Dement et al., 1978). Because sleepiness is inherently a state of physiological drive, sleepiness always occurs when enough sleep is lost. Consistently reducing one's sleep time produces a cumulative amount of sleep loss known as sleep debt (Carskadon & Dement, 1981). The larger one's sleep debt becomes, the greater the drive to sleep. In fact, the correct physiological explanation for "sleeping in" on weekends and holidays is that such sleep reduces sleep debt. The effects of even a large sleep debt may go unnoticed (i.e., the level of subjective sleepiness is low) if one's external environment provides intense enough stimulation or muscular activity. However, if one removes the stimulation or activity, overwhelming drowsiness occurs almost immediately.

Sleep Quality

Patients who report sleeping approximately 8 hours each night may still have a sleep debt if their sleep quality is poor. Sleep quality is compromised when sleep is disrupted or fragmented. Sleep disturbances that affect sleep quality can originate either externally or internally. External influences stem from the sleeping environment and can include high levels of noise or extreme ambient room temperatures. Internal influences are related to physiological conditions, such as obstructive sleep apnea, chronic pain, or periodic limb movement disorder.

Time-of-Day Factors

The probability for experiencing sleepiness is also related to the time of day. During our 24-hour alertness–sleep cycle (i.e., circadian rhythm), there is a bimodal tendency for sleep (Broughton, 1989; Richardson, Carskadon, Orav, & Dement, 1982). The major peak in sleep tendency occurs between 11 p.m. and 6 a.m. A smaller second peak in the tendency to fall asleep occurs in the mid-afternoon between approximately 1 and 4 P.M. (Lavie, 1989). There is a corresponding alertness cycle where the ability to fall asleep is lowest. This alertness cycle has an early morning peak and a mid-evening peak. During the time period in which the physiological tendency to sleep is at its highest (between the hours of 1 and 4 a.m.), vehicular accidents and industrial disasters are reported to occur most frequently (Mitler et al., 1988). To accommodate the mid-afternoon tendency for sleep, various societies have initiated rituals in their culture, such as siestas and closing businesses between 1 and 4 p.m. "Tea-time" rituals, which traditionally occur between 3 and 4 p.m., might also be indirect attempts to counteract afternoon sleepiness. The existence of this mid-afternoon peak in sleepiness is unrelated to the amount of a prior night's sleep (though lack of sleep can potentiate its effects), the timing of the midday meal, or age (Richardson et al., 1982). In addition to recognizing sleep quantity, sleep quality, and circadian rhythm as contributing factors for daytime sleepiness, the ability to differentiate normal from pathological sleepiness enables the clinician to clarify further a complaint of excessive daytime sleepiness.

Defining Sleepiness

A quantitative distinction exists between pathological sleepiness associated with an underlying pathological condition and sleepiness manifested as a normal physiological occurrence caused by circadian factors. Pathological sleepiness can be identified by the marked susceptibility to falling asleep in situations that are commonly not soporific. The woman who falls asleep at her son or daughter's wedding and the man who must actively fight sleep while eating a meal are both experiencing pathological sleepiness. More commonly reported events, such as falling asleep or dozing while driving a car, are also considered markers for excessive sleepiness. Moderate sleepiness exists when an individual feels compelled to sleep during the daytime, but if requested, can remain awake. (Because of the possible serious ramifications, special attention should be paid to the complaint of a school-aged child having difficulty remaining awake during such passive situations as reading or listening to a lecture.) Common mild sleepiness occurs when one is sleepy during low stimulation events, such as late afternoon meetings, evening concerts, or while riding as a passenger during a long car trip. Sometimes qualitative distinctions in sleepiness are difficult to make; therefore, various tools have been used to assess the subjective experience and the objective evidence for excessive daytime sleepiness.

Subjective Estimates of Excessive Sleepiness

The subjective report of sleepiness can assist in understanding the severity of the complaint. Unfortunately, semantics can make this task difficult. For example, two individuals may complain of feeling tired during the daytime. However, on closer examination, one person falls asleep while driving and the other has low ambition and listlessness. This illustrates the critical distinction between sleepiness and fatigue. Individuals with symptoms of fatigue complain of feeling tired, "achy," or "washed out," although they do not actually sleep. (Fatigue is often a complaint of those suffering from insomnia; less commonly is sleepiness reported with insomnia.) In an attempt to assess accurately an individual's level of energy, ability to function, desire for sleep, and the temporal aspect of alertness, several interview and questionnaire techniques have been developed. Among the best known of these questionnaire techniques is the Stanford Sleepiness Scale (SSS; Hoddes, Zarcone, Smythe, Phillips, & Dement, 1973). Patients choose from one of the following seven statements to describe their current level of sleepiness: (a) feeling active and vital, alert, wide awake; (b) functioning at a high level, but not at peak; able to concentrate; (c) relaxed, awake, not at full alertness, responsive; (d) a little foggy, not at peak, let down; (e) fogginess, beginning to lose interest in remaining awake, slowed down; (f) sleepiness, prefer to be lying down, fighting sleep, woozy; and (g) almost in reverie, sleep-onset soon, hard to stay awake. The major strengths of the SSS are that it can be administered many times each day, it reflects the effects of sleep loss, and it correlates well with standard measures of performance (Hoddes et al., 1973). However, throughout the 24-hour day, all levels of the SSS have been endorsed by individuals without sleep disorders, experimentally sleep-deprived though otherwise healthy individuals, and individuals with sleep disorders. Thus, there is no clear gauge for determining what is typical and what is atypical sleepiness on the SSS. Furthermore, in patients with sleep apnea Dement and colleagues (1978) have documented glaring discordancies between high SSS ratings of 1 or 2 and gross behavioral indicators of sleep such as closed eyes and snoring. They suggest that such discordancies stem either from an individual's loss of a proper frame of reference for normal alertness or from a simple denial of sleepiness. Another possible explanation for the discordance between one's subjective report and witnessed behavior may be that the SSS and behavioral indicators of sleep simply reflect different things.

Another common self-report instrument is the Epworth Sleepiness Scale (ESS; Johns, 1991). The ESS asks individuals to rank from 0 to 3 (*never, slight, moderate,* and *high*) the likelihood they would fall asleep in eight different situations: (a) sitting and reading; (b) watching TV; (c) sitting, inactive in a public place (i.e., a theater); (d) as a car passenger for an hour without a break; (e) lying down to rest in the afternoon when circumstances permit; (f) sitting and talking to someone; (g) sitting quietly after lunch without alcohol; and (h) in a car, while stopping for a few minutes in traffic. An ESS score ranges from 0 to 24. The ESS statistically distinguishes between individuals with sleep disorders (characterized by the symptom of excessive sleepiness) and those without such disorders, and it also correlates well with both daytime and nocturnal electroencephalographically determined sleep latencies (Johns, 1992). However, the ESS is not designed for use on multiple occasions during the day or in the presence of short-term conditions that might influence sleep tendency, such as acute sleep loss.

Objective Estimates of Excessive Sleepiness

In addition to subjective measures for determining the level of perceived sleepiness, identifying what occurs when external factors (e.g., environmental stimulation, physical activity, and to a lesser extent, personal motivation) are removed is helpful in ascertaining the extent of an individual's sleepiness. One of the most widely used objective measures to diagnose pathological sleepiness is the Multiple Sleep Latency

Test (MSLT; Mitler et al., 1979; Richardson et al., 1978; Thorpy, 1992), an electroencephalographically-based, well-validated clinical and research tool. The MSLT measures the daytime level and captures the afternoon rise in sleep tendency by providing approximately 5 separate 20-minute opportunities to sleep. The MSLT distinguishes between excessively sleepy individuals and those who are not sleepy and can also detect the daytime carry-over effects of long-acting sleeping medications (Mitler et al., 1984). A variant of the MSLT is the Maintenance of Wakefulness Test (MWT; Mitler, Gujavarty, & Browman, 1982), which was originally devised to obviate some of the interpretative and conceptual problems of the MSLT (Poceta et al., 1992). Early MWT studies demonstrated a prolonged sleep latency as a result of the instruction to remain awake, compared with asking the individual to go to sleep, as is done in the MSLT (Erman, Beckman, Gardner, & Roffwarg, 1987; Hartse, Roth, & Zorick, 1982; Sangal, Thomas, & Mitler, 1992). However, both the MSLT and the MWT are only available through a sleep disorders center. Therefore, prior to making such a referral the assessment of excessive daytime sleepiness should begin with a clinical sleep interview.

The Clinical Sleep Interview

Initial Evaluation

A structured clinical sleep interview identifies specific factors related to the complaint of excessive daytime sleepiness. The evaluation begins with a statement from the patient regarding the nature of the complaint and how the patient has coped with it. A thorough history of the patient's psychiatric and medical status, including medication, alcohol, and illicit drug use, is also obtained. In addition, any family history of sleep disorders aids in identifying a possible vulnerability to certain pathological conditions, such as narcolepsy. A physical examination and (if possible) a neurological examination should also be requested. During the clinical sleep interview, an attempt is made to clarify the presenting complaint by soliciting information about situations associated with sleep episodes. The following three areas offer clues into the etiology of the complaint and help determine the severity of the problem: (a) sleep habits and behaviors, (b) work and school schedules, and (c) the physical parameters of the bedroom.

Sleep Habits and Behaviors

Questions related to sleep habits and behaviors attempt to elicit information regarding the patient's approach to going to sleep (e.g., one's usual lights-out time and the time of the final awakening). It is also helpful to ask patients how many hours of sleep they think they need to function well during the day. (For example, someone who claims to need 9 hours of sleep per night but is receiving only 6 is probably suffering from insufficient sleep syndrome.) How long does the patient estimate it takes to fall asleep and what is the number and time of awakenings during the night? These questions help determine whether the complaint of excessive daytime sleepiness is related to difficulty falling asleep (which shortens total sleep time), fragmented sleep, or the possible early-morning awakening symptom of depression. Are there any events in the night that are noteworthy, such as nightmares, night terrors, or sleep walking? Are there any significant variations in their weekday versus weekend sleep schedules? (Sleep time that is significantly extended during the weekends suggests that the individual receives insufficient sleep during the week.) Is there a typical adverse bedtime routine, such as watching television until falling asleep and then awakening in the night to turn it off, or drinking a large amount of fluid at bedtime and waking later to void? Both of these behaviors can contribute to disrupted or fragmented sleep.

Many sleep problems such as sleep apnea are not evident to the patient. Therefore, it is often helpful to determine what the bed partner reports regarding the patient's sleep behavior. Questions to ask the bed partner that could indicate the presence of obstructive sleep apnea would include the following: Does the patient snore loudly or toss and turn excessively during the night? Does the patient stop breathing or breathe very shallowly while asleep? Does the patient seem confused or disoriented on awakening (e.g., walks into the closet rather than the bathroom during the night)? Does the patient consistently wake in the morning complaining of a poor night's sleep?

Work or School Schedules

An important area to investigate is the influence of the patient's work or school schedule on sleep. Shift workers, especially those assigned the "graveyard shift," find it difficult to sleep during daylight hours. Though their work schedule allows for sufficient sleep time, they often take only "cat naps" of 2 to 3 hours' duration. Parents of small children who work evening shifts (4 p.m. to 12 a.m.) often must wake early in the morning to monitor their children (after receiving only 4 to 5 hours of sleep). They can accumulate a large enough amount of sleep debt to exhibit signs of excessive daytime sleepiness. (Such individuals may then be diagnosed with insufficient sleep syndrome). A child who struggles with bedtime but has difficulty waking for school in the morning may be an "owl" or "night person," as opposed to a "lark" or "morning person" (Horne & Ostberg, 1976) or may be suffering from a delayed sleep phase. Delayed sleep phase syndrome is the extreme of being a night person and indicates that the circadian rhythm of alertness and sleep has been shifted in such a manner that the sleep tendency peak occurs much later in the night (Roehrs & Roth, 1994). High school and college students often suffer from a delayed sleep phase. The corollary to delayed sleep is an advanced sleep phase syndrome, in which individuals who find themselves falling asleep too early in the evening awake fully alert in the early-morning hours. This is often a complaint in geriatric populations.

Physical Parameters of the Bedroom

In addition to sleep habits, nocturnal conditions, and the influences of daytime schedules, the specifics of the sleep setting are also important to identify. The sleep environment must be conducive for sleeping—otherwise, sleep may be light, fragmented, or disrupted. Questions to ask to elicit information regarding specific sleeping conditions would include the following: Does the patient live near an airport, railway line, or busy thoroughfare or have loud neighbors? Is the temperature of the bedroom sufficiently comfortable? Is the bedroom too light or dark? Is the sleep surface uncomfortable or are certain awkward sleep positions being enforced by an infirmity, such as a leg cast or surgical wound? Does the bed partner's activities cause sleep disturbance? (Bed partners who snore or make excessive movements are often disruptive to the other's sleep.) Once the basic elements regarding sleep behaviors, daytime schedules, and environmental conditions of the bedroom have been established, and no clear cause has emerged, questions directed at specific clinical conditions such as obstructive sleep apnea or narcolepsy should be addressed.

Clinical Conditions Associated
With Excessive Daytime Sleepiness

Obstructive Sleep Apnea

Obstructive sleep apnea is a respiratory disturbance characterized by repetitive episodes of upper airway resistance or blockage during sleep. The obstructive episodes are accompanied by loud gasps, snorts, and snores, which lead to brief arousals. These arousals alternate with episodes of silence in which there is a cessation in breathing that can last approximately 20 to 40 seconds (Thorpy, 1990). Excessive daytime sleepiness is the most common presenting complaint. A bed partner's observations of these respiratory events are very helpful in determining whether obstructive sleep apnea is present. Questions to ask the individual include whether he or she snores (and typically in all sleeping positions), ever wakes up gasping for breath or air, or has morning headaches. Obstructive sleep apnea may present as an insomnia complaint; the respiratory arousals can occur immediately upon sleep onset, causing patients to feel they have never fallen asleep (Erman & Poceta, 1993). Therefore, it is also helpful to ask whether the individual wakes repeatedly during the night or has difficulty falling asleep.

Narcolepsy

Narcolepsy is a relatively common (about 1 in 1,000) central nervous system condition involving a classic tetrad of symptoms: excessive daytime sleepiness, cataplexy, sleep paralysis, and hypnogogic hallucinations (Mitler, Hajdukovic, Erman, & Koziol, 1990).

Cataplexy is an episodic loss of muscle tone in response to a strong emotion, such as surprise, laughter, or anger. The muscle weakness may involve a mild head or jaw droop, buckling of the knees, or a complete loss of bilateral muscle tone resulting in a fall to the ground. Frequently sleep follows a cataplectic event. An individual often volunteers a problematic history related to cataplectic episodes. Reports of being unable to move, speak, or breathe deeply while falling asleep or on awakening are indicative of sleep paralysis. Often these episodes of sleep paralysis can provoke great anxiety and fear of death. Hypnogogic hallucinations are sleep-onset phenomena associated with vivid hallucinations involving visual, auditory, kinetic, or tactile stimuli. The content of these hallucinations often consist of experiencing the presence of someone or something accompanied by a feeling of fear or dread.

One should suspect narcolepsy if an individual presenting with the complaint of excessive daytime sleepiness also answers affirmatively to any questions related to cataplexy (e.g., "do you find your muscles getting weak or do you fall down when surprised or angry?"), sleep paralysis (e.g., "do you often feel you cannot move just as you're falling asleep or when you wake up?"), or hypnogogic hallucinations (e.g., "do you ever have visions of people or things just as you're falling asleep?").

Periodic Limb Movement Disorder

Periodic limb movement disorder (PLMD) or nocturnal myoclonus is characterized by stereotypic, periodic, and repetitive episodes of leg movements (e.g., jerks, twitches) during sleep (Thorpy, 1990). These movements frequently produce partial arousals from sleep. Nonrestorative sleep or daytime sleepiness may be the presenting complaint. Though the patient may be unaware of the leg movements or sleep disruptions, an associative complaint of restless leg syndrome often presents at sleep onset. In addition, reports of leg movements witnessed by a bed partner can aid in the diagnosis. This limb movement disorder is unrelated to what is known as *sleep starts*, which typically occur only during drowsiness before sleep onset and with no regularity. PLMD, on the other hand, occurs with regular periodicity throughout most NREM stages of sleep (Fredrickson & Krueger, 1994).

Idiopathic Hypersomnia

Idiopathic hypersomnia or idiopathic central nervous system (CNS) hypersomnolence is a condition of constant excessive daytime sleepiness. Nocturnal sleep episodes are greater than 8 hours and daytime naps are excessive in duration and usually unrefreshing (Guilleminault, 1994). Associated physical symptoms related to this autonomic nervous system dysfunction include dull headaches, mild to moderate fainting episodes, lightheadedness upon standing, and peripheral vascular complaints (e.g., cold hands and feet; Thorpy, 1990). The condition has no clear etiology, but a history of a past viral infection such as mononucleosis is sometimes present.

Sleepiness Secondary to Medical Disorders

Various medical, biochemical, and neurological disorders can cause or promote excessive sleepiness. For example, pathological sleepiness can occur in medical conditions that disturb sleep, such as congestive heart failure or chronic obstructive pulmonary disease, and in medical conditions treated with drugs that have sedating side effects (e.g., Dilantin). An exhaustive listing of such conditions and medications is not possible here; however, Table 1 provides a list of exemplary conditions associated with excessive daytime sleepiness. If any of the listed physiological conditions are suspected, prompt referral to a sleep disorders specialist is in order. To facilitate such referrals, most accredited sleep disorders centers are equipped with brief questionnaires that contain questions suggestive of various sleep pathologies. Contacting a sleep center in your area and requesting such a questionnaire can encourage a helpful liaison between the psychologist, sleep disordered individual, and sleep diagnostician.

Sleepiness Associated With Psychological Disorders

Though most patients with major depression complain of insomnia (usually early-morning awakening problems), a subgroup of depressed patients may present with excessive daytime sleepiness (Benca, 1994). Patients with bipolar depressive episodes or seasonal affective disorder typically experience symptoms of hypersomnia. It is this long sleep duration that often extends into the daytime that can be mistaken for excessive daytime sleepiness. Dysthymic individuals may complain of fatigue and attempt to compensate for their malaise through daytime napping. Because sleepiness is a manifestation of sleep tendency—a physiological drive state—it is important to note that the sleepiness in depression may be related more to a social withdrawal mechanism than a physiological need to sleep. Individuals suffering from depression may not necessarily be fighting a sleep drive but rather feel compelled consciously or unconsciously to escape their psychic pain through sleep. In fact, objective testing of sleep tendency demonstrated no abnormal physiological sleepiness in depressed patients (Nofzinger, Thase, & Reynolds, 1991). Depression may also be secondary to alcoholism, which can create a state of excessive sleepiness independent of the mood disorder. Psychological objective assessment such as the Minnesota Multiphase Personality Inventory can assist in uncovering an explicit personality pathology or mood disorder which can help explain the complaint of excessive daytime sleepiness.

Table 1

Conditions Associated With Excessive Daytime Sleepiness

Sleep Disruption
   Obstructive sleep apnea
   Periodic limb movement disorder
   Sleep stage abnormality
   Nightmares
   Sleep deprivation (total or partial)
   Age (childhood to adulthood)
   Insufficient sleep in a long sleeper

Circadian Rhythm
   Time of day (sleep tendency)
   Delayed sleep phase syndrome
   Advanced sleep phase syndrome

Neurologic Disorders
   Narcolepsy
   Idiopathic hypersomnia syndrome
   Psychomotor epilepsy
   Klein–Levin syndrome
   6–18 months post-head trauma
   Early symptom of progressive hydrocephalus
   Intracranial space-occupying lesions

Psychological Disorders
   Depression
   Malingering
   Somatoform disorders

Biomedical–Physical Disorders
   Hypoglycemia
   Myotonic dystrophy
   Hypothyroidism
   Alcoholism
   Prader–Willi syndrome
   Drug withdrawal (especially from central nervous system stimulants)
   Long half-lives of sedatives
   Chronic obstructive pulmonary disease
   Congestive heart failure

Malingering should be considered if the complaint of excessive day-time sleepiness presents opportunities for significant secondary gain, such as exemption from particular duties, disability leave, or possible access to stimulant medication.

The possibility of a somatoform sleep disorder must also be considered. Individuals with this type of pathology attempt to gain attention, sympathy, or credibility by receiving a medical diagnosis characterized by the symptoms of excessive sleepiness. Often, such patients state that they have had "narcolepsy for years." In addition, a sleep-related medical diagnosis can provide a rational for social failure and vocational underachievement. Differentiating the psychological motivation from actual physiological sleep tendency requires documentation through objective physiological assessment.

Conclusion

Excessive daytime sleepiness is the most common sleep-related reason for a person to seek professional help. This is thought to be due to excessive daytime sleepiness-related caused inability to fulfill work and social responsibilities. Appropriate diagnosis and treatment of excessive daytime sleepiness will significantly improve the patient's quality of life. In fact 90% of all excessive daytime sleepiness complaints involve medically treatable conditions such as sleep apnea, narcolepsy, and CNS hypersomnia. The chances of patients with clinically significant excessive daytime sleepiness being successfully identified and treated increases with the ability of their mental health professionals to discern normal from pathological sleepiness.

REFERENCES

Benca, R. M. (1994). Mood disorders. In M. H. Kryer, T. Roth, & W. C. Dement (Eds.), *Principles and practices of sleep medicine* (2nd ed., pp. 899–913). Philadelphia: W. B. Saunders.

Broughton, R. J. (1989). Chronobiological aspects and models of sleep and napping. In D. F. Dinges & R. J. Broughton (Eds.), *Sleep and alertness: Chronobiological, behavioral and medical aspects of napping* (pp. 71–98). New York: Raven Press.

Carskadon, M. A. (1990). Patterns of sleep and sleepiness in adolescents. *Pediatrician, 17,* 5–12.

Carskadon, M. A., & Dement, W. C. (1981). Cumulative effects of sleep restriction on daytime sleepiness. *Psychophysiology, 18,* 107–113.

Carskadon, M. A., & Dement, W. C. (1982). Nocturnal determinants of daytime sleepiness. *Sleep, 5*(Suppl.), 73–81.

Carskadon, M. A., Dement, W. C., Mitler, M. M., Guilleminault, C., Zarcone, V. P., & Spiegel, R. (1976). Complaint versus sleep laboratory findings in 122 drug-free subjects with a complaint of chronic insomnia. *American Journal of Psychiatry, 133,* 1382–1388.

Carskadon, M. A., Harvey, K., Duke, P., Anders, T. F., Litt, I. F., & Dement, W. (1980). Pubertal changes in daytime sleepiness. *Sleep, 2,* 453–460.

Dement, W. C., Carskadon, M. A., & Richardson, G. S. (1978). Excessive daytime sleepiness in the sleep apnea syndrome. In C. Guilleminault & W. C. Dement (Eds.), *Sleep apnea syndromes* (pp. 23–46). New York: Alan R. Liss.

Erman, M. K., Beckman, B., Gardner, D., & Roffwarg, H. (1987). The Modified Assessment of Sleepiness Test (MAST). *Sleep Research, 16,* 550.

Erman, M. K., & Poceta, J. S. (1993). Obstructive sleep apnea presenting as insomnia. *Sleep Research, 22,* 194.

Findley, L., Weiss, J. W., & Jabour, E. R. (1991). Serious automobile crashes caused by undetected sleep apnea. *Archives of Internal Medicine, 151,* 1451–1452.

Fredrickson, P. A., & Krueger, B. R. (1994). Insomnia associated with specific polysomnographic findings. In M. H. Kryer, T. Roth, & W. C. Dement (Eds.), *Principles and practices of sleep medicine* (2nd ed., pp. 523–534). Philadelphia: W. B. Saunders.

Guilleminault, C. (1994). Idiopathic central nervous system hypersomnia. In M. H. Kryer, T. Roth, & W. C. Dement (Eds.), *Principles and practices of sleep medicine* (2nd ed., pp. 562–566). Philadelphia: W. B. Saunders.

Guilleminault, C., Eldridge, F., Simmons, F., & Dement, W. C. (1976). Sleep apnea in eight children. *Pediatrics, 58,* 23–30.

Hartse, K. M., Roth, T., & Zorick, F. J. (1982). Daytime sleepiness and daytime wakefulness: The effect of instruction. *Sleep, 5*(Suppl.), 107–118.

Hoddes, E., Zarcone, V. P., Smythe, H., Phillips, R., & Dement, W. C. (1973). Quantification of sleepiness: A new approach. *Psychophysiology, 10,* 431–436.

Horne, J. A., & Ostberg, O. A. (1976). A self-assessment questionnaire to determine morningness-eveningness in human circadian rhythms. *International Journal of Chronobiology, 4,* 97–110.

Johns, M. W. (1991). A new method for measuring daytime sleepiness: The Epworth Sleepiness Scale. *Sleep, 14,* 540–545.

Johns, M. W. (1992). Reliability and factor analysis of the Epworth Sleepiness Scale. *Sleep, 15,* 376–381.

Lavie, P. (1989). To nap, perchance to sleep: Ultradian aspects of napping. In D. F. Dinges & R. J. Broughton (Eds.), *Sleep and alertness: Chronobiological, behavioral and medical aspects of napping* (pp. 99–120). New York: Raven Press.

Mitler, M. M. (1991). Two-peak 24-hour patterns in sleep, mortality and error. In J. H. Peter, T. Penzel, T. Podszus, & P. von Wichert (Eds.), *Sleep and health risk* (pp. 65–77). Berlin: Springer-Verlag.

Mitler, M. M., Carskadon, M. A., Czeisler, C. A., Dement, W. C., Dinges, D. F., & Graeber, R. C. (1988). Catastrophes, sleep and public policy. *Sleep, 11,* 100–109.

Mitler, M. M., Gujavarty, K. S., & Browman, C. P. (1982). Maintenance of Wakefulness Test: A polysomnographic technique for evaluating treatment in patients with excessive somnolence. *Electroencephalography and Clinical Neurophysiology, 53,* 658–661.

Mitler, M. M., Gujavarty, K. S., Sampson, M. G., & Browman, C. P. (1982). Multiple daytime nap approaches to evaluating the sleepy patient. *Sleep,* 5(Suppl.), 119–127.

Mitler, M. M., Hajdukovic, R. M., Erman, M. K., & Koziol, J. A. (1990). Narcolepsy. *Journal of Clinical Neurophysiology, 7,* 93–118.

Mitler, M. M., Seidel, W. F., Van den Hoed, J., Greenblatt, D. J., & Dement, W. C. (1984). Comparative hypnotic effects of flurazepam, triazolam and placebo: A long-term simultaneous nighttime and daytime study. *Journal of Clinical Psychopharmacology, 4,* 2–13.

Mitler, M. M., Van den Hoed, J., Carskadon, M. A., Richardson, G. S., Park, R., Guilleminault, C., & Dement, W. C. (1979). REM sleep episodes during the Multiple Sleep Latency Test in narcoleptic patients. *Electroencephalography and Clinical Neurophysiology, 46,* 479–481.

Nofzinger, E. A., Thase, M. E., & Reynolds, C. F. (1991). Hypersomnia in bipolar depression: A comparison with narcolepsy using the multiple sleep latency test. *American Journal of Psychiatry, 148*(9), 1177–1181.

Poceta, J. S., Timms, R. M., Jeong, D., Ho, S., Erman, M. K., & Mitler, M. M. (1992). Maintenance of Wakefulness test in obstructive sleep apnea syndrome. *Chest, 101,* 893–897.

Richardson, G. S., Carskadon, M. A., Flagg, W., Van den Hoed, J., Dement, W. C., & Mitler, M. M. (1978). Excessive daytime sleepiness in man: Multiple sleep latency measurement in narcoleptic and control subjects. *Electroencephalography and Clinical Neurophysiology, 45,* 621–627.

Richardson, G. S., Carskadon, M. A., Orav, E. J., & Dement, W. C. (1982). Circadian variation in sleep tendency in elderly and young adult subjects. *Sleep,* 5(Suppl.), 82–92.

Roehrs, T., & Roth, T. (1994). Chronic insomnia associated with circadian rhythm disorders. In M. H. Kryer, T. Roth, & W. C. Dement (Eds.), *Principles and practices of sleep medicine* (2nd ed., pp. 477–481). Philadelphia: W. B. Saunders.

Sangal, R. B., Thomas, L., & Mitler, M. M. (1992). Maintenance of Wakefulness Test and Multiple Sleep Latency Test: Measurement of different abilities in patients with sleep disorders. *Chest, 101,* 898–902.

Thorpy, M. J. (Ed.). (1990). *The international classification of sleep disorders: Diagnostic and coding manual.* Minneapolis, MN: American Sleep Disorders Association.

Thorpy, M. J. (1992). Report from the American Sleep Disorders Association. The clinical use of the Multiple Sleep Latency Test. *Sleep, 15,* 268–276.

8

The Polysomnogram

Sonia Ancoli-Israel

Polysomnography

S leep is something all people do and all people have observed others do. We assume someone is asleep when his eyes are closed and he is unresponsive. However, to understand what is going on during sleep, one needs to record the physiological aspects of sleep. The physiological study of sleep has roots as early as the 1930s, when the first electroencephalographic (EEG) studies were performed (Carskadon, 1982). In the 1950s, Kleitman, Aserinsky, and Dement discovered eye movements during sleep, and in 1957 Kleitman and Dement published a description of the EEG and eye movements during sleep, a condition they labeled rapid eye movement (REM) sleep (Dement & Kleitman, 1957). In the late 1960s, the study of sleep turned from basic research to clinical application. The first center for the diagnosis and treatment of sleep disorders was accredited in 1976. Today there are over 200 accredited sleep disorders centers and as many as 600 unaccredited centers conducting sleep studies as part of the clinical evaluation of

Supported by National Institute on Aging AG02711, National Institute on Aging AG08415, National institute on Mental Health MH49671, National Heart, Lung, and Blood Institute HL44915, the Research Service of the Veterans Affairs Medical Center, and the Sam and Rose Stein Institute for Research on Aging.

sleep disorders. Over 100,000 sleep studies are performed in the United States each year. Additionally, the sleep study or *polysomnogram*, remains an important research tool.

Sleep is defined by brain waves measured by electroencephalography (EEG); eye movements, recorded by electrooculography (EOG); and muscle tension, ascertained by electromyography (EMG). The combination of these three channels of information allows the determination of the different levels, or stages, of sleep. The recording of these variables is called *polysomnography*, meaning "many sleep writings" (Carskadon, 1993). The machine that records these functions is called a *polygraph*. The electrical signal (such as the EEG, EOG, or EMG) recorded from the person being tested flows through cables to the polygraph, where it is amplified (enlarged) and filtered (cleaned of unwanted noisy signals).

By reading the EEG, EOG, and EMG, a trained polysomnographer (sleep specialist) can glean much information about sleep. Sleep is divided into five stages. Each stage is characterized by the amplitude and frequency of brain waves and the presence or absence of eye movements and muscle tension. These stages are described fully in chapter 1 but are briefly reviewed here. A description of how sleep is evaluated will follow.

The first stage of sleep, Stage 1, is transitional sleep, the point when most people find themselves drifting off, realizing they are not fully asleep but no longer fully alert. Stage 1 sleep is defined by a decrease in alpha EEG activity (7–12 cycles per second) and an increase in theta brain waves (4–7 cycles per second). There is high activity in the chin muscle, and there may be some slow rolling eye movements.

Stage 2 sleep is most often considered the official onset of sleep. It is characterized by sleep spindles (brief periods of activity in the 12–14 cycles per second range), with low muscle tension and increased amounts of slow rolling eye movements. Stages 3 and 4 are progressively deeper, with Stage 4 being the deepest level of sleep. Stages 3 and 4 are sometimes combined and called *deep sleep* or *slow wave sleep*. Both Stages 3 and 4 are characterized by delta brain waves (1–4 cycles per second). In Stage 3 sleep, 20–50% of the time is spent in delta wave activity. In Stage 4 sleep, greater than 50% of the time is spent in delta activity. These four stages of sleep together are called *nonrapid eye movement sleep*, or non-REM (NREM).

The fifth stage of sleep, REM sleep, is defined by low-voltage, fast-frequency EEG and rapid eye movements. The EMG during REM sleep is essentially flat, because except for the eyes and respiration, the body is paralyzed during this stage of sleep. Because about 85% of dreams take place during REM sleep, this paralysis is believed to be a protective mechanism that keeps us from acting out our dreams.

About 25% of the night is spent in REM sleep and 75% in NREM sleep. NREM sleep is distributed with 5% in Stage 1, 45% in Stage 2, and 25% in Stages 3 and 4. As the night progresses, people cycle in and out of the different stages of sleep. This cycling is called the *sleep architecture*.

Sleep begins in Stage 1 and progresses through Stage 2 to Stages 3 and 4. It then goes back through Stage 2 into the first REM period, generally 90–100 minutes after sleep onset. One continues to cycle in and out of the different stages throughout the night. Most of deep sleep occurs in the first third of the night and most of REM sleep occurs in the last third of the night, in the morning hours.

By reading the EEG, EOG, and EMG, a polysomnographer can determine if sleep architecture is appropriate, how long each individual spends in each stage of sleep, how long it takes to fall asleep (sleep-onset latency), how long the person sleeps at night (total sleep time [TST]), how much time is spent awake during the night (wake after sleep onset [WASO]), how much time is spent in bed (total sleep period [TSP]), latency to the first REM period, and number of REM periods. All this information is used to determine whether sleep is normal and, if not, what is wrong with it.

Sleep Disorders Clinic Recordings

In the sleep clinic, doctors are usually interested in more than just the stage or the amount of sleep. Other physiological systems in the body are also active during sleep. During NREM sleep, heart rate and breathing slow down and become quite regular. EMG decreases but stays at a steady state. During REM, however, many parts of the autonomic nervous system (e.g., heart rate, respiration, blood pressure) become extremely irregular, speeding up and slowing down almost at random. During REM, control of body temperature is also lost, so that an individual is more likely to get cold if the room is cold or feel warm if the room is hot.

During REM sleep, it is normal for men to experience erections. The erections have nothing to do with dreaming or with sexual desire but are part of the physiological process of REM sleep. There is also a female counterpart, in which women experience vaginal and clitoral swelling during REM sleep.

There are two types of REM behaviors. The first is called *tonic*, referring to behaviors that occur throughout the REM period. Tonic behaviors include the suppressed EMG, elevated brain temperature, and erections. The second type of activity is called *phasic*, referring to behaviors that occur periodically throughout the REM period. These include the rapid eye movements, tongue movements, some muscle or limb twitches, and variable heart rate and blood pressure. For clinical recordings, sensors (electrodes) also are used to monitor respiration and airflow, heart rate, blood oxygen saturation levels, leg muscle tension, carbon dioxide, blood pressure, body temperature, penile tumescence, and any other physiological system that can be measured and may add information about sleep. These physiological parameters are measured continuously throughout the patient's sleep, often for 8–10 continuous hours.

In the sleep disorders clinic, the polysomnogram is also recorded during the day to evaluate daytime sleepiness. Two tests are used, the Multiple Sleep Latency Test (MSLT; Carskadon et al., 1986; Carskadon & Dement, 1987) and the Maintenance of Wakefulness Test (MWT; Mitler, Gujavarty, & Browman, 1982), to evaluate how sleepy a patient really is during the day (see chapter 9 for more detailed information on these tests). These tests are especially useful in patients suspected of narcolepsy or sleep apnea. In the MSLT, a patient is asked to go to sleep four to five times at 2-hour intervals. Patients are allowed to stay in bed for only 20 minutes, and then they arise, whether or not they have fallen asleep. When patients do fall asleep, they are allowed to sleep for only a few minutes. The purpose of the test is to test their sleep latency: how long it takes them to fall asleep when left in a dark room.

The MWT tests sleepiness by having patients seated in a dark room five times at 2-hour intervals. However, instead of being told to go to sleep, patients are asked to stay awake. This test is especially helpful in determining the effect of treatments on a patient's ability to control daytime sleepiness and to stay awake in quiet environments.

A Typical Sleep Evaluation

All sleep clinic evaluations begin with an interview with the patient and, when possible, the patient's bed partner. The doctor begins by asking questions about medical history, drug use (including prescription, over-the-counter, and illicit drugs), sleep habits, daytime activities, diet, and use of nicotine and alcohol. Some sample questions are listed in Exhibit 1. Sleep-related questions are intended to establish the patient's sleep pattern and whether the chief complaint is related to insomnia, excessive daytime sleepiness (hypersomnia), or some other medical or psychiatric problem. In addition, there are questions that help identify any symptoms that occur either at night or during the day that suggest a specific sleep problem such as sleep-disordered breathing, narcolepsy, or periodic limb movements in sleep.

The doctor may also have blood pressure, weight, and height measured. If the complaints and symptoms are suggestive of sleep-disordered breathing, the patient's airway will need to be examined to identify signs of redness or enlarged structures (such as a long soft palate, a long uvula, a large tongue, or large tonsils). Sometimes special tests need to be done to examine and take measurements of the airway.

Once the history and physical examination are completed, a date and time are scheduled for the sleep recording. Sleep laboratories or clinics are furnished with at least one room that houses the polygraphs—the large machines that record data concerning the physiological systems of interest—and computers. Each clinic also has at least one, but usually multiple, bedrooms in which patients sleep. The bedrooms often look more like attractive hotel rooms than hospital rooms. Infrared video cameras are set up so that patients can be observed as well as recorded.

A Night in the Sleep Disorders Clinic or Laboratory

In sleep disorders clinics and laboratories throughout the world, the same basic methods are used to study sleep. Study participants or patients arrive at the sleep clinic about 1 or 2 hours before their normal bedtime. Once the patient has gotten ready for bed, electrodes (special sensors) are placed in standardized locations on the head for the EEG, around the eyes for the EOG, and under the chin for the EMG. EEG is generally recorded from either the left or right central portion of the head, with one side actually recorded and the other acting as a backup in case the first set of electrodes becomes disconnected.

For the placement of the EEG electrodes to be reliable at each application, the international 10–20 placement system is used (Jasper, 1958). This system requires measurement of distances from set points on the

Exhibit 1

Sample Sleep Interview Questions

How long does it take you to fall asleep at night?
How many times do you wake up during the night?
Are you aware of what wakes you during the night?
Do you ever wake up at night short of breath or choking?
Do you ever wake up at night confused?
Do you have difficulty falling back to sleep?
What time do you wake up in the morning?
How do you feel when you wake up in the morning?
Do you wake up with a headache in the morning?
Are you aware of or have you been told that you snore?
How loudly do you snore? Can your snoring be heard outside your bedroom?
Are you aware of or have you been told that you stop breathing at night?
What position do you normally sleep in? Is your snoring worse in certain body positions? Is your snoring better in certain body positions?
Are you sleepy during the day? Do you take naps on purpose? How often and how long do you nap on purpose?
Do you find yourself falling asleep without meaning to? Do you fall asleep reading, watching television, at meetings at work, while sitting with friends, at the movies?
Have you ever had a near-miss automobile accident due to sleepiness?
Have you ever had an automobile accident due to sleepiness?
How much alcohol do you drink? How often do you drink? What time of day do you drink?
Has your weight changed? Did your sleep problem, snoring, or sleepiness get better, worse, or stay the same as your weight changed?
What medications do you take? Do you ever take any sleeping pills or other medication to help you sleep?
Does anyone in your family (your father, mother, brother, sister, or other relative) snore or have other symptoms like yours?
Have you been told or are you aware that your legs kick or twitch at night?
Do you ever experience episodes of muscular weakness during the day? Does anything special trigger this weakness?
Do you ever experience hypnagogic hallucinations or sleep paralysis on falling asleep?
[FOR MEN] Do you wake up with an erection in the morning?

head to determine the exact location of the electrodes. Electrodes are placed at intervals of 10% or 20% of the distance between the set points, hence the name, the 10–20 system. The standardization guarantees that electrodes are always placed in the same spot on each head by each technician.

The scalp and skin must be cleaned to reduce skin resistance, and special electrode paste or jelly is used both to help the electrodes adhere to the skin and to help in conductivity of the signals. For EEG electrodes, gauze soaked in collodion (an adhesive substance) is placed over the electrodes to help seal them in place. The collodion is usually dried with air blown from an air compressor.

The reason for recording EOG data is to identify the slow rolling eye movements that accompany sleep onset and the rapid eye movements of REM sleep. EOG is recorded by taping small electrodes to the side of each eye, with one slightly higher than the other. Traditionally, two channels of eye movement are recorded, although both the rolling eye movements and rapid movements can be identified from a single channel.

The purpose of recording chin EMG is to identify the muscle relaxation or paralysis that accompanies REM sleep. EMG is recorded by placing three electrodes beneath the chin, over the submental muscle. Two electrodes are needed for the recording, and the third is a backup in case one electrode disconnects. Although other muscles could be recorded, the submental is particularly easy to access.

Depending on the complaints, other variables may be recorded, but not all are necessarily recorded in all patients. Heart rate is recorded by placing electrodes in standardized electrocardiographic (ECG) locations. Respiration may be recorded in several ways, although it always includes airflow and chest (thoracic) and abdominal (diaphragmatic) breathing. The more common ways of recording respiration include use of strain gauges, plethysmography (which records respiratory effort), and electromyography (muscle tone) of intercostal muscles. Airflow is recorded with a thermistor (heat sensor) placed either in each nostril or under the nose and over the mouth; this measurement aids in the determination of respiratory abnormalities. In addition, blood oxygen saturation level is measured with ear or finger pulse oximetry, which measures the amount of oxygen in the blood by shining a light through the ear or finger and measuring the wavelength of light that passes through the hemoglobin molecules. The amount of carbon dioxide being exhaled and inhaled may also be measured.

Blood pressure can be measured with a standard blood pressure cuff that automatically inflates at set intervals. Body temperature is generally monitored by a rectal thermistor. Penile tumescence is measured with a plethysmograph, which records the changes in the size of the penis. Because men normally experience penile erections during sleep, recording nocturnal penile tumescence affords the ability to distinguish between physiological impotence (i.e., no erections would occur during REM) and psychological impotence (erections would occur during REM).

The sensors all attach to a cable that passes through a hole in the wall and connects to the polygraph machine. Patients who sleep in the laboratory are monitored all night by a sleep technologist, who makes sure the polygraph is operating properly, paper does not jam, ink does not run out, electrodes do not disconnect, and most important, the patient is sleeping comfortably. Once the patient is all hooked up and in bed, the technologist begins a calibration period. This is the time to make sure all the electrodes are recording properly and all the filters and amplifiers on the polygraph are set correctly.

In the morning, when the patient awakens, all electrodes are removed and the patient is free to leave the clinic. The work then begins for the sleep technologist. The polysomnograms are usually run at speeds that result in each page representing 20 or 30 seconds. Therefore, a sleep period of 8 hours often takes a quarter of a mile of polysomnograph paper. Each page of the polysomnogram must be read and scored, a process that can take many hours, depending on how abnormal the recording is. The sleep technologist must score sleep stages using standardized rules (Rechtschaffen & Kales, 1973) and examine each other channel recorded (e.g., count respiratory events, count leg jerks, and examine the ECG for abnormalities). The results of this recording are then used to make the diagnosis.

Computerized Polysomnography

Traditional polysomnography requires many hours of recording, scoring, and interpreting records and large amounts of space to store the paper records. Computerized polysomnography saves time, money, and space, yet many sleep researchers and clinicians have not made the leap to this advanced technology. Part of the problem lies in the great difficulty of scoring clinical records. No computer program has yet been able to score these complicated records accurately; however, many programs allow the user to define default parameters or to hand score the records, and the computer program adds up the totals.

In one of the few reliability studies, Orr, Eiken, Pegram, Jones, and Rundall (1994) found that one automatic scoring system's sensitivity and specificity for diagnosing obstructive sleep apnea were high; however, correlations for sleep staging were not accurate. Hirshkowitz and Moore (1994) reviewed the complex issues involved in computerized polysomnography. There are multiple computerized systems on the market, all of varying quality and with varying levels of testing. An ideal system needs to have screens with high resolution so that EEG records can be easily scored, on-line record review so that past pages can be easily examined, and display speed equal to that of manual page turning. These systems need to be tested for reliability and validity and compared with traditional polysomnography. Carskadon and Rechtschaffen, (1989) suggested that automatic scoring systems must meet the following requirements before they are acceptable: validation against the gold standard of conventional polysomnography, validation for the particular patients that will be monitored, validation for particular age groups, compatibility with available laboratory hardware, availability of raw data, overriding of automatic scoring with hand scoring, flexibility for future applications, and availability of consultants. As more research is done on these systems, more and more laboratories and clinics will find themselves switching to computerized polysomnographs.

Portable Polysomnography

Although the all-night laboratory polysomnogram is considered the gold standard, there are times when recording sleep in the patient's home or on hospital wards may be preferable. Portable recorders have the advantages of being less intrusive and easier for some patients to tolerate, recording sleep in a more natural environment (i.e., the patient's bedroom), running for longer time periods to enable recording of napping or other daytime behaviors, accommodating patients who are unable to come to the laboratory, and being less expensive to operate (Ancoli-Israel, 1989). In addition, it is easier to do multiple recordings, follow-up studies, and studies of treatment efficacy. The main disadvantage is that no personnel are available to correct problems that might arise during the night. A full review of the different applications of portable recordings can be found in a book by Miles and Broughton (1990).

The typical portable or ambulatory recorder is self-contained and includes physiological amplifiers, filters, sensors, and data storage. Data must be transferred to a larger computer for analysis. There are many portable recorders now available on the commercial market. Some are completely ambulatory, powered by batteries; others, brought to the patient's home or bedside in the hospital by technologists, are miniaturized versions of the systems used in sleep disorders centers, recording 10 or more physiological parameters simultaneously. Other systems record only some of the variables. Most portable recorders do not measure EOG or EEG because they do not contain sufficient storage space.

The type of recorder used and the variables recorded depend completely on the patient's presenting complaints. For patients with complaints suggestive of sleep apnea, a recorder capable of recording four to six channels of physiological data, including respiratory effort, airflow, heart rate, and oximetry, is often used. These recordings are especially helpful for follow-up studies to evaluate the efficacy of treatment for sleep apnea.

For patients complaining of insomnia or circadian rhythm problems, a wrist-worn device that measures sleep–wake activity for consecutive 24-hour periods is preferable (Brooks, Friedman, Bliwise, & Yesavage, 1992; Buck, Tobler, & Borbely, 1989; Hauri & Wisbey, 1992; Sadeh, Sharkey, & Carskadon, 1994). Studies have shown that when they are awake, people tend to move their wrists, and when they are asleep, their wrists tend to be still. Wrist actigraphs transform the wrist movements into signals that are digitized and stored in memory for days, weeks, or months. They are generally small, watchlike devices. The long recording periods allow information to be gained not only about nighttime behavior but also about napping and normal daytime behavior. Although these devices are cost-efficient, they do not add any information about stage of sleep or the underlying mechanisms of the sleep disturbances seen, such as apnea. A second device, the Actillume, records both wrist movement and exposure to light (see Figure 1). This device is especially useful for studying problems in circadian rhythms or seasonal affective disorder (Cole, Kripke, Gruen, Mullaney, & Gillin, 1992).

Ambulatory monitors have been used to study many sleep disorders. Broughton (1989) has used portable recorders to study narcolepsy. He reported that the advantages include gaining information about sleep throughout the 24 hours, including amount of daytime alertness. Underlying circadian rhythm problems can be identified; combined with sleep logs, this information adds to the knowledge about cata-

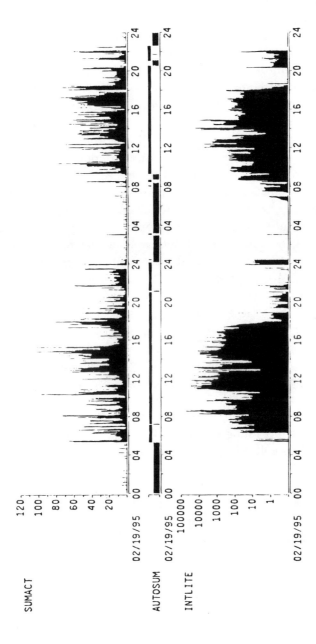

Figure 1.   Actillume recording (Ambulatory Monitoring, Inc., Ardsley, New York) of a 23-year-old woman. SUMACT refers to the average activity recorded per minute. AUTOSUM is the automatic scoring of wakefulness (upper line) and sleep (lower line). Note that it is very clear when this person went to sleep and when she awoke, including a brief awakening in the middle of the night and a brief nap from 2030h to 2100h. INTLITE refers to the lux level of light recorded per minute. Notice that one can see the light slowly increasing as the sun rises in the morning and light filters into the bedroom.

plexy and sleep paralysis. Ambulatory monitoring is also useful in studying the response of sleep to medication. Broughton reported a repeat rate owing to technical problems of less than 5%. Marsh and McCall (1989) suggested that ambulatory recordings can be helpful in studying sleep in patients with psychiatric diseases such as schizophrenia, anxiety, and depression. Radtke, Hoelscher, and Bragdon (1989) concluded that ambulatory monitoring is sufficient for diagnosing periodic limb movements in sleep, although they suggested that more validation studies were needed.

Surprisingly few studies have looked at the reliability of portable recorders when compared with the traditional polysomnogram. Studies that are available have compared either sleep staging or reliability of respiratory and leg movement counts. Emsellem et al. (1990) and Decker, Redline, Arnold, Masny, and Strohl (1991) examined the validity and reliability of detecting sleep apnea with the Edentrace (which records nasal and oral airflow, chest wall movement, heart rate, and oximetry) when compared with the polysomnograph and found high sensitivity (95%) and specificity (96–100%). Ancoli-Israel, Kripke, Mason, and Messin (1981) tested the modified Medilog/Respitrace system (which records thoracic and abdominal respiration, tibialis EMG, and wrist activity) and found a sensitivity of 100% and specificity of 97% for detecting sleep apnea. Correlations were as follows: for apnea index, $r = .94$ ($p < .01$); for total sleep time, $r = .69$ ($p < .01$); and for myoclonus index, $r = .64$ ($p < .005$). Gyulay tested the Vitalog system and found a sensitivity of 100% and specificity of 83% (Gyulay et al., 1987). A fourth system commonly used is the MESAM system, which monitors heart rate, breathing sounds, oximetry, and body position. Stoohs and Guilleminault (1990) found that using information from all available channels prevented any false-positive identification of obstructive sleep apnea.

A more detailed review of other studies can be found in a recently published article by the American Sleep Disorders Association Committee on Standards of Practice. In addition to the review, criteria for using portable recorders in assessing patients with suspected obstructive sleep apnea are presented (Ferber et al., 1994; Standards of Practice Committee of the American Sleep Disorders Association, 1994). This group reported that there have not been enough validation studies done and that different types of equipment available on the market are not comparable. Nevertheless, there are many advantages to using portable systems, including greater accessibility, lower cost, and increased convenience, as discussed earlier. For clinical purposes, portable recorders should have a minimum of four channels of information, including airflow, respiratory effort, heart rate, oximetry, and some measure of wakefulness and sleep. The authors concluded that, given the state of the art, portable equipment should be used in cases of symptoms suggestive of severe obstructive sleep apnea; when instigation of treatment is urgent and standard polysomnography is not available; for patients who are unable to sleep in the laboratory; and for follow-up studies to test the efficacy of treatment.

Conclusion

The current state of technology is such that sleep data can be collected in the laboratory, using computerized equipment, or in the home with unattended monitoring. With each of these recordings of sleep, evaluations of sleep problems can be made and proper treatment initiated. It is up to each individual sleep professional to decide which approach best suits the needs of the patient.

REFERENCES

Ancoli-Israel, S. (1989). Ambulatory cassette recording of sleep apnea. In J. S. Ebersole (Ed.), *Ambulatory EEG monitoring* (pp. 299–315). New York: Raven Press.

Ancoli-Israel, S., Kripke, D. F., Mason, W., & Messin, S. (1981). Comparisons of home sleep recordings and polysomnograms in older adults with sleep disorders. *Sleep, 4*, 283–291.

Brooks, J. O., III, Friedman, L., Bliwise, D.L., & Yesavage, J.A. (1992). Use of the wrist actigraph to study insomnia in older adults. *Sleep, 16*, 151–155.

Broughton, R. J. (1989). Ambulatory sleep-wake monitoring in the hypersomnias. In J. S. Ebersole (Ed.), *Ambulatory EEG monitoring* (pp. 277–298). New York: Raven Press.

Buck, A., Tobler, I., & Borbely, A. A. (1989). Wrist activity monitoring in air crew members: A method for analyzing sleep quality following transmeridian and north-south flights. *Journal of Biological Rhythms, 4*(1), 93–105.

Carskadon, M. A. (1982). Basics for polygraphic monitoring of sleep. In C. Guilleminault (Ed.), *Sleeping and waking disorders: Indications and techniques* (pp. 1–16). Menlo Park CA: Addison-Wesley.

Carskadon, M. A. (Ed.). (1993). *Encyclopedia of sleep and dreaming*. New York:

Macmillan Publishing Co.

Carskadon, M. A., & Dement, W. C. (1987). Daytime sleepiness: Quantification of a behavioral state. *Neuroscience and Biobehavioral Reviews, 11*, 307–317.

Carskadon, M. A., Dement, W. C., Mitler, M. M., Roth, T., Westbrook, P. R., & Keenan, S. (1986). Guidelines for the Multiple Sleep Latency Test (MSLT): A standard measure of sleepiness. *Sleep, 9*, 519–524.

Carskadon, M. A., & Rechtschaffen, A. (1989). Monitoring and staging human sleep. In M. H. Kryger, T. Roth, & W. C. Dement (Eds.), *Principles and practice of sleep medicine* (pp. 665–683). Philadelphia: Saunders.

Cole, R. J., Kripke, D. F., Gruen, W., Mullaney, D. J., & Gillin, J. C. (1992). Automatic sleep/wake identification from wrist activity. *Sleep, 15*, 461–469.

Decker, M. J., Redline, S., Arnold, J. L., Masny, J., & Strohl, K. P. (1991). Normative values of oxygen saturation over time. *Journal of Ambulatory Monitoring, 4*, 297–304.

Dement, W. C., & Kleitman, N. (1957). Cyclic variations in EEG during sleep and their relation to eye movements, body motility, and dreaming. *Electroencephalography and Clinical Neurophysiology, 9*, 673–690.

Emsellem, H. A., Corson, W. A., Rappaport, B. A., Hackett, S., Smith, L. G., & Hausfeld, J. N. (1990). Verification of sleep apnea using a portable sleep apnea screening device. *Southern Medical Journal, 83*, 748–752.

Ferber, R., Millman, R., Coppola, M., Fleetham, J., Murray, C. F., Iber, C., McCall, V., Nino-Murcia, G., Pressman, M., Sanders, M., Strohl, K., Votteri, B., & Williams, A. (1994). Portable recording in the assessment of obstructive sleep apnea. *Sleep, 17*, 378–392.

Gyulay, S., Gould, D., Sawyer, B., Pond, D., Mant, A., & Saunders, N. A. (1987) Evaluation of a microprocessor based portable home monitoring system to measure breathing during sleep. *Sleep, 10*, 130–142.

Hauri, P. J., & Wisbey, J. (1992). Wrist actigraphy in insomnia. *Sleep, 15*, 293–301.

Hirshkowitz, M., & Moore, C.A. (1994). Issues in computerized polysomnography. *Sleep, 17*, 105–112.

Jasper, H. H. (1958). The ten twenty electrode system of the International Federation. *Electroencephalography & Clinical Neurophysiology 10*, 371–375.

Marsh, G. R., & McCall, W. V. (1989). Sleep disturbances in psychiatric disease. In J. S. Ebersole (Ed.), *Ambulatory EEG monitoring* (pp. 331–348). New York: Raven Press.

Miles, L. E., & Broughton, R. J. (1990). *Medical monitoring in the home and work environment*. New York: Raven Press.

Mitler, M. M., Gujavarty, K. S., & Browman, C. P. (1982). Maintenance of Wakefulness Test: A polysomnographic technique for evaluating treatment efficacy in patients with excessive somnolence. *Electroencephalography & Clinical Neurophysiology, 53*, 658–661.

Orr, W. C., Eiken, T., Pegram, V., Jones, R., & Rundall, O. H. (1994). A laboratory validation study of a portable system for remote recording of sleep-related respiratory disorders. *Chest, 105(1)*, 160–162.

Radtke, R. A., Hoelscher, T. J., & Bragdon, A. C. (1989). Ambulatory evaluation of periodic movements of sleep. In J. S. Ebersole (Ed.), *Ambulatory EEG monitoring* (pp. 317–330). New York: Raven Press.

Rechtschaffen, A., & Kales, A. (Eds.) (1973). *A manual of standardized terminology, techniques and scoring system for sleep stages of human subjects.* Los Angeles: Brain Information Service, Brain Research Institute, UCLA.

Sadeh, A., Sharkey, K. M., & Carskadon, M. A. (1994). Activity-based sleep-wake identification: An empirical test of methodological issues. *Sleep, 17,* 201–207.

Standards of Practice Committee of the American Sleep Disorders Association. (1994). Practice parameters for the use of portable recording in the assessment of obstructive sleep apnea. *Sleep, 17,* 372–377.

Stoohs, R., & Guilleminault, C. (1990). Investigations of an automatic screening device (MESAM) for obstructive sleep apnoea. *European Respiratory Journal, 3,* 823–829.

The Significance
and Interpretation
of the Polysomnogram

Richard P. Allen

At the heart of sleep disorders medicine lies the polysomnogram (PSG). This objective test procedure in large part both defines and enables the practice of sleep disorders medicine. The term itself derives from the Greek *poly* for "many" plus the Latin *somni* for "sleep" plus the Greek *gramma* for "anything written or drawn" to describe the *many* pen *drawings* from *sleep* on chart paper made by several channels of different physiological recordings. As the sleep disorders field has developed, PSG has expanded to include recording not only from sleep but also from the transition between wake and sleep as well as alertness in the awake state and the rhythm of wake and sleep. The PSG now draws on paper as well as on digitized computer bytes of memory and on magnetic and optical media such as disks or tapes. The drawings may find their way into cyberspace, traveling from patients' homes to central recording laboratories or between laboratories.

The purpose of PSG, whether recorded on magnetic tapes, worn on a patient's waist, or printed on long stacks of folded paper, is principally to aid in the diagnosis and evaluation of sleep disorders. The information required to support diagnoses, therefore, also defines the PSG. Electroencephalography (EEG), electrooculography (EOG; eye movement recording), and electromyography (EMG; muscle activity recording from the chin or neck) determine the sleep and wake states. Respiratory measures of airflow, respiratory effort, and blood oxygen saturation are used in the diagnosis of sleep-disordered breathing. EMG from the legs assesses movement disorders, and temperature recordings follow the biological circadian rhythm of sleep and waking. These essential ingredients and others constitute the PSG. Without this test, recognition of some of the basic sleep disorders would never have occurred and diagnosis of others would be difficult.

This is not to say that every patient with a suspected sleep disorder needs a PSG. This chapter first discusses indications for ordering the procedure. The clinical sleep disorders specialist must decide what type of a PSG, if any, should be done for each patient. The referring clinician often participates in this decision, but as with most diagnostic tests, the thoughtful and restrained use of the test provides the best patient care. The doctor must determine in advance what diagnostic information is needed and how this information effects treatment. The data collected for each polysomnogram will therefore vary somewhat depending on the diagnostic and therapeutic questions asked. The interpretation is made after the PSG recording has been reduced to a data form that presents the essential physiological information. A PSG involves obtaining the physiological data, reducing the data to a set of numbers and graphs, and interpreting these reduced data. The PSG report generally includes the critical reduced data from the procedure and a written interpretation. Understanding the basis for interpreting the data aids in deciding when to refer patients for a PSG and in implementing treatment on the basis of the results of the a PSG.

This chapter provides a basic introduction to the interpretation of PSG data. PSG data collection and reduction issues, such as EEG sleep stages are not discussed because they are primarily technical issues too complex to be covered here (see chapter 1); instead, it is assumed that these data are available as part of the PSG report. The problem of interpretation involves making sense out of these data in relation to the clinical problems and status of the patient. The interpretation of the PSG follows from the clinical decision to order the PSG and cannot be made without definition of both the clinical problem and the conditions of the PSG study. The chapter contains guidelines concerning the major components of the PSG: indications for ordering the test, test and patient conditions, sleep EEG, circadian rhythms, leg movements, respiration, sleep behaviors, and the Multiple Sleep Latency Test (MSLT) nap test.

Indications for Ordering a PSG

A PSG in 1997 cost between $1,100 and $3,000, which is not particularly expensive when compared with other diagnostic studies. Nonetheless, this cost and the inconvenience to patients need to be justified. Several guidelines have been published concerning when it is appropriate to order a PSG, some by those who have to pay for the study and others by those who receive the payments. Unavoidable and often unconscious bias introduced by these financial issues affect the guidelines. The following is intended to strike a balance between these conflicting approaches. Although they are not exhaustive, these guidelines provide one framework for the clinical decision to obtain a PSG and the subsequent interpretation of results. These items have been listed in Table 1.

Excessive sleepiness often results from a serious sleep disorder indicating a need for a PSG. Before a PSG is done, a sleep log like that shown in chapter 6, Figure 2, should be kept by the patient for 1 week and reviewed to ensure that the patient is spending enough time in bed trying to sleep. Short sleep periods of less than 7 hours a night are likely to produce excessive sleepiness. When this pattern is observed, a therapeutic trial with longer sleep periods should occur, and a PSG should be ordered only if the excessive sleepiness persists despite sleep periods of at least 8 hours per night or longer. Excessive sleepiness should be distinguished from fatigue or feeling tired, run down, and sluggish. A sleepy patient generally reports feeling a need, even a desire or craving, to sleep and usually reports falling asleep easily even if sleep is only momentary. These patients usually also benefit from the MSLT, which can be performed the day after the nocturnal PSG to assess objectively the degree of daytime sleepiness.

Sleep apnea or other respiratory disturbances often accompany excessive sleepiness. When the patient reports loud snoring or other signs of respiratory disturbance during sleep, a PSG is worth considering. This is particularly the case if the patient also has excessive sleepiness. If there is no indication for excessive sleepiness or if the sleep apnea is suspected to be severe, an MSLT is not needed; otherwise, an MSLT is always advised.

Narcolepsy has several features in addition to excessive sleepiness that, if present, strongly indicate a need for PSG and MSLT evaluation. The most significant features are (a) sudden loss of muscle control during wake time, usually brought on by an emotional event; (b) reported brief restoration of wakefulness after a very short (5–15 minutes) nap;

Table 1

Indications for Obtaining a Polysomnogram With and Without a Multiple Sleep Latency Test

Clinical signs	Action
Excessive daytime sleepiness	Obtain sleep log, check medication use.
	Check for other narcoleptic symptoms.
If cataplexy reported	Order PSG with MSLT.
If short normal sleep (<7 hr per night)	Extend sleep to 8+ hours per night.
	Remove or reduce sedating medications if any.
If excessive sleepiness persists	Order PSG with MSLT.
Loud snoring or observed sleep apneas	Check for excessive sleepiness as above.
	Check weight, blood pressure.
If significantly overweight and adult	Order PSG.
If elevated blood pressure	Order PSG (also order MSLT unless mild severity).
Abnormal movements in legs	Check for day symptoms of restless legs
If restless legs signs	Order PSG to confirm diagnosis and extent of PLM.
If no restless legs signs	Check for pattern—better sleep in a.m.
If pattern is unclear or correct	Order PSG for diagnosis of significant PLM.
If pattern is wrong	Treat as insomnia (or obtain ambulatory activity monitor).
Abnormal behaviors during sleep	Check for excessive sleepiness as above.
	Check for risk of injury.
	Check for indications of seizure disorder.
If seizure indication	Neurology consult—EEG evaluations.
If not seizure and injury is a concern	Review for arousal disorder.
If arousal disorder	Trial on benzodiazepine.

Clinical signs	Action
If not successful on benzodiazepine and injury still a concern	Order PSG.
Intractable insomnia	Check for adequate insomnia treatment trial and check for possible depressive disorder.
If no depressive disorder and adequate prior treatment failed	Order PSG. Add temperature probe if any indication of circadian rhythm disturbance.

Note. PSG = polysomnography; MSLT = Multiple Sleep Latency Test; PLM = periodic limb movements.

and (c) active vivid dreaming occurring shortly after sleep onset. If any of these are present or if profound dreamlike images occur either at sleep onset (hypnagogic) or on awakening (hypnopompic), sometimes with transitory paralysis, then the PSG and MSLT should be ordered, even if the sleep log shows mildly reduced sleep times. EWS with normal sleep times in the sleep log should be further evaluated with a PSG.

Excessive movements in sleep indicate a possible neurological movement disorder, either periodic leg movements (PLM) in sleep or the restless legs syndrome. Diagnosis of either of these can be difficult except for extreme cases. A PSG is specifically required to confirm the diagnosis of PLM suspected from a bed partner's report or the patient's description of the disruption of bed sheets that occurs during sleep. It is important to note that this disorder is related to restless behavior during sleep and not during waking, even when waking occurs during the night. For patients with clear afternoon or evening symptoms of restless legs, a nocturnal PSG is important to determine the need to treat the associated PLM during sleep.

Abnormal, injurious behavior during sleep can stem from seizure disorders, arousal disorders from nonrapid eye movement (NREM) sleep, rapid eye movement (REM) behavior disorders, or various psychiatric disorders. Sometimes the history suffices for the diagnosis, but when there is uncertainty and the behavior poses a safety or health risk, a

PSG should be done. The PSG may need to include extra EEG leads or a planned partial awakening during deeper NREM sleep (to trigger an event), depending on the question being asked.

Intractable insomnia and ambiguous circadian rhythm problems are conditions for which PSG is likely to be beneficial to determine both presence and severity of the disorder. It is particularly useful when improvements in sleep hygiene and other behavioral treatments have failed to resolve the problem. In some cases, the underlying circadian rhythm cannot be clearly discerned from the sleep log. The PSG may help in these instances, and may require a continuous rectal temperature recording and extended sleep period in the morning.

Interpreting the Data in the PSG Report

Much of the interpretation of the PSG results depends on the clinical question being asked and the indication for doing the study. The following overview discusses the general nature of the information gained; it is not exhaustive or definitive. Nonetheless, it suffices for most common clinical situations in which PSG is deemed appropriate.

Although the PSG interpretation usually follows directly from the data provided on the PSG report, additional information is sometimes provided by a board-certified sleep disorders specialist. It is important to emphasize that this final, written interpretation of the PSG should always be made by a sleep disorders specialist certified by the American Board of Sleep Disorders Medicine who has reviewed the raw data from the PSG. This ensures the quality control that is needed for any complex and expensive diagnostic test.

In many cases, the information from the PSG is inadequate to make a diagnosis without added clinical information. In these situations, the interpretation includes lists of options and may specifically reference the need for clinical correlation with the interpretation. The major items to be considered when interpreting the PSG are discussed in the following sections.

Test Conditions

The environment of the testing should be conducive to sleep. A quiet, private, cool (e.g., 68°F) room with a reasonably comfortable and large bed (at least the standard twin size) is preferred. If the recording equipment makes any noise or disturbing flashes of lights, it should not be in the same room as the patient. These conditions are not always described in the PSG report, but if the study is from a fully accredited sleep disorders center, they can be assumed. If the place where the PSG is done is not an accredited sleep disorders center, some comment about the facilities should be requested to accompany the PSG report.

The time of this sleep test should match the preferred bedtime of the patient being evaluated. Reference to sleep logs completed by the patient before the study suffices to determine this time. Particular attention should be paid to the bedtime, because it may vary, particularly if technical difficulties occur in setting up the patients that night. Similarly, the final wake time and the total time in bed both should be carefully noted. These should correspond with values from the sleep log, and total time in bed should be at least 7, and preferably 8, hours. Shorter times produce more sleepiness the next day, reducing the accuracy of the MSLT. The general physical status of the patient is noted if it is significantly abnormal. The medications the patient is taking are listed, with appropriate comments in the interpretation regarding any that affect sleep or alertness. The medication list also includes comments about any medications that have been discontinued within the past week, particularly any discontinued within the day or two before the study. Similarly, any special treatment the patient is receiving is noted either with the PSG data or in the interpretative report.

Subjective Reports

The patient's subjective impression of the sleep during the PSG is recorded and included in the PSG report. This generally includes at least the patient's overall impression of how long he took to fall asleep, how long he slept, and how well he slept. Sometimes the patient is asked to comment on how the sleep during the PSG compared with his normal sleep. These subjective impressions become particularly important when they differ from the objective sleep data or when sleep during the night of the PSG is reported to differ significantly from the patient's usual sleep.

Physiological EEG Sleep

The amount of time in the basic sleep stages should be specified in the report as minutes and as percentages of total sleep time. The minutes required to fall asleep after "lights out" (referred to as *sleep latency*) and the percentage of time in bed during which physiological sleep occurred (referred to as *sleep efficiency*) should also be recorded on the PSG report.

A reasonable rule of thumb is that sleep latency should not be more than 30 minutes. The total sleep time should exceed 6 hours, with values less than this considered clearly abnormal; however, values of 7–8 hours are preferred if an MSLT for sleepiness is planned the next day. The sleep efficiency is one of the more important variables and should exceed age-adjusted normal limits. This measure is only significant when it is too low, because the normal range includes the maximum of 100%.

Among the sleep stages, the most relevant clinical information is provided by amounts of deep sleep (the combination of Stage 3 and Stage 4 sleep, usually referred to as *slow wave sleep*) and of very light sleep (referred to as Stage 1 sleep). Too little slow wave sleep suggests poor sleep quality, whereas too much suggests possible chronic insufficient sleep the week before the study or a propensity for deep sleep, particularly characteristic of patients with arousal disorders from sleep such as sleepwalking or night terrors. The amount of Stages 3 and 4 has to be carefully interpreted, given the strong age effects on these stages. When the percentage of Stage 1 sleep exceeds a generous normative range, it also suggests poor quality sleep. Table 2 presents suggested age-corrected normal limits for Stages 3–4, and sleep efficiency, but these norms may be adjusted on the basis of local laboratory standards and experience.

Table 2

Suggested Age-Adjusted Normal Range for Measurements of Sleep

Age	Minimum of normal range	
	Slow wave sleep (min)	Sleep efficiency (%)
10–20	83	92
20–30	58	92
30–40	30	92
40–50	12	87
50–60	0	74
60+	0	58

These five sleep parameters (total sleep time, sleep latency, sleep efficiency, slow wave sleep, and Stage 1 sleep) carry most of the clinically relevant sleep stage information. Other measures are useful in special circumstances. The cycles of sleep stages should also be noted. Ideally, a sleep histogram or similar chart is printed with the report, giving the flow of sleep stages across the night (see Figure 1). For the normal adult, slow wave sleep occurs more frequently in the first part of the night, and Stage 1 occurs more frequently in the last part. There should be 3–5 cycles of sleep, each ended by an REM sleep period and each about 90 minutes long. For young children, the first cycle ending with the first REM period is likely to be very long, and for the elderly, the first cycle up to the first REM period is likely to be somewhat shorter. REM sleep itself should occur more in the last part of sleep than at the beginning of sleep, and this tendency is more marked for younger patients. Wake time after sleep onset should be spread fairly evenly over the night, occurring somewhat more in the latter part of sleep. Very long awakenings (greater than 15 min) should be noted in relation to when they occur in the sleep pattern. Any premature awakening (a long awakening in the early morning without a return to sleep) deserves special attention. Awakenings predominately in the later part of sleep and a premature awakening indicate a need for clinical inquiry regarding depression or sleep phase advance.

Several qualitative features of physiological sleep are noted by the sleep specialist interpreting the PSG, and any unusual features generally are included in the official interpretation of the report. These features are too many and varied and often too infrequent to justify inclusion in a checkoff list in the official PSG report. Most of these are somewhat technical in nature and at times are important. For example, reduced or disrupted atonia (absence of muscle tone) during REM sleep occurs with the REM behavior disorder (Schenck, Bundlie, Ettinger, & Mahowald, 1986), and excessive EEG spindles occur with recent benzodiazepine use (Gaillard, 1994). The qualitative nature of these features and their importance indicate the need to ensure that the final PSG interpretation has been made by an experienced board-certified sleep disorders specialist.

Circadian Rhythms

Circadian rhythm disorders produce characteristic marked skewing of wake times during the PSG period to either the first or last part of sleep, provided the bedtimes are at the customary 10:30–11:30 p.m. (Roehrs & Roth, 1994). *Sleep phase delay* produces somewhat long sleep onset and

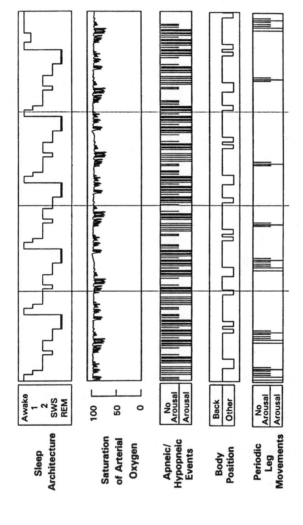

Figure 1.   Histogram showing data from a polysomnogram. SWS = slow wave sleep; REM = rapid eye movements.

increased wake time in the first half of the sleep period, with better sleep (less waking) in the second half of sleep. Slow wave sleep may even be delayed, with most occurring after the first REM period. Conversely, *sleep phase advance* produces shorter sleep-onset times, with poor sleep (excessive waking) in the last part of the sleep period. Depressive disorders tend to show the sleep advance pattern.

If a continuous core temperature recording is obtained, preferably rectal temperature, the timing of the nadir of the temperature curve and the amount of variation should be noted. The normal low point should occur between 2:00 and 5:00 a.m. Any significant variation from this norm suggests either an advanced or a delayed sleep cycle disturbance. These values need to be carefully interpreted, however, because they are affected by the amount and timing of wakefulness during the sleep period and by the amount of physical activity in sleep, which increases with respiratory, movement, and anxiety disorders. Wake time, in particular, leads to increases in temperature, masking the circadian rhythm and often obscuring the real nadir of the temperature curve.

The sleep log taken the week before PSG is obtained should provide another major source of information regarding circadian patterns of sleep. Comparing the sleep log with the PSG pattern is essential for consideration of circadian rhythm disturbances of sleep.

Movements in Sleep

Leg movements in sleep are routinely recorded during PSG using EMG of the anterior tibialis of one or both legs. Slow repeated movements (4 or more movements, each lasting 0.5–5 sec and separated by 4–90 sec without movement) noted on the report as "periodic," should occur no more than 5 times per hour during NREM sleep (Coleman, 1982). It is essential that this density be noted for NREM and not for REM sleep, because the atonia and muscle twitching of REM sleep represent a distinctly different phenomenon. Periodic movements of 5–15 per hour are considered to be minimally disturbing to sleep and probably not clinically significant, but at greater than 15 per hour, they should be noted as a potentially significant disturbance of sleep. These movements are reported along with the percentage that cause arousal from sleep; when arousal from sleep occurs more than once every 6 minutes (10 per hr), significant sleep disruption is likely. It is important to emphasize that it is the arousal rate from sleep that matters the most for determining the clinical severity of the movement disorder. Moreover, some patients appear to be disturbed by these frequent brief arousals, whereas others appear to have no adverse effects from them (Bixler et al., 1982; Coleman et al., 1983). The periodic movements associated with the primary disorders of periodic leg movements in sleep and the restless legs syndrome occur much more frequently in the first part of sleep and abate, sometimes dramatically, in the early-morning sleep. Leg movements, even when periodic, should not be considered clinically significant unless they follow this pattern or markedly disturb sleep with associated arousal rates of greater than 10 per hour.

Respiratory abnormalities are also periodic and can produce leg movements with arousals. The leg movements associated with sleep-disordered breathing should be removed from the count of periodic leg movements.

Respiration in Sleep

The primary respiratory analyses involve counting the number of episodes of apnea (cessation of breathing) or hypopnea (significantly decreased breathing) lasting, for adults, at least 10 seconds and usually resulting in transitory decreases in oxygen saturation. The combined rate (number per hour of sleep) of episodes of apnea and hypopnea is sometimes loosely referred to as the *sleep apnea rate* but more correctly represents the rate of sleep-disordered breathing events. The normal range has been estimated at 5 per hour or less (Guilleminault, 1994; Guilleminault & Dement, 1978). Rates of 15 or fewer per hour can be considered a mild disturbance and not a clinically significant abnormality. Rates between 15 and 30 per hour indicate moderate sleep apnea, and rates above 30 per hour indicate severe sleep apnea. The decrease in oxygen saturation is often presented as both the average of the low points for all of the events and the lowest value observed. Average oxygen saturation decreases above 90% indicate only mild decreases, whereas decreases of 85–90% can be considered moderate, and those below 80%, severe. This severity rating reflects the rapid changes in PO_2 with oxygen saturation decreases of below 90%.

Decreases in oxygen saturation are sometimes presented as the number of events with decreases below a fixed criterion such as 90 or 80% or, alternatively, the amount of time with decreases below a criterion value. These provide a statistically less satisfactory measure than the average decrease, but they can be easier to calculate, particularly if the PSG record is being scored by hand. Thus, the rate (number per hour) and the average low oxygen saturation are used to determine clinical judgment about the severity of sleep-disordered breathing. These values are classified as REM versus NREM sleep and in terms of events occurring while the patient is sleeping on the back versus the side or stomach. They are also classified by type of apnea into central (lack of effort to breathe), obstructive (breathing efforts blocked by closed or partially closed airway, usually associated with snorting), and a mixture of central and obstructive apnea. The overall severity can be determined by either the rate for all of sleep or the rate for NREM sleep only. The rates are usually higher in REM than in NREM sleep; a pattern of REM rates dramatically lower than NREM rates indicates an atypical sleep apnea condition, such as apnea occurring mostly during transition between waking and sleep. Because REM sleep is usually less than 20% of the total sleep time, sleep apnea that occurs mostly or only in REM is generally considered to be of limited clinical significance unless it is extreme. The patient produces the highest sleep apnea rates when lying on the back. If the rate when on the back is significantly greater than for the other positions, separate clinical severity rating for body position should be noted; otherwise, clinical severity can be set by the rate for all of NREM sleep.

Other sleep-related respiratory problems that occur are noted in the PSG interpretation. In particular, reduced baseline oxygen saturation (less than 90%) may occur during sleep and should be noted in the report. The baseline oxygen saturation values are generally provided with the PSG data in the report. Cheyne–Stokes respiration, delays in circulation times, and problems with upper airway resistance (Guilleminault & Stoohs, 1991) may also be detected from the PSG; the information should be provided in the interpretation of the report.

Behaviors in Sleep

For patients with reported abnormal behaviors during sleep, part of the PSG evaluation includes visual observation of the patient's behavior, using a low-illumination video camera in the patient's bedroom and, if possible, a video recording of the movements. The occurrence of unusual behaviors is generally noted by time of night and sleep stage at the start of the behavior. The two most important clinical distinctions involve discriminating between NREM arousal disorder (Broughton, 1968) and REM behavior disorder (Schenck et al., 1986) and between seizures and nonepileptic behaviors (Kavey, Whyte, Resor, & Gidro-Frank, 1990). The first of these distinctions is clear from the sleep stage during which the event occurs. Excluding seizures in sleep can be more complicated and may require more elaborate EEG recordings during sleep than are usually provided on the PSG. The need for this type of recording is determined by the overall clinical history (Shouse, 1994).

The Multiple Sleep Latency Test

This test is commonly done in association with the nocturnal PSG to assess both daytime sleepiness and abnormalities of rapid onset of REM sleep during a nap. The test consists of four or five nap opportunities spaced 2 hours apart, each lasting at least 20 minutes; if sleep occurs, the nap time may be extended to ensure it includes the next 15–20 minutes, provided sleep continues during that time. (Carskadon, Dement, & Mitler, 1986). Overall sleepiness is assessed by the median (or average) of the sleep latencies from each of the tests. Pathological sleepiness occurs with a median sleep latency of 5 minutes or less, whereas a median of 5–8 minutes is often considered to indicate moderate sleepiness, 8–10 minutes to represent mild sleepiness, and above 10 to be normal (Richardson et al., 1978).

Sleep-onset REM (REM sleep occurring within the first 15 min of sleep) occurs fairly commonly for patients with narcolepsy (Mitler, van den Hoed, & Carskadon, 1979), severe sleep apnea, and marked disturbances of the normal circadian rhythm. When circadian rhythms and sleep-related respiration are normal and there are no medication effects related to REM sleep, the occurrence of two or more REM onset naps on an MSLT, combined with a median sleep latency of 5 minutes or less, is a reasonably specific diagnostic indicator for narcolepsy. Any other diagnosis requires further explanation in the interpretation.

Using the PSG Interpretation

The interpretation of the PSG as provided by the sleep disorders specialist can be largely confirmed by checking with the PSG data, as noted previously. This report provides the essential basis for diagnosis and treatment recommendations. The final treatment considerations require integrating this interpretation with the clinical information to treat the patient, not the test result. Interpretation of polysomnographic data is a complicated process requiring extensive knowledge of sleep, sleep disorders, and laboratory recording techniques and practices.

Conclusion

The clinical evaluation of the sleep disorder patient starts with the initial diagnostic interview when basic diagnostic questions should be formed. The polysomnogram and the multiple sleep latency tests provide important information to support diagnosis and guide treatment, but the type of polysomnogram and the interpretation of the results depends upon the conceptual framework developed from the initial clinical evaluation. Following the guidelines in this chapter should lead to a reasonable use and interpretation of the polysomnogram. It is important, however, to emphasize avoiding three errors commonly made when interpreting the polysomnogram: First common error, the polysomnogram is ordered because it is unclear what else to do. As noted the polysomnogram must follow from the clinical questions and like other diagnostic tests should not be used without clinical indications for the test. It can not substitute for the clinical diagnostic evaluation. Second common error, looking at the polysomnogram data during only the sleep times. All of the night's recording should be analyzed including the periods of wakefulness; where possible the recording should be kept running continuously during the sleep time. The analysis should also incorporate information about the patient's sleep patterns for the past week before the study and should include some comparison of the pattern in the lab with that at home. Final common error, values from normal subjects for sleep characteristics are often used for comparison with the patient data without making allowances for the general health of the patient and the often less than ideal circumstances under which the test occurs. Following the guidelines in this chapter should help avoid these three common errors. When correctly used the polysomnogram will provide you the best information possible to help solve your patient's sleep problems.

REFERENCES

Bixler, E., Kales, A., Soldalos, C. R., & Vela-Bueno, A. (1982). Nocturnal myoclonus and nocturnal myoclonic activity in a normal population. *Research Communications in Chemistry, Pathology and Pharmacology, 36,* 129–140.

Broughton, R. (1968). Sleep disorders: Disorders of arousal. *Science, 159,* 1070–1078.

Carskadon, M., Dement, W., & Mitler, M. (1986). Guidelines for the Multiple Sleep Latency Test (MSLT): A standard measure of sleepiness. *Sleep, 9,* 519–524.

Coleman, R. (1982). Periodic movements in sleep (nocturnal myoclonus) and restless legs syndrome. In C. Guilleminault (Ed.), *Sleeping and waking disorders: Indications and techniques* (pp. 265–296). Menlo Park, CA: Addison-Wesley.

Coleman, R., Bliwise, D., Sajben, N., deBruyn, L., Boomkamp, A., Menn, M., & Dement, W. (1983). Epidemiology of periodic movements during sleep. In C. Guilleminault & E. Lugaresi (Eds.), *Sleep/wake disorders: Natural history, epidemiology, and long-term evolution* (pp. 217–229). New York: Raven Press.

Gaillard, J. (1994). Benzodiazepines and GABA-ergic transmission. In M. Kryger, T. Roth, & W. C. Dement (Eds.), *Principles and practice of sleep disorders medicine* (2nd ed., pp. 349–354). Philadelphia: Saunders.

Guilleminault, C. (1994). Clinical features and evaluation of obstructive sleep apnea. In M. Kryger, T. Roth, & W. C. Dement (Eds.), *Principles and practice of sleep disorders medicine* (2nd ed.). Philadelphia: Saunders.

Guilleminault, C., & Dement, W. (1978). Sleep apnea syndromes and related sleep disorders. In R. Williams & I. Karacan (Eds.), *Sleep disorders: Diagnosis and treatment*. New York: Wiley.

Guilleminault, C., & Stoohs, R. (1991). The upper airway resistance syndrome. *Sleep Research, 20,* 250.

Kavey, N., Whyte, J., Resor, S., & Gidro-Frank, S. (1990). Somnambulism in adults. *Neurology, 40,* 749–750.

Mitler, M., van den Hoed, J., & Carskadon, M. (1979). REM sleep episodes during the Multiple Sleep Latency Test in narcoleptic patients. *Electroencephalography and Clinical Neurophysiology, 46,* 479–481.

Richardson, G., Carskadon, M., Flagg, W., van den Hoed, J., Dement, W., & Mitler, M. (1978). Excessive daytime sleepiness in man: Multiple sleep latency measurement in narcoleptic and control subjects. *Electroencephalography and Clinical Neurophysiology, 45,* 621–627.

Roehrs, T., & Roth, R. (1994). Chronic insomnias associated with circadian rhythm disorders. In M. Kryger, T. Roth, & W. C. Dement (Eds.), *Principles and practice of sleep medicine* (2nd ed., pp. 477–482). Philadelphia: Saunders.

Schenck, C., Bundlie, S., Ettinger, M., & Mahowald, M. (1986). Chronic behavior disorders of human REM sleep: A new category of parasomnia. *Sleep, 9,* 293–308.

Shouse, M. (1994). Epileptic seizure manifestations during sleep. In M. Kryger, T. Roth, & W. Dement (Eds.), *Principles and practice of sleep medicine* (2nd ed., pp. 801–814). Philadelphia: Saunders.

The Measurement
of Daytime Sleepiness

Sidney D. Nau

Because the desire to sleep is an everyday occurrence, the possible negative consequences of excessive sleepiness are easy to picture. Everyone has experienced how compelling strong sleepiness feels. It can have the potency of a powerful drug and can undermine vigilance, perception, thinking, judgment, and emotional control. Excessive sleepiness is suspected to have been a factor in the Chernobyl nuclear catastrophe (Dinges, Graeber, Carskadon, Czeisler, & Dement, 1989; Mitler et al., 1988). The accurate measurement of excessive daytime sleepiness serves the attainment of valid diagnosis and treatment planning. A fundamental goal is to prevent the unfortunate outcomes that can occur because of undocumented and untreated disorders of excessive sleepiness.

The present chapter is about the goal of accurate sleepiness measurement. The clinical benefits of formal sleepiness testing are explained. The inconsistent relationship between the subjective and physiological aspects of sleepiness is highlighted because of its importance to clinical decision making. There is significant risk for inaccurate clinical judgments when depending solely on patient self-descriptions of sleepiness. Current clinical and research measures of daytime sleepiness and standard procedures for directly recording the physiological tendency to fall asleep are reviewed in detail. The future is touched on in a closing discussion about the assessment of treatment outcome. Some of the information presented suggests the future is rich with potential research opportunities for creating and refining approaches with sleepiness measurement.

The Nature of Sleepiness

The need for sleep is considered a basic drive by many researchers (Dement & Carskadon, 1982), and sleepiness is the reflection of unmet need. Sleepiness, therefore, is a hypothetical underlying physiological need state, somewhat similar to thirst or hunger. Sleepiness is a universal daily experience. Each individual requires a personal minimum amount of relatively sound sleep each day to maintain alertness during the waking portion of the circadian sleep–wake cycle.

Subjectively, sleepiness is the desire for sleep; it involves associated features such as tendency to stay at rest, difficulty keeping eyes open, slowness, and difficulty concentrating. The experience of sleepiness includes the feelings, physiological shifts away from arousal, changes in mental status, and specific behaviors that increase as the time since last sleep increases. Behaviorally and physiologically, sleepiness is often defined as the *tendency to fall asleep, physiological sleep tendency*, or simply, *sleep tendency* (Carskadon & Dement, 1977).

When sleepiness as a subjective experience is strong, it is correlated with sleepy appearance and behavior and the tendency to fall asleep. The strength of correlation is less with mild and moderate sleepiness. The variability in correlation limits the value of subjective clinical data in the evaluation of sleepiness. When subjective sleepiness is moderate, mild, or within normal limits, it has inconsistent accuracy as a predictor of behavior or physiological sleep tendency. For example, many individuals with moderate sleepiness, who fall asleep unintentionally on a daily basis during sedentary activities, do not complain about difficulty staying awake. They maintain a self-perception of normalcy, even though physiological testing may show a significantly increased sleep tendency. When a person has strong sleepiness, she or he will feel drowsy, appear listless, and tend to fall asleep whenever inactive.

The Importance of Formal Sleepiness Assessment

The functional significance of excessive sleepiness is strong. It is more dangerous than other sleep disorder symptoms. It characterizes the most common severe sleep disorders or severely disturbed sleep: the conditions that are most significant in terms of compromising ability to function. The best examples are obstructive sleep apnea and narcolepsy. The histories of patients of sleep disorders centers indicate the seriousness of excessive sleepiness in their lives. Nearly one-half of patients with excessive sleepiness report automobile accidents, over half report accidents at work, and many have lost jobs because of their sleepiness (Broughton et al., 1981; Guilleminault & Carskadon, 1977). Because of the importance of wakefulness for adaptation and survival, treatment is consistently recommended for persistent excessive sleepiness.

Clinical judgments of sleepiness deal with key issues of need for treatment, symptom severity, benefits of therapy, and whether resolution of excessive sleepiness has been achieved. The measurement of sleepiness helps to shape decisions about whether the severity of a sleepiness symptom justifies treatment. Recommendations about aggressiveness of therapy may also be influenced when clinicians face questions such as the following: Does a patient need a prescription for lifelong stimulant therapy for narcolepsy, require surgery for obstructive apnea, or need nasal continuous positive airway pressure (CPAP) for obstructive apnea? Sleepiness measurement is sometimes needed to decide whether a patient is ready to return to work following treatment.

Subjective ratings can help with the clinical assessment of sleepiness, but accuracy is variable. Sleep specialists often note that patients resist acknowledging a history of excessive sleepiness. Clinicians have reported that patients may rate themselves as alert (e.g., on the Stanford Sleepiness Scale; Hoddes, Zarcone, Smythe, Phillips, & Dement, 1973) even while observed falling asleep. Also, Stanford scale ratings have not shown a consistent relationship with physiological measures of sleepiness (Johnson, Freeman, Spinweber, & Gomez, 1991). Assessment through interview alone must be done cautiously. Objective testing is advisable because patients frequently underestimate and sometimes overestimate sleepiness. A comprehensive assessment of sleepiness with subjective and standardized physiological measures is generally recommended for important clinical decisions.

Types of Sleepiness Assessment

There are four categories of sleepiness assessment, including (a) history taking, which typically involves a sleep history with associated observations of appearance and behavior as well as a mental status examination and medical history to aid in differential diagnosis; (b) subjective–introspective assessment with logs, rating scales, and questionnaires; (c) performance measurement to observe for decrements related to decreased alertness; and (d) physiological measurements (some directly assess sleep tendency, whereas others examine a variety of physiological changes known to fluctuate with general level of sleepiness).

History Taking

Behavior observation. Observations of sleepy behavior are most commonly obtained indirectly through a thorough sleep history. The information is generally in the form of the patient's self-observations concerning past events or reports from family or friends. Display of sleepy behaviors during history taking is the exception because the behavioral signs and indicators of sleepiness tend to have a relatively high threshold. An individual can be very sleepy before appearing sleepy. Severely somnolent patients occasionally are found in the waiting room nodding or sound asleep. Facial appearance with unresponsiveness, particularly in the eyes, may project sleepiness during history taking, with or without eye closures, nodding, and lapses. Sleepy patients rarely volunteer how sleepy they feel even when their behavior makes it obvious. Yawning and behaviors intended to fend off sleepiness may also be present (e.g., lip biting, fidgeting, nonstop talking). Severely sleepy patients do not bring caffeinated beverages to sleep history interviews. Perhaps they are too proud or defensive to acknowledge their problem by acting it out that way.

Sleep history interview. The International Classification of Sleep Disorders (ICSD; Diagnostic Classification Steering Committee, 1990) provides guidelines for interpretation of patient history and behavior to estimate severity of daytime sleepiness. These guidelines focus on the frequency of unintentional sleep. Patients should be asked about a variety of common situations that can unmask sleepiness (e.g., sitting at work or in church, reading, watching TV, riding in a car, watching a movie, driving, talking on long telephone calls). Asking individuals if they ever have periods of "having to fight sleepiness" during the daytime can be a good entry question, but it is less threatening to ask about sleepiness in specific situations. It is important to obtain information about morning, afternoon, and evening activities. The goal is to include a variety of routine questions presented in a matter-of-fact manner that will reliably reveal evidence of physiological sleepiness, because many sleepy patients flatly deny or try to explain away excessive sleepiness and avoid talking about it. Some tell the practitioner that they have trouble staying awake only when they are relatively inactive. They may deny the significance of their sleepiness because it is only irresistible when they are sitting. It is desirable for patients to bring someone who lives with them to the sleep history interview to report their observations, ideally a spouse, parent, or similar observer.

Introspective Measures

Sleep logs. Daily sleep logs and sleep diaries (Hauri, 1990) typically include information about daytime sleepiness–alertness (such as logging of naps or self-ratings of fatigue) in addition to valuable data about sleep schedule and estimated amount of sleep. They can also contain information about sleep hygiene and other contributing factors. This brief, practical measure can be started at the time of the first patient contact to aid in the initial evaluation and can be continued for monitoring and evaluating response to treatment.

Visual Analogue Scale. Some patients and research participants are asked to monitor their own sleep tendency with multiple subjective ratings of general level of sleepiness. Each rating is for sleepiness at a specific time. The Visual Analogue Scale is a simple 100-mm line with the end points *very alert* and *very sleepy*. The patient marks present level of alertness or sleepiness, and the response is scored in millimeters going from one end to the point marked.

Stanford Sleepiness Scale. The Stanford Sleepiness Scale (Hoddes et al., 1973) is a seven-option rating scale in which each point is defined with adjectives that provide an introspective assessment of sleepiness. Although ratings from the scale have been shown to correlate significantly with measurements of how rapidly the individual falls asleep while being monitored in the laboratory (Dement, 1976), some patients and research participants have rated themselves not sleepy on the Stanford scale while being observed to be falling asleep (Dement, Carskadon, & Richardson, 1978). The correlation between scores on the scale and physiological measures of daytime sleepiness, therefore, have not consistently been significant.

Epworth Sleepiness Scale. The Epworth Sleepiness Scale (ESS; Johns, 1993) is a newer self-rating scale that incorporates some of the features of sleep interviews. The participant or patient is asked to rate the chance of falling asleep in eight situations commonly encountered in daily life. The initial validity study (Johns, 1991) showed a significant correlation between Epworth scores and sleep latency during daytime sleepiness testing and nocturnal polysomnography. There were also significant differences between scores of nonpatients and of patients with sleepiness disorders, and in a later study, between scores of patients who had obstructive sleep apnea syndrome and those who had simple snoring (Johns, 1993).

Comments on the use of introspective measures. Rating scales and logs measure subjective sleepiness to obtain predictors of overt sleepiness that have face validity. Factors that can decrease the likelihood of subjective sleepiness in spite of high physiological need for sleep include high motivation; competing needs (e.g., thirst, hunger); excitement (surprise, anxiety, anger, and other emotions); physical exertion; environmental stimulation; and individual differences. For example, a severely sleepy individual who is a conscientious assembly line employee in trouble because of falling asleep at work may feel alert owing to fear of job loss and threat to self-esteem, as well as close observation by a supervisor, but still may doze off while working. Also, introspective measures can be rather easily faked in a positive or negative direction. They are widely used in research protocols but are mainly for description. They do not stand alone for establishing diagnosis in clinical settings.

Performance Measures

Laboratory performance tasks or task simulations provide indirect measures of sleepiness. Because sleepy individuals can sustain adequate performance in short bursts, performance testing must be lengthy (60 min or longer) to provide a sample of negative consequences that are due to sleepiness.

Wilkinson Vigilance Test. The Wilkinson Vigilance Test assesses vigilance with a signal detection task (Wilkinson, 1968). The dependent variable is the proportion of correct responses to a series of repetitive stimuli. The detection rate improves with increased wakefulness (Valley & Broughton, 1983).

Simulation. Task simulations (such as simulated driving or flying) have become increasingly used in response to improvements in technology and enhanced concern about safety and sleepiness in public transportation (French, Bisson, Neville, Mitcha, & Storm, 1994; Stampi & Heitmann, 1993). Simulations of manufacturing tasks have also been used to evaluate the consequences of sleepiness (Schweitzer, Muehlbach, & Walsh, 1992). Any lengthy repetitive task is a potential subject for simulation.

Actual performance. The performance and physiology of transportation workers can be recorded electronically during work. For example, transoceanic airline pilots have been monitored for sleep, alertness, and performance while on duty (Dinges, Graeber, Connell, Rosekind, & Powell, 1990). This methodology can be used to evaluate therapeutic interventions such as prophylactic naps for airline crew members.

Physiological Measures of Sleepiness

Multiple Sleep Latency Test. The Multiple Sleep Latency Test (MSLT; Carskadon & Dement, 1977) is a series of nap opportunities during which the patient is monitored for speed of falling asleep. Physiological sleepiness is defined as propensity to fall asleep (Dement & Carskadon, 1982). The MSLT is the simplest standardized direct measure of overt sleep tendency.

This widely used test was validated in a series of carefully selected populations anticipated to show variations from normal in sleepiness (Carskadon & Dement, 1982; Dement, Carskadon, & Richardson, 1978; Reynolds, Coble, Kupfer, & Holzer, 1982; van den Hoed et al., 1981; Zorick et al., 1982). It is considered the only electrophysiological test scientifically validated as able to detect varying degrees of daytime sleepiness (Thorpy, 1992). Test–retest reliability has been documented (Scrima, Hartman, Johnson, Thomas, & Hiller, 1990; Zwyghuizen-Doorenbos, Roehrs, Schaefer, & Roth, 1988).

The MSLT involves a series of four or five 20-minute rest periods in a quiet, dark room. The patient lies in bed wearing loose-fitting street clothes. The subtests are begun at 2-hour intervals starting 1.5–3.0 hours after the patient ends the nocturnal polysomnographic procedure that is performed before daytime testing. At the time of "lights out" that begins each nap test, the patient is given standard instructions to lie quietly with eyes closed and try to sleep (or is told to allow sleep to occur). The same instructions are repeated at the start of each subtest.

The results of each MSLT subtest are basically two pieces of data: If the patient fell asleep, how long to sleep onset in minutes was it, and if the patient showed rapid eye movement (REM) sleep, how long it took after sleep onset to reach the beginning of REM. A mean sleep latency is reported for the set of naps and number of REM periods. A mean sleep latency of 5 minutes or less is considered to show a severe or pathological degree of daytime sleepiness, and two or more REM periods within the series of four of five 20-minute rest periods is characteristic for a narcolepsy disorder.

Indications for the MSLT are presented in the American Sleep Disorders Association guide to clinical use of the test (Thorpy, 1992). They are reprinted here with permission of the editors and publishers of *Sleep*:[1]

1. *Narcolepsy*. An MSLT is indicated for all patients suspected of narcolepsy to confirm the diagnosis and to determine the severity of sleepiness; it should be performed before commencing treatment with stimulant medications.

2. *Obstructive sleep apnea syndrome.* The MSLT is indicated in patients with mild to moderate obstructive sleep apnea syndrome who complain of moderate to severe sleepiness; it may be indicated also in patients with moderate to severe obstructive sleep apnea syndrome, especially if severe sleepiness is unappreciated or denied.

3. *Other causes of sleepiness.* An MSLT is indicated in the evaluation of patients suspected of having idiopathic hypersomnia or periodic limb movement disorder, as well as those in whom the cause of excessive sleepiness in unknown.

4. *Insomnia.* The MSLT is indicated when the presence of moderate to severe excessive sleepiness is suspected.

5. *Circadian rhythm sleep disorders.* The MSLT may be useful in documenting sleepiness in some circadian rhythm disorders, but adequate scientific validation is not yet available.

6. *Assessment of treatment effects.* The MSLT is indicated to assess the response to treatment following effective therapy for disorders that cause sleepiness when an additional sleep disorder that produces sleepiness is suspected, or if confirmation of relief of sleepiness is required to ensure occupational safety.

7. *Repeat MSLT testing.* Repeat MSLT testing is indicated in the following situations: (a) when the initial test is believed to be an invalid representation of the patient's status; (b) when ambiguous or uninterpretable MSLT findings occur; (c) when the response to treatment needs to be ascertained; and (d) when more than one sleep disorder is suspected.

Maintenance of Wakefulness Test. The Maintenance of Wakefulness Test (MWT) is a variation on the MSLT procedure (Mitler, Gujavarty, & Browman, 1982). It is performed under the same testing conditions as the MSLT, except the patient is semireclining in a chair in a dimly lit room and the instructions are to attempt to remain awake for 40 minutes. A

---

[1]Copyright 1992 American Sleep Disorders Association and Sleep Research Society.

similar technique, the Repeated Test of Sustained Wakefulness, uses the same instruction but maintains more of the standard MSLT setting to favor falling asleep; specifically, the patient lies in bed in a darkened room (Hartse, Roth, & Zorick, 1982).

The MWT is used less frequently than the MSLT; it has been adopted mainly as a method to assess improved alertness following treatments. The MWT has been reported to be sensitive to the alerting effects of stimulant medications (Mitler, Hajdukovic, Erman, & Koziol, 1990). MSLT studies of narcolepsy treatment outcome have not reliably demonstrated significant reduction in sleepiness with stimulant medication at clinically effective doses. These findings suggest a different effect of stimulant medication on ability to remain awake when one is motivated to do so. The MWT differs when compared with some MSLT studies that have shown an absence of significant change in physiological sleep tendency using pre- and posttreatment MSLT evaluations, where patients are asked to try to fall asleep during a rest period (van den Hoed et al., 1981).

Other physiological measures.

Pupillometry. An early physiological measure of sleepiness, pupillometry (Lowenstein, Feinberg, & Loewenfeld, 1963) has been used to assess daytime somnolence in narcolepsy (Yoss, Moyer, & Ogle, 1969). This technique uses variations in pupil size that are associated with decreased alertness. Because pupil diameter and stability of pupil size both decrease with level of wakefulness, reaction to a light flash that stimulates pupil constriction can be used to measure sleepiness. Pupil size and stability have shown some divergence in their relationship with daytime sleepiness (Pressman et al., 1984), but norms for pupillometry have not been established. A small number of sleep disorders centers regularly use pupillometry in clinical evaluations. Generally, however, its use has been limited to research studies on daytime somnolence.

Average evoked EEG response. The average evoked response shows consistent changes in waveform related to stage of sleep (Williams, Tepas, & Morlock, 1962). Several studies have shown relationships between averaged EEG response and levels of daytime alertness (Pressman, Spielman, Pollak, & Weitzman, 1982). The technique has not been widely adopted or evaluated in clinical settings.

Ambulatory 24-hour monitoring. Ambulatory monitoring of sleep and wakefulness provides a capability for extended recording of multiple physiological measures. Twenty-four-hour and multiple-day recordings can be obtained in the patient's home at relatively low expense (Broughton et al., 1988). Because of the unique features of ambulatory sleep monitoring, it has been recommended that a large normative database be obtained with comparison data for common diagnostic groups (McCall, Erwin, Edinger, Krystal, & Marsh, 1992).

Actigraphy. The use of activity-level monitoring for sleep–wake evaluation has achieved a significant degree of acceptance and use among researchers and clinical sleep specialists. Actigraphs provide a cost-effective method to perform field studies of sleep, including use of extended-duration recordings of sleep and wakefulness (Cole, Kripke, Gruen, Mullaney, & Gillin, 1992). Actigraphic estimates of total sleep time have shown an acceptable correlation with polysomnographic recordings (Newman, Stampi, Dunham, & Broughton, 1988).

Context of a Sleepiness Evaluation

In addition to the primary cause of an individual problem with excessive sleepiness, there are other determinants that influence whether a person will show overt sleepiness. These contextual factors relate to situations, physiological state, psychological influences, health status, behavioral issues, individual differences, and biological rhythms. When patients are evaluated for physiological sleep tendency, there are behavioral issues (including health habits) that are basic to accurate assessment, such as insufficient amount of sleep, prescription medication use, use of alcohol and drugs, and sleep hygiene. In addition, circadian rhythms of sleep and wakefulness come into play.

An extreme example is a professional who must awaken for emergencies and manage them with phone calls during the nocturnal sleep period or a shift worker returning to a night job after a weekend living on a day-shift schedule with his or her family. These individuals are forced to perform during the sleepiness phase of their day. Tests of excessive sleepiness should be performed in synchrony with patients' sleep–wake schedules. This might dictate testing some night-shift workers during their usual work hours. However, almost all midnight shift workers revert to sleeping at night when they are off work, and available MSLT norms are for day testing.

Context of Sleepiness Measurements

When evaluating a primary disorder of excessive sleepiness, it is necessary to evaluate context before measuring sleepiness. This must be done because situational factors may be present that alter the client's pattern of sleep and wakefulness or increase severity of sleepiness (e.g., negative sleep hygiene behaviors such as use of alcohol as a sleep aid). In addition to the standardized procedures of the MSLT, guidelines have been recommended by the American Sleep Disorders Association for preparing a person for daytime somnolence testing and preparing the setting for the test (Carskadon et al., 1986; Thorpy, 1992). For example, failure to withdraw a patient from heavy caffeine use can contribute to false-negative measurements. Without specific instructions on how to prepare for testing, some patients intentionally deprive themselves of sleep time on the nights before a sleep study to ensure ease of falling asleep in the sleep laboratory. To move beyond a patient's tiredness complaint and sleepiness symptoms toward standardized physiological measurements, there is a need to assess the patient in a prescribed context and take steps to control some of the important independent variables that contribute to overall level of sleepiness. As an example, published guidelines state that "drugs known to affect sleep latency (e.g., tricyclic antidepressants, monoamine oxidase inhibitors, amphetamines) will influence the test results and should be withdrawn for 2 weeks before MSLT testing" (Carskadon et al., 1986, p. 520).

Physiological Measures of Change in Sleepiness

Because of the recent growth of sleep disorders medicine, the need to evaluate treatment results is also growing. Measuring the benefits of treatment has been an area of clinical assessment with limited activity. When physiological measurement has been attempted, those assessing treatment outcome have repeated the tests used to diagnose excessive sleepiness (the MSLT and, to a lesser extent, the MWT).

The Standard Measure of Sleepiness Severity

The MSLT is the only validated objective test of physiological sleep tendency that has been demonstrated to be a sensitive test of excessive daytime sleepiness. Its criterion validity stands above that of other physiological measures. In contrast a newer test designed to measure the ability to stay awake (Mitler, Gujavarty, & Browman, 1988) does not reliably show significant differences in the alertness of normal controls when composed to the MSLT. The MSLT helps define some sleep disorder diagnoses (e.g., the sleep-onset REM periods that characterize test results of patients with narcolepsy; ICSD; Diagnostic Classification Steering Committee, 1990) and is valuable for documenting severity of sleepiness.

How does the MSLT stand in relation to other types of physiological measurement? This is a question that leads to some exciting possibilities. MSLT and MWT relationships are interesting and have potential clinical importance. The MWT appears to be more sensitive to the benefits of stimulant medication for patients with narcolepsy. This possible strength relative to the MSLT may establish a complementary assessment relationship for the two measures. Because the clinical usefulness of the MWT is not well established at present, its use is not widespread.

Differing Goals of the Two Sleep Tendency Tests

The MSLT is designed to see how fast a person falls asleep when conditions are designed to remove impediments to falling asleep. It is a relatively pure measure of physiological tendency to fall asleep. Patients undergoing MSLT testing are instructed to "lie still, keep your eyes closed," and "try to fall asleep" or alternatively, to "let yourself fall asleep" (Carskadon et al., 1986, p. 521). The absence of strong task demands or pressure and the efforts to limit confounding variables favor achievement of the simple, parsimonious measurement that was the aim of the MSLT developers: the unimpeded expression of the sleepiness drive (Carskadon & Dement, 1977).

The MWT instructs the patient to remain awake as long as possible (Mitler, Gujavarty, & Browman, 1982). Measuring the capacity to stay awake when motivated to do so potentially offers a unique tool to add to the MSLT for documenting physiological sleep tendency in research and clinical settings. The physiological sleepiness that is reflected in the MSLT results is only one of the factors that influence capacity to maintain wakefulness. The face validity of the MWT testing conditions as representative of life's daily demands for wakefulness also adds to its potential generalizability.

For example, consider the following hypothetical assessment activities. If a battery of occupational tests to assess alertness, sleepiness, and ability to maintain wakefulness in a work situation were developed in the future, it might benefit from inclusion of the MWT. Such a battery might also include nocturnal polysomnography and the MSLT.

Practical measures of sleepiness such as pupillometry might also fit in the battery, perhaps as preliminary screening tools to identify individuals who appeared to be excessively sleepy and in need of more in-depth testing. Repeated testing with performance measures may be useful for identifying impairment related to sleepiness. The MSLT may be the key test for documenting significant excessive sleepiness. The MWT may meet the need to show the benefit of specific pharmacotherapies.

Assessment of Treatment Outcome

The use of the MSLT in the assessment of response to treatment is less well defined than its use for determining a baseline level of physiological sleepiness and for diagnosis. The question of when to repeat the MSLT for examining treatment response often depends on the need to document that the patient is safe. Most patients do not require MSLT evaluation of treatment response when improvement in the sleep disorder is considered clinically optimal.

As noted previously, some patients with narcolepsy show little improvement on the MSLT during subjectively successful treatment with stimulant medication. With a severe and chronic disorder of excessive sleepiness such as narcolepsy, the MWT may be a better test of treatment effects than the standard MSLT.

The MSLT and MWT have been shown to be capable of documenting improved alertness following treatment of obstructive sleep apnea. However, after resolution of obstructive sleep apnea by treatment with tracheostomy or CPAP, some patients continue to have excessive sleepiness (Lamphere et al., 1989). These patients may have more than one sleep disorder, or the currently available physiological testing may not be sensitive to the improvements that have occurred with treatment.

The evaluation of treatment outcome for disorders of excessive sleepiness may benefit from new ideas and techniques. The need for sleep disorder treatments helped to stimulate the beginning of the field of sleep medicine in the 1970s. The expansion of the field in the 1980s and 1990s, with its rapid growth in the availability of treatment, has caused a mushrooming need for treatment evaluation tools. The ideal measure would be a practical, repeatable physiological test of sleepiness that cannot be faked, akin to checks of blood pressure and body temperature. Such an ideal measure would be an extraordinary sleepiness test, but it may be unreasonable to expect such characteristics from any single instrument because of the multiply determined nature of physiological sleep tendency. Currently, the MSLT stands as the only established standard test of physiological sleep tendency.

Conclusion

Sleepiness is familiar to everyone because of the daily need for sleep. Excessive sleepiness has potential negative consequences that also are easy to appreciate, yet subjective information about degree of sleepiness has limited validity, unless sleepiness is extremely strong. Sleepiness feelings, behavior, and physiology are rather weakly correlated except when the need for sleep is strong. Therefore, the subjective description of one's own sleepiness experience may disagree with measurements of physiological sleep tendency. Formal sleepiness measurement is important for accurate identification of disorders of excessive sleepiness because dependence on subjective clinical information involves significant risk for error. This error includes underestimation of sleepiness because of patient denial plus the risk of overestimation that is inherent in potentially biased patient self-descriptions.

The importance of formal sleepiness assessment is also related to the high functional significance of excessive sleepiness and treatment decisions related to the management of sleepiness. It is more dangerous than other sleep disorder symptoms. Clinical decisions about sleepiness deal with issues of symptom severity, need for treatment, and resolution of excessive sleepiness. Evaluations that include the objective measurement of sleepiness can increase the accuracy of diagnosis and treatment recommendations.

There are laboratory techniques that directly measure various features of physiological sleep tendency, such as speed of falling asleep when trying to nap and ability to maintain wakefulness when motivated. There are also a variety of techniques to assess physiological correlates of sleepiness and document its effects on ability to perform tasks. Evaluations generally begin with commonsense interview probes, and an initial diagnostic workup may use history taking, rating scales, and sleep logs, as well as observation of appearance and behavior. Performance measures to assess the consequences of excessive sleepiness are used in research. There are physiological tests for evidence of sleepiness, which include pupillometry and average evoked EEG response. The MSLT and MWT directly measure tendency to fall asleep. The MSLT is the only direct measure of sleep tendency that has been validated and standardized for clinical and research use. The continuing search for monitoring methods is providing a wealth of potentially useful measures, which may be as simple as a wrist acti-graph or as rich as 24-hour multichannel physiological monitoring of sleep and wakefulness.

When conducting formal measurement of sleepiness, it is important to assess the independent variables that influence sleep tendency and attempt to control important ones to increase measurement accuracy.

Testing to document improvement in sleepiness after treatment is an area of growing concern. The expansion of treatment availability caused by the new sleep medicine field has created a need for more out-come testing and an opportunity for researchers.

REFERENCES

Broughton, R., Dunham, W., Newman, J., Lutley, K., Duschesne, P., & Rivers, M. (1988). Ambulatory 24 hour sleep-wake monitoring in narcolepsy cata-plexy compared to matched controls. *Electroencephalography and Clinical Neurophysiology, 70,* 473–481.

Broughton, R., Ghanem, Q., Hishikawa, Y., Sugita, Y., Nevsimalova, S., & Roth, B. (1981). Life effects of narcolepsy in 180 patients from North America, Asia and Europe compared to matched controls. *Canadian Journal of Neurological Science, 8,* 299–304.

Carskadon, M. A., & Dement, W. C. (1977). Sleep tendency: An objective mea-sure of sleep loss. *Sleep Research, 6,* 200.

Carskadon, M. A., & Dement, W. C. (1982). The Multiple Sleep Latency Test: What does it measure? *Sleep, 5*(Suppl. 2), S67–S72.

Carskadon, M. A., Dement, W. C., Mitler, M. M., Roth, T., Westbrook, P. R., & Keenan, S. (1986). Guidelines for the Multiple Sleep Latency Test (MSLT): A standard measure of sleepiness. *Sleep, 9,* 519–524.

Cole, R. J., Kripke, D. F., Gruen, W., Mullaney, D. J., & Gillin, J. C. (1992). Automatic sleep/wake identification from wrist activity. *Sleep, 15,* 461–469.

Dement, W. (1976). Daytime sleepiness and sleep "attacks." In C. Guilleminault, W. Dement, & P. Passouant (Eds.), *Narcolepsy* (pp. 17–42). New York: Spectrum Publications.

Dement, W. C., & Carskadon, M. A. (1982). Current perspectives on daytime sleepiness: The issues. *Sleep, 5*(Suppl. 2), S56–S66.

Dement, W. C., Carskadon, M. A., & Richardson, G. S. (1978). Excessive day-time sleepiness in the sleep apnea syndrome. In C. Guilleminault & W. C. Dement (Eds.), *Sleep apnea syndromes* (pp. 23–46). New York: Alan R. Liss.

Diagnostic Classification Steering Committee, Thorpy, M. J., Chairman. (1990). *ICSD International classification of sleep disorders. Diagnostic and coding manual.* Rochester, MN: American Sleep Disorders Association.

Dinges, D. F., Graeber, R. C., Carskadon, M. A., Czeisler, C. A., & Dement, W. C. (1989). Attending to inattention. *Science, 245,* 342.

Dinges, D. F., Graeber, R. C., Connell, L. J., Rosekind, M. R., & Powell, J. W. (1990). Fatigue-related reaction time performance in long-haul flight crews. *Sleep Research, 19,* 117.

French, J., Bisson, R. U., Neville, K. J., Mitcha, J., & Storm, W. F. (1994). Crew fatigue during simulated, long duration B-1B bomber missions. *Aviation Space and Environmental Medicine, 65*(Suppl. 5), A1–A6.

Guilleminault, C., & Carskadon, M. (1977). Relationship between sleep disorders and daytime complaints. In W. P. Koella & P. W. Oevin (Eds.), *Sleep 1976* (pp. 95–100). Basel, Switzerland: Karger.

Hartse, K. M., Roth, T., & Zorick, F. J. (1982). Daytime sleepiness and daytime wakefulness: The effect of instruction. *Sleep, 5*(Suppl. 2), S107–S118.

Hauri, P., & Linde, S. (1990). *No more sleepless nights.* New York: Wiley.

Hoddes, E., Zarcone, V., Smythe, H., Phillips, R., & Dement, W. (1973). Quantification of sleepiness: A new approach. *Psychophysiology, 10,* 431–436.

Johns, M. W. (1991). A new method for measuring daytime sleepiness: The Epworth Sleepiness Scale. *Sleep, 14,* 540–545.

Johns, M. W. (1993). Daytime sleepiness, snoring and obstructive sleep apnea: The Epworth Sleepiness Scale. *Chest, 103*(1), 30–36.

Johnson, L. C., Freeman, C. R., & Spinweber, C. L., & Gomez, S. A. (1991). Subjective and objective measures of sleepiness: Effect of benzodiazepine and caffeine on their relationship. *Psychophysiology, 26,* 65–71.

Lamphere, J., Roehrs, T., Wittig, R., Zorick, F., Conway, W. A., & Roth, T. (1989). Recovery of alertness after CPAP in apnea. *Chest, 96,* 1364–1367.

Lowenstein, O., Feinberg, R., & Loewenfeld, I. E. (1963). Pupillary movements during acute and chronic fatigue: A new test for the objective evaluation of tiredness. *Investigative Ophthalmology, 2,* 138–157.

McCall, W. V., Erwin, C. W., Edinger, J. D., Krystal, A. D., & Marsh, G. R. (1992). Ambulatory polysomnography: Technical aspects and normative values. *Journal of Clinical Neurophysiology, 9*(1), 68–77.

Mitler, M. M., Carskadon, M. A., Czeisler, C. A., Dement, W. C., Dinges, D. F., & Graeber, R. C. (1988). Catastrophes, sleep and public policy: Consensus report. *Sleep, 11,* 100–109.

Mitler, M. M., Gujavarty, S., & Browman, C. P. (1982). Maintenance of Wakefulness Test: A polysomnographic technique for evaluating treatment efficacy in patients with excessive somnolence. *Electroencephalography and Clinical Neurophysiology, 53,* 658–661.

Mitler, M. M., Hajdukovic, R., Erman, M., & Koziol, J. A. (1990). Narcolepsy. *Journal of Clinical Neurophysiology, 7,* 93–118.

Newman, J., Stampi, C., Dunham, D. W., & Broughton, R. (1988). Does wrist-actigraphy approximate traditional polysomnographic detection of sleep and wakefulness in narcolepsy-cataplexy? *Sleep Research, 17,* 343.

Pressman, M. R., Spielman, A. J., Korczyn, A. D., Rubenstein, A. E., Pollak, C. P., & Weitzman, E. D. (1984). Patterns of daytime sleepiness in narcoleptics and normals: A pupillometric study. *Electroencephalography and Clinical Neurophysiology, 57,* 1984.

Pressman, M. R., Spielman, A. J., Pollak, C. P., & Weitzman, E. D. (1982). Long-latency auditory evoked responses during sleep deprivation and in narcolepsy. *Sleep, 5*(Suppl. 2), S147–S156.

Reynolds, C. F., Coble, P. A., Kupfer, D. J., & Holzer, B. C. (1982). Application of the multiple sleep latency test in disorders of excessive sleepiness. *Electroencephalography and Clinical Neurophysiology, 53,* 443–452.

Schweitzer, P. K., Muehlbach, M. J., & Walsh, J. K. (1992). Countermeasures for night work performance deficits: The effects of napping or caffeine on performance at night. *Work and Stress, 6,* 355–365.

Scrima, L., Hartman, P. G., Johnson, F. H., Thomas, E. H., & Hiller, F. C. (1990). The effects of gamma-hydroxybutyrate on the sleep of narcolepsy patients: A double blind study. *Sleep, 13,* 479–490.

Stampi, C., & Heitmann, A. (1993). Truck driver alertness as a function of cab vibration levels. *Sleep Research, 22,* 390.

Thorpy, M. J. (1992). The clinical use of the Multiple Sleep Latency Test. *Sleep, 15,* 268–276.

Valley, V., & Broughton, R. (1983). The physiological (EEG) nature of drowsiness and its relation to performance deficits in narcoleptics. *Electroencephalography and Clinical Neurophysiology, 55,* 243–251.

Van den Hoed, J., Kraemer, H., Guilleminault, C., Zarcone, V. P., Miles, L. E., Dement, W. C., & Mitler, M. M. (1981). Disorders of excessive somnolence: Polygraphic and clinical data for 100 patients. *Sleep, 4,* 23–37.

Wilkinson, R. T. (1968). Sleep deprivation: Performance tests for partial and selective sleep deprivation. *Progress in Clinical Psychology, 8,* 28–43.

Williams, H. L., Tepas, D. I., & Morlock, H. C. (1962). Evoked responses to clicks and electroencephalographic stages of sleep in man. *Science, 138,* 685–686.

Yoss, R. E., Moyer, N. J., & Ogle, K. N. (1969). The pupillogram and narcolepsy: A method to measure decreased levels of wakefulness. *Neurology, 19,* 921–928.

Zorick, F., Roehrs, T., Koshorek, G., Sicklesteel, J., Hartse, K., Wittig, R., & Roth, T. (1982). Patterns of sleepiness in various disorders of excessive daytime somnolence. *Sleep, 5*(Suppl. 2), S165–S174.

Zwyghuizen-Doorenbos, A., Roehrs, T., Schaefer, M., & Roth, T. (1988). Test-retest reliability of the MSLT. *Sleep, 11,* 562–565.

III

Sleep Disorders
and Their Treatment

Delayed Sleep Phase Syndrome and Related Conditions

Gary K. Zammit

Sleep is governed by a circadian rhythm that influences the occurrence, timing, and duration of sleep episodes that take place during each 24-hour day. This rhythm is the primary factor that promotes the recurrence of sleep at regular and appropriate intervals. It is thought to be an endogenous biological rhythm (i.e., occurring within the organism) and may be genetically determined (Roehrs & Roth, 1994). Although its pacemaker is influenced by environmental factors (e.g., light), the circadian rhythm is quite powerful and normally sustains its influence over sleep timing in the absence of external time cues (Moore, 1978; Wever, 1979), even when sleep is otherwise disrupted by medical, psychiatric, or sleep disorders. The circadian rhythm is believed to be among the strongest determinants of sleep, alongside age, gender, and prior sleep debt.

Circadian rhythm sleep disorders are diagnosed when the timing of sleep episodes becomes misaligned with the sleep period that is desired or regarded as the societal norm (American Sleep Disorders Association [ASDA]; 1990). This misalignment represents a lack of coherence between the endogenous rhythm and the external environment. The occurrence of sleep episodes may be shifted to an earlier time

I would like to thank Dr. Stephen Lund for reviewing the manuscript.

(phase advanced) or a later time (phase delayed; see Figure 1), or the timing may be irregular or not based on a 24-hour (circadian) cycle. The effects of high-speed air travel and shift work have resulted in additional categories of circadian rhythm sleep disorders that address problems associated with time zone changes (jet lag) and sleep disorders related to shift work (see chapter 12 for discussion of shift work).

Disturbances of sleep timing are common in a variety of illnesses. Insomnia is frequently associated with difficulty falling asleep at the desired time, as well as with the early morning or late termination of sleep. Obstructive sleep apnea, narcolepsy, or shift work can result in irregular sleep patterns that may be identical to those seen in circadian rhythm sleep disorders. Certain medical conditions such as congenital blindness and psychiatric disorders such as major depression can also result in marked changes in sleep timing. Consequently, it is difficult to determine the prevalence of circadian rhythm sleep disorders in the general population. Currently available data suggest that these disorders are rare. Studies of diagnoses made at sleep disorders centers in the United States indicate that 2% or less of the patient population are likely to have a diagnosis of circadian rhythm sleep disorder (Coleman et al., 1982).

Although circadian rhythm sleep disorders are not common, they present serious problems for patients, who frequently suffer from clinically significant, severe symptoms. Circadian rhythm sleep disorders may be associated with psychological problems or impairments in cognitive, social, or occupational functioning, and as a result they may come to the attention of a mental health professional. The purpose of this chapter is to define the characteristics of circadian rhythm sleep disorders, discuss the features of these disorders that may be relevant to the practice of health psychologists, and briefly outline treatment.

Delayed Sleep Phase Syndrome

Delayed sleep phase syndrome (DSPS) is characterized by (a) sleep-onset and wake times that are consistently and intractably later than desired, (b) sleep-onset times at nearly the same daily clock hour, (c) little or no reported difficulty in maintaining sleep once sleep has begun, (d) extreme difficulty awakening at the desired time in the morning, and (e) a relatively severe to absolute inability to advance the sleep phase to earlier hours by enforcing conventional sleep and wake

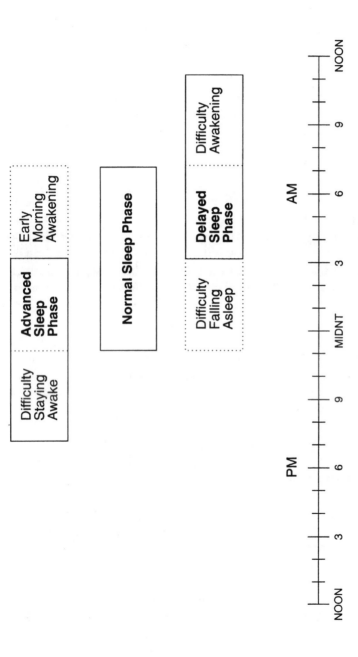

Figure 1.   The horizontal base axis indicates time in hours. Graphic images identify the position, relative to clock time, of advanced sleep phase, normal sleep phase, and delayed sleep phase patterns. The bold-lined rectangles indicate actual sleep tendency in comparison to the normal sleep phase (dotted-lined rectangles). Comments denote the types of complaints reported by individuals who attempt to remain awake or sleep at times other than those favored by each phase.

times (ASDA, 1990). DSPS is thought to affect approximately 1.2% of patients who present to a sleep disorders center and to represent 39.1% of circadian rhythm sleep disorder diagnoses (Coleman et al., 1982). It frequently begins in childhood and may be most common in adolescents, with 7.3% of 12- to 19-year-olds reporting symptoms consistent with DSPS diagnostic criteria (Pelayo, Thorpy, & Glovinsky, 1988). Figure 1 provides a graphic illustration of the circadian rhythm of sleep and wakefulness in patients with DSPS.

Typically, individuals with DSPS feel best and function at peak during the late evening and night hours (ASDA, 1990). However, they often complain of the inability to fall asleep before 2:00 a.m., with sleep onset sometimes so delayed that it occurs just before the desired rise time. Once asleep, the individual sustains an uninterrupted sleep period. Spontaneous awakenings usually occur in the late morning or afternoon. Attempts to awaken earlier with the aid of an alarm clock or other means can be successful but often fail. Consequently, individuals often adapt to DSPS by securing employment or adopting other lifestyle changes that allow their absence during the morning hours. Several cases have been reported of individuals with DSPS who have adapted their schedules and functioned quite well in a variety of home, academic, and work situations (Weitzman et al., 1981). When such accommodations cannot be made, the individual may have difficulty sustaining employment or personal relationships and may experience grossly impaired functioning in many other life circumstances (Alvarez, Dahlitz, Vignau, & Parkes, 1992).

Sleepiness during the morning hours is common in DSPS. Individuals who force themselves to rise to meet social or occupational obligations often suffer from sleepiness, fatigue, memory and concentration impairment, and diminished productivity, especially in the hours just after awakening (Thorpy, Korman, Speilman, & Glovinsky, 1988). Morning sleepiness is probably a consequence of two primary factors (Wagner, 1990): Individuals with DSPS who rise early are terminating the sleep during their endogenous "night," when there is a circadian rhythm tendency to maintain sleep. They are also terminating the nighttime sleep period before sufficient sleep has been obtained, leaving them in a sleep-deprived state. Repeated nights of insufficient sleep can markedly increase sleepiness during the morning hours and throughout the day. It is common for patients with DSPS to seek professional help when problems in daytime functioning become severe or when their employment status is jeopardized by sleepiness.

There is a clear distinction between DSPS and insomnia. Patients with DSPS may deliver the presenting complaint of insomnia and may characterize their symptoms in a way that is consistent with sleep-onset insomnia (Weitzman et al., 1979). This is especially true when patients attempt to normalize their sleep schedule by retiring at earlier bedtimes, only to lie awake tossing and turning. These patients differ from patients with insomnia in that they characteristically have (a) a chronic and stable pattern of sleep phase delay, (b) continuous and undisturbed sleep, (c) normal amounts of daily sleep, and (d) failure of response to conventional treatments for insomnia, including sedative–hypnotic medication (Roehrs & Roth, 1994; Wagner, 1990). The differential diagnosis of DSPS versus insomnia often is made with the help of sleep logs that provide a record of bedtimes and rise times over an extended period. Figure 2 provides examples of sleep log data obtained from one patient with DSPS and another patient with insomnia.

DSPS is sometimes confused with the lifestyle choice to remain awake late into the night. Television and radio programming and the late hours of businesses that make goods and provide services, including recreation, around the clock have helped to make this lifestyle choice possible. Distinct from those who suffer from DSPS, individuals who maintain a late-night lifestyle usually do so by desire, can fall asleep earlier than usual, and are able to arise at socially acceptable hours. Although the distinction between DSPS and lifestyle choice is clear, it is important to acknowledge that some patients with DSPS report that their difficulties began following a period during which they stayed awake late at night (ASDA, 1990). University students who fall into a pattern of late-night television viewing and studying, delayed bedtime and rise time, and afternoon or evening classes can experience extreme difficulty when daytime job opportunities arise or when new class schedules require morning attendance. Shift work and changes in the photoperiod (the pattern of daily exposure to light) can have similar effects in contributing to the development of DSPS.

Psychopathology has been reported in approximately half of adult patients with DSPS (Weitzman et al., 1981). The psychopathology is varied in type and severity, but depression appears to be the most common finding. One study of 22 adolescents with DSPS found that 36% had features of depression and that an additional 27% had a history of prior treatment for depression (Thorpy et al., 1988). The relationship between DSPS and mood disorders is not well understood. DSPS may give rise to depression, or there may be a primary mood disorder that

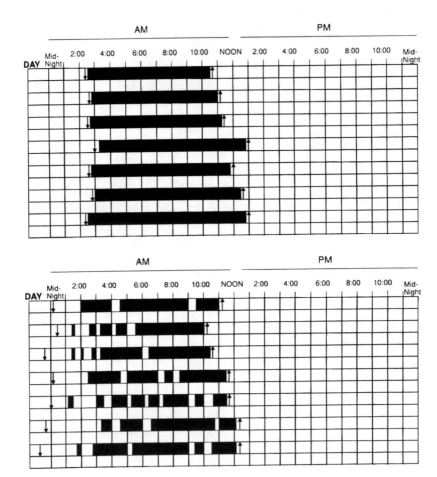

Figure 2. Sleep log data from an individual with delayed sleep phase syndrome (DSPS; upper graphic) and one with insomnia (lower graphic). The individual with DSPS retires consistently between 2:20 a.m. and 3:00 a.m., falls asleep quickly, and remains asleep for the duration of the sleep period. Rise time is late, occurring between 10:45 a.m. and 1:00 p.m. Sleep efficiency is generally high and within normal limits. In contrast, the individual with insomnia experiences long sleep latencies, irrespective of bedtime, and experiences multiple and/or long awakenings during the sleep period. Sleep efficiency is below the normal limit.

evokes symptoms that are characteristic of DSPS. Psychosocial problems also have been evident in subgroups of these patients, who may
be mistakenly viewed as lazy, unmotivated, or mentally ill (Wagner,
1990). These findings dictate that psychiatric symptoms be evaluated in
patients who present with symptoms that are consistent with DSPS.

Polysomnographic studies of individuals with DSPS who select their
bedtimes and rise times have shown that sleep onset is delayed, reducing overall sleep efficiency. However, once asleep, DSPS patients tend
to have normal sleep architecture and normal total daily amounts of
sleep (between 7 and 9 hours; Weitzman et al., 1981). If bedtimes and
rise times are shifted to an earlier, socially accepted time, sleep latency
is markedly increased. Once sleep is initiated, however, it is generally
maintained throughout the balance of the sleep period. Findings
obtained from the Multiple Sleep Latency Test (MSLT) in adolescent
patients with DSPS revealed shorter latency to sleep onset during
morning naps compared with afternoon naps (Thorpy et al., 1988).

The pathophysiology of DSPS is not well defined. Neural and
endocrine mechanisms that serve as pacemakers for the circadian system have been identified (Harrington, Rusak, & Mistlberger, 1994;
Jacklet, 1985). The suprachiasmatic nucleus (SCN), an organ that is
about the size of the head of a pin and located in the hypothalamus, is
known to play a key role in maintaining the circadian rhythm. It has
been hypothesized that the SCN is involved in the abnormalities of the
sleep–wake rhythm seen in DSPS. It has also been suggested that individuals with DSPS have a limited ability to advance their sleep–wake
rhythm in response to normal environmental cues. Transient sleep
phase delays due to lifestyle choice or environmental demands that are
not problematic for most people may unmask DSPS in individuals who
are prone to the condition (ASDA, 1990).

Advanced Sleep Phase Syndrome

Advanced sleep phase syndrome (ASPS) is a condition in which the
sleep period occurs at a time that is earlier than desired or acceptable
(see Figure 1). It is characterized by an intractable and chronic inability
to delay the onset of evening sleep or extend sleep later into the morning hours by enforcing conventional bedtimes and rise times (ASDA,
1990). Individuals with ASPS typically retire before 9:00 p.m. and
awaken between 3:00 and 5:00 a.m. They may report the presenting

complaints of excessive evening sleepiness, early-morning awakening, or both. There have been only two cases of ASPS extensively described in the literature. One case concerned a 63-year-old female who habitually retired at 9:00 p.m. and rose at 6:00 a.m. (Kamei, Hughes, Miles, & Dement, 1979), and the other concerned a 62-year-old male with obstructive sleep apnea who was excessively sleepy during the day (Moldofsky, Musisi, & Phillipson, 1986). Partly because these cases of ASPS may have been secondary to normal aging or another sleep disorder and because of the difficulty in identifying new cases, some authors have suggested that the symptoms of ASPS may not represent a distinct syndrome (Roehrs & Roth, 1994).

Individuals with ASPS usually have difficulty functioning in the evening. If unable to retire at the usual bedtime, they may fall asleep despite their best efforts, especially when involved in quiet, sedentary situations. They may adapt by excusing themselves from social or other activities in order to sleep, altogether avoiding evening or late-night commitments. It is possible that ASPS often fails to come to the attention of professionals because such adaptations are considered socially acceptable and the functional impairments associated with this disorder are not as public as in DSPS. Sleepiness that occurs as a result of ASPS is likely to occur in the evening, when the individual is apt to have fewer social and occupational commitments, so that impairment in functioning may not be reported.

Early-morning awakenings are another common symptom of ASPS (Moldofsky et al., 1986). The sleeper awakens feeling fully alert and is unable to return to sleep, even though environmental conditions favor continued sleep. Some patients complain that early-morning awakenings are frustrating and contribute to the feeling that they are "out of step" with the rest of the world. Others develop adaptive lifestyles in which they fill early-morning hours with productive activity. They may consider their ability to rise early as an asset, being the first to arrive at work in the morning or having accomplished many tasks before others start their day.

Patients with ASPS may report the presenting complaint of terminal insomnia (Roehrs & Roth, 1994). However, as in DSPS, there are no sleep-maintenance problems associated with the disorder. When bedtimes are delayed to a later time, early-morning awakenings persist, indicating that there is an abnormality of sleep timing rather than a simple impairment in the ability to sustain sleep. It is important to distinguish early-morning awakenings that are associated with ASPS from those that occur secondary to depression; early-morning awakenings are well known to occur in major depressive disorder (Diaz-Guerrero, Gottlieb, & Knott, 1946; Gresham, Agnew, & Williams, 1965). Therefore, underlying primary mood disorders must be ruled out when one considers the diagnosis of ASPS.

It has been suggested that the characteristics of sleep in the elderly are consistent with ASPS. Elderly individuals are known to retire and awaken earlier than young and middle-aged adults. The circadian rhythm of body temperature is also advanced and in phase with the sleep–wake rhythm. However, these changes are normal variations in sleep that occur as people get older. They do not indicate chronobiological abnormalities consistent with ASPS. Normal aging is frequently associated with a decline in evening activities, a reduction of total nightly sleep time, fragmented nighttime sleep, and an increase in daytime napping.

Polysomnography performed during the habitual sleep period of patients with ASPS reveals that the total awake time in bed is elevated (Kamei et al., 1979), with possible abnormal duration and architecture of sleep (Moldofsky et al., 1986). When more than one night of polysomnography is performed, early awakenings may be observed. The MSLT may reveal normal levels of alertness during the morning hours, with alertness diminishing later in the day. The pathophysiology of ASPS is not known, although it is presumed to be the converse of the putative underlying pathophysiology in DSPS.

Non-24-Hour Sleep–Wake Syndrome

The non-24-hour sleep–wake syndrome, also known as the *hypernyc-themeral syndrome* (Kokkoris et al., 1978), is characterized by sleep onset and rise times that occur at a period of 25 hours or longer. This pattern is similar to that observed in individuals living in isolation from time cues. Such individuals tend to have sleep onset and rise times that are progressively delayed each day, so that the sleep period is continuously moving forward. The delay of the sleep period is usually about 2 hours or less per day, although longer delays have been reported (Mikami, Sugita, Teshima, & Iijima, 1987). The sleep period travels in and out of phase with the desired or socially acceptable hours for sleep, such that it is periodically and temporarily normal (see Figure 3). However, the progressive delay of the sleep period

TIME OF DAY

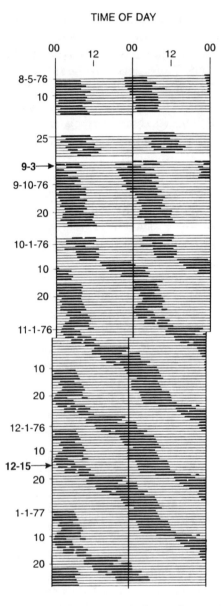

Figure 3. Raster plot depicting non-24-hour-sleep-wake syndrome in one individual. The horizontal axis indicates time of day. The vertical axis indicates the month, day, and year of recording. Solid bars denote the individual's daily sleep period, revealing progressively later bed times and rise times each day. This results in a pattern in which the sleep period progressively transitions "around the clock," taking it from desirable and acceptable times to undesirable and inappropriate times.

over time invariably results in complaints of difficulty sleeping at night and difficulty sustaining alertness during the day. Individuals with this syndrome report severe impairment in functioning, which is interrupted by periods during which they are asymptomatic (ASDA, 1990).

Individuals with non-24-hour sleep–wake syndrome have great difficulty responding to conventional time cues that normally entrain the circadian rhythm of sleep and wakefulness. They may attempt to enforce wakefulness during the day with the use of loud or multiple alarm clocks, caffeinated beverages, or other stimulant substances. They may attempt to induce sleep at desired times by using over-the-counter or prescription drugs, especially hypnotics, which do not result in reentrainment of the circadian rhythm. The strategies used by patients with this disorder and the gradual evolution of poor sleep hygiene often contribute to the chronicity of this condition. The marginal success of reentrainment strategies also may result in sleep deprivation, compounding sleepiness and its associated functional impairments (Kamgar-Parsi, Wehr, & Gillin, 1983). Some patients eventually abandon their attempts to synchronize their sleep to conventional hours (Weber, Cary, Connor, & Keyes, 1980).

The prevalence of non-24-hour sleep–wake syndrome is low, but it may be more frequent in blind persons than in the general population. Studies of blind individuals have shown that 75% complain of sleep disturbance (Miles & Wilson, 1977), possibly owing to free-running (i.e., non-24-hour) circadian rhythms. It has been shown that the circadian rhythms of sleep, body temperature, alertness, performance, cortisol secretion, and urinary electrolyte excretion may assume periods of greater than 24 hours in a blind individual (Miles, Raynal, & Wilson, 1977). These tendencies may first appear during childhood. One study of four congenitally blind mentally retarded children revealed irregular sleep–wake rhythms as early as 4 years of age (Okawa et al., 1987). The endogenous circadian pacemaker in blind persons may drive the system so strongly that attempts at entrainment using nonphotic time cues may not be successful (Klein et al., 1993).

The pathophysiology of non-24-hour sleep–wake syndrome in blind individuals is thought to be related to the absence of photic entrainment cues that result from the perception of light or the light–dark cycle. It is thought that diminished afferent stimulation of the SCN from retinal ganglion cells via the retinohypothalamic tract leads to a reduction in entrainment to photic stimuli (Czeisler & Allan, 1988). The pathophysiology of this syndrome in sighted individuals is not known, although a defect in entrainment mechanisms has been postulated (Kokkoris et al., 1978). Psychiatric and personality factors may play an important role. There may be a conscious or unconscious failure to acknowledge entrainment cues that may provide secondary gain. Avoidance of routine and other anxiety-provoking situations must be considered.

Irregular Sleep–Wake Pattern

Irregular sleep–wake pattern is characterized by temporally disorganized and variable episodes of sleep and wakefulness despite normal 24-hour total sleep time. Unlike DSPS, ASPS, and non-24-hour sleep–wake syndrome, in this disorder there is no recognizable ultradian or circadian pattern of sleep and wakefulness. Multiple sleep episodes are obtained each day, and the duration of these episodes is extremely variable (ASDA, 1990). The occurrence of sleep episodes is not related to any known precipitant or entrainment cue, making it virtually impossible to predict when the individual will be asleep or awake. The timing of all daily activities, including grooming, dressing, and meals, may become irregular and dependent on the sleep schedule. The disorder is rare and may be more common in elderly demented institutionalized patients than in the general population or nondemented elderly (Allen, Seiler, Stahlen, & Spiegel, 1987).

Many patients with irregular sleep–wake pattern present with the complaint of insomnia, frequent daytime napping, or both. Cognitive impairment and sleepiness are common during periods of wakefulness, and patients may complain of intense frustration concerning their inability to manage their sleep schedule. Lassitude or mood disturbance may be present, and it is important to differentiate these states from underlying depressive disorders that may be the primary cause of irregularities in the sleep–wake pattern. Polysomnographic studies of elderly demented individuals with irregular sleep–wake pattern have revealed fragmented sleep, less Stage 2 and REM sleep at night, and more slow wave sleep (SWS) and shifts to wakefulness during daytime sleep episodes when compared with controls (Allen et al., 1987).

The pathophysiology of irregular sleep–wake pattern is unknown. It has been suggested that diffuse brain disease is one predisposing factor. An association has been observed between Alzheimer's disease and irregular patterns of sleep and wakefulness. However, one must also consider the impact of environment in elderly patients, especially those who are institutionalized. The absence of important time cues may contribute to the development of this disorder. Constant lighting, interruptions by staff and other residents at night, and irregular schedules of toileting or other activities may promote irregular sleep patterns. The disorder may also occur in otherwise healthy or younger patients. These patients may have a history of difficulty responding to or a disregard for entrainment cues that leads to chronic and intractable schedule irregularities.

Time Zone Change (Jet Lag) Syndrome

Time zone change (jet lag) syndrome is characterized by difficulty initiating or maintaining sleep, excessive sleepiness, decrements in daytime alertness and performance, and somatic symptoms following rapid travel across multiple time zones. These symptoms arise primarily as a result of the desynchrony between the individual's endogenous circadian rhythm of sleep and wakefulness and external time cues in the new time zone (ASDA, 1990). The nature and severity of the symptoms experienced by an individual depend on a number of factors, including the direction of travel and the number of time zones that are crossed. Most individuals experience jet lag as a minor inconvenience. Others find its symptoms to be severe and associated with significant functional impairments owing to sleepiness or fatigue. The prevalence of jet lag is not known, although it is a common transient problem experienced by air travelers. Individuals over 50 years of age are more likely to experience jet lag than those under 30 years of age.

Rapid travel across multiple time zones results in a misalignment between the individual's internal biological rhythms and the external world (Nicholson, Pascoe, Spencer, & Benson, 1993). Following westward travel, the endogenous circadian rhythm is *phase advanced* relative to local time. The circadian rhythm favors sleep onset and rise times that are earlier than normal relative to local time. For example, the circadian rhythm of an individual traveling from New York to Los Angeles (crossing three time zones and losing 3 hours) who typically retires at 11:00 p.m. and rises at 7:00 a.m. Eastern Standard Time (EST) promotes sleep onset at 8:00 p.m. and sleep termination at 4:00 a.m. in the new time zone. Consequently, the individual is likely to report evening fatigue and early-morning awakenings. Following eastward travel, the endogenous circadian rhythm is *phase delayed* relative to local time. Sleep-onset and rise times that are later than normal relative to local time are favored. For example, the circadian rhythm of an individual traveling from Los Angeles to New York (crossing three time zones and gaining 3 hours) who typically retires at 11:00 p.m. and rises at 7:00 a.m. Pacific Standard Time promotes sleep onset at 2:00 a.m. and sleep termination at 10:00 a.m. in the new (EST) time zone. This person is likely to complain of sleep-onset insomnia and excessive morning or daytime sleepiness.

In addition to desynchronization with the external world, rapid travel results in internal desynchronization (Graeber, 1994). There are many biological rhythms that work in harmony with the circadian rhythm of sleep and wakefulness, including the daily rhythms of body temperature and endocrine secretion. When the circadian rhythm of sleep and wakefulness is out of phase owing to travel across time zones, the rhythm naturally shifts in order to realign with local time. The speed with which this rhythm shifts may be different from the speed of the shift of other biological rhythms. This difference creates internal desynchrony, which may contribute to the occurrence or severity of jet lag symptoms. It also appears that it is easier for the sleep–wake rhythm to adapt to the new time zone following westward than eastward flights, indicating that it is easier to delay rather than advance the rhythm.

Sleep loss and sleepiness are not uncommon in jet lag. Sleep loss may originate before the trip if the individual deprives him- or herself of sleep while preparing for travel. Transient insomnia, sometimes owing to stress associated with anticipated travel, may also result in sleep loss. Following arrival at the destination in the new time zone, the traveler may have schedule demands that do not allow adequate sleep. Westward travelers may have evening obligations that interfere with their desire to retire early, and eastward travelers may have morning obligations that prevent sleeping late into the morning. The pressure to reentrain rhythms to the new time zone compels travelers to deprive themselves of sleep during the days immediately following travel, which may contribute to the severity of symptoms and malaise experienced in jet lag. Sleep following air travel is often fragmented and shortened (Nicholson, 1994), and excessive sleepiness may also be present (Dement, Seidel, Cohen, Bliwise, & Carskadon, 1986).

Individuals who frequently travel across time zones may experience chronic sleep disturbances and symptoms of jet lag (Wagner, 1990).

Studies of aircrew members who fly long-haul trips have shown that sleep is divided into two major episodes and that there is a decrease in sleep quality and an increase in daytime sleepiness during layover (Gander, Graeber, Connel, & Gregory, 1991; Graeber, Lauber, Connel, & Gander, 1986). Similar problems may be experienced by aircraft passengers who do not remain in the destination time zone long enough for reentrainment of the circadian rhythm. Reentrainment following a single trip usually occurs within several days of arriving in the new time zone. Several studies have suggested that the rate of readjustment is dependent on the direction of the flight. Travelers adjust at a rate of about 1.5 hours per day following westward flights and 1 hour per day following eastward flights (Graeber, 1994). Therefore, an individual flying from New York to Los Angeles is likely to readjust within 2 days, whereas 3 days may be required for the return trip.

Polysomnography has been performed following travel across multiple time zones. These studies have shown that sleep is fragmented and there is a greater percentage of Stage 1 sleep following travel (Nicholson, Pascoe, Spencer, Stone, & Green, 1986; Sasaki, Kurosaki, Mori, & Endo, 1986). There is also an irregularity both in the duration of sleep episodes and in the time of day during which they occur following flight (Nicholson, 1994). Although jet lag is presumed to impose its effects immediately after arrival in the new time zone, the direction of travel as well as the delay to first rest period following travel have an impact on sleep quality, duration, and architecture. Polysomnographic evaluation has shown that no significant effect of jet lag may be observed during the first night following travel but that subsequent nights may be disturbed (Nicholson, Pascoe, Spencer, Stone, et al., 1986).

Jet lag is associated with dry itching eyes, irritated nasal passages, muscle cramps, headaches, nausea, abdominal distention, dependent edema, and dizziness; however, these symptoms are believed to be a function of aircraft cabin conditions rather than jet lag. Menstrual abnormalities have been reported in women who frequently fly across multiple time zones. In healthy individuals, serious psychological problems rarely are a result of jet lag. However, low mood or depression has been reported in some travelers (ASDA, 1990). It is also well known that a period of sleep loss, such as might occur with jet lag, may provoke or exacerbate an episode of mania. Alcohol ingestion immediately before, during, or after the flight may contribute to the malaise experienced during jet lag, and travelers should not be encouraged to use alcohol as a sedative or to induce sleep during or after the flight.

Chronotherapy

Chronotherapy was specifically designed to treat patients with DSPS (Czeisler et al., 1981; Weitzman et al., 1981). It takes advantage of the previously discussed natural tendency for the biological clock to drift to a later time in the absence of normal time cues. To reset the internal biological clock, patients are requested to stay up 3 hours later and to awaken 3 hours later each day until they have literally delayed around the clock to the preferred bedtime and wake time. The patient essentially lives on a 27-hour day for the 4–7 days it typically takes to complete chronotherapy. For example, a patient who complains of an inability to fall asleep before 5:00 a.m. but sleeps normally for 8 hours would be told to start chronotherapy by remaining awake on Day 1 to 8:00 a.m. and sleeping until 4:00 p.m. On Day 2 of treatment, the patient would remain awake until 11:00 a.m. and then sleep until 7:00 p.m. On Day 3 of treatment, the patient would remain awake until 2:00 p.m. and then sleep until 10:00 p.m. On Day 4 of treatment, the patient would stay awake until 5:00 p.m. and sleep until 1:00 a.m. On Day 5 of treatment, the patient would stay awake until 8:00 p.m. and sleep until 4:00 a.m. At this point, the clinician and patient would decide what the usual bedtime and waketime are to be and adjust the final day of treatment accordingly.

During the course of chronotherapy, patients are usually instructed not to nap. Once the new sleep–wake schedule is established, patients are instructed to maintain the schedule on weekdays and weekends and not to vary the schedule by more than an hour. Any major variations even for a day or two may result in the sleep phase becoming delayed again, with return of the original presenting symptoms. Patients who are compliant with chronotherapy and follow-up instructions often report complete elimination of their sleep problems.

Light Therapy

Exposure to bright light is known to be an important modulator of biological rhythms (Terman et al., 1995). Circadian rhythms appear not to respond significantly to indoor light with a brightness of 150 lux, but they do respond to lights with the brightness of outdoor light of 2500–10,000 lux. When bright light is administered at certain times of the day and is blocked at other times of the day, shifts in the sleep–wake rhythm may be achieved (Eastman, Stewart, Mahoney, Liu, & Fogg, 1994). To "phase advance" a sleep–wake rhythm (move to an earlier time), bright light is administered for up to 2 hours immediately on awakening and is avoided for several hours before bedtime. To phase delay a sleep–wake rhythm, bright light is administered for up to 2 hours before the usual bedtime and avoided at other times. Bright light is usually administered through commercially available light boxes similar to those used for treatment of seasonal affective disorder. Duration of exposure is determined by the brightness of the light and other characteristics of the light box. Light therapy has been shown to be useful for treating both DSPS and ASPS. There may be additional application for light therapy in treating jet lag and disorders of sleep and wakefulness caused by shift work (Czeisler & Allan, 1987; Czeisler, Johnson, Duffy, Brown, & Kronauer, 1990).

Conclusion

Sleep occurs in the context of a regular and recurrent circadian rhythm. Circadian rhythm sleep disorders reflect a primary abnormality of, or are associated with, this rhythm. Circadian rhythm sleep disorders can result in marked abnormalities of sleep timing, duration, and architecture; severe physical symptoms; and significant impairment in functioning. Psychopathology may contribute to the occurrence of these disorders, but it may also be their result, warranting the careful clinical evaluation of patients who present for treatment. The features of circadian rhythm sleep disorders discussed here highlight the importance of understanding the impact of biological rhythms in the pathophysiology of sleep and psychological disorders. Health psychologists play an important role in clarifying the nature and epidemiology of these disorders as well as their relationship to psychopathology. Health psychologists may also serve to refine behavioral interventions further; behavioral interventions are currently regarded to be the most effective treatments for circadian rhythm disorders.

REFERENCES

Alvarez, B., Dahlitz, M. J., Vignau, J., & Parkes, J. D. (1992). The delayed sleep phase syndrome: Clinical and investigative findings in 14 subjects. *Journal of Neurology, Neurosurgery, and Psychiatry, 55,* 665–670.

American Sleep Disorders Association. (1990). *The international classification of sleep disorders.* Rochester, MN: Author.

Coleman, R. M., Roffwarg, H. P., Kennedy, S. J., Guilleminault, C., Cinque, J., Cohn, M. A., Karacan, I., Kupfer, D. J., Lemmi, H., Miles, L., Orr, W. C., Phillips, E. R., Roth, T., Sassin, J. F., Schmidt, H. S., Weitzman, E. D., & Dement, W. C. (1982). Sleep-wake disorders based on a polysomnographic diagnosis. *Journal of the American Medical Association, 247,* 997–1003.

Czeisler, C. A., & Allan, J. S. (1987). Acute circadian phase reversal in man via bright light exposure: Application to jet lag. *Sleep Research, 16,* 605.

Czeisler, C. A., & Allan, J. S. (1988). Pathologies of the sleep-wake schedule. In R. L. Williams, I. Karacan, & C. A. Moore (Eds.), *Sleep disorders: Diagnosis and treatment* (pp. 109–130). New York: Wiley.

Czeisler, C. A., Johnson M. P., Duffy, J. F., Brown, J. M., & Kronauer, R. F. (1990). Exposure to bright light and darkness to treat physiologic maladaptation to night work. *New England Journal of Medicine, 322,* 1253–1257.

Czeisler, C. A., Richardson, G. S., Coleman, R. M., Zimmerman, J. C., Moore-Ede, M. C., Dement, W. C., & Weitzman, E. D. (1981). Chronotherapy: Resetting the circadian clocks of patients with delayed sleep phase insomnia. *Sleep, 4,* 1–21.

Dement, W. C., Seidel, W. F., Cohen, S. A., Bliwise, N. G., & Carskadon, M. A. (1986). Sleep and wakefulness in aircrew before and after transoceanic flights. *Aviation, Space, and Environmental Medicine, 57*(Suppl.), B14–B28.

Diaz-Guerrero, R., Gottlieb, J. S., & Knott, J. R. (1946). The sleep of patients with manic-depressive psychosis, depressive type. *Psychosomatic Medicine, 8,* 399–404.

Eastman, C. I., Stewart, K. T., Mahoney, M. P., Liu, L., & Fogg, L. F. (1994). Dark goggles and bright light improve circadian rhythm adaptation to night-shift work. *Sleep, 17.*

Gander, P. H., Graeber, R. C., Connel, L. J., & Gregory, K. B. (1991). *Crew factors in flight operations: VIII. Factors influencing sleep timing and subjective sleep quality in commercial long-haul flight crews.* NASA Technical Memorandum 103852.

Graeber, R. C. (1994). Jet lag and sleep disruption. In M. H. Kryger, T. Roth, & W. C. Dement (Eds.), *Principles and practice of sleep medicine* (2nd ed., pp. 463–470). Philadelphia: Saunders.

Graeber, R. C., Lauber, J. K., Connel, L. J., & Gander, P. H. (1986). International aircrew sleep and wakefulness after multiple time zone flights: A cooperative study. *Aviation, Space, and Environmental Medicine, 57*(Suppl.), B3–B9.

Gresham, S., Agnew, H., & Williams, R. (1965). The sleep of depressed patients. *Archives of General Psychiatry, 13,* 503–507.

Harrington, M. E., Rusak, B., & Mistlberger, R. E. (1994). Anatomy and physiology of the mammalian circadian system. In M. H. Kryger, T. Roth, & W. C. Dement (Eds.), *Principles and practice of sleep medicine* (2nd ed.). Philadelphia: Saunders.

Jacklet, J. W. (1985). The neurobiology of circadian rhythm generators. *TINS, 8,* 69–73.

Kamei, R., Hughes, L., Miles, L., & Dement, W. C. (1979). Advanced sleep phase syndrome studied in a time isolation facility. *Chronobiologia, 6,* 115.

Kamgar-Parsi, B., Wehr, T. A., & Gillin, J. C. (1983). Successful treatment of human non-24-hour sleep-wake syndrome. *Sleep, 6,* 257–264.

Klein, T., Martens, H., Derk-Jan, D., Kronauer, R. E., Seely, E. W., & Czeisler, C. A. (1993). Circadian sleep regulation in the absence of light perception: Chronic non-24-hour circadian rhythm sleep disorder in a blind man with a regular 24-hour sleep-wake schedule. *Sleep, 16,* 333–343.

Kokkoris, C. P., Weitzman, E. D., Pollak, C. P., Speilman, A. J., Czeisler, C. A., & Bradlow, H. (1978). Long-term ambulatory temperature monitoring in a subject with a hypernycthemeral sleep-wake cycle disturbance. *Sleep, 1,* 177–190.

Mikami, A., Sugita, Y., Teshima, Y., & Iijima, S. (1987). A 48-hour sleep-wake schedule in a patient with parkinsonism. *Sleep Research, 16,* 625.

Miles, L. E., Raynal, D. M., & Wilson, M. A. (1977). Blind man living in normal society has circadian rhythms of 24.9 hours. *Science, 198,* 421–423.

Miles, L. E. M., & Wilson, M. A. (1977). High incidence of cyclic sleep/wake disorders in the blind. *Sleep Research, 6,* 192.

Moldofsky, H., Musisi, S., & Phillipson, E. A. (1986). Treatment of a case of advanced sleep phase syndrome by phase advance chronotherapy. *Sleep, 9,* 61–65.

Moore, R. Y. (1978). Central neural control of circadian rhythms. In W. F. Ganong & L. Martini (Eds.), *Frontiers in neuroendocrinology.* New York: Raven Press.

Nicholson, A. N. (1994). Aircrew and their sleep. In J. Ernsting & P. King (Eds.), *Aviation medicine.* (pp. 576–584). London: Butterworth.

Nicholson, A. N., Pascoe, P. A., Spencer, M. B., & Benson, A. J. (1993). Jet lag and motion sickness. *British Medical Bulletin, 49,* 285–304.

Nicholson, A. N., Pascoe, P. A., Spencer, M. B., Stone, B. M., & Green, R. L. (1986). Nocturnal sleep and daytime alertness of aircrew after transmeridian flights. *Aviation, Space, and Environmental Medicine, 57*(Suppl.), B42–B52.

Nicholson, A. N., Pascoe, P. A., Spencer, M. B., Stone, B. M., Roehrs, T., & Roth, T. (1986). Sleep after transmeridian flights. *Lancet, 2,* 1205–1208.

Okawa, M., Nanami, T., Wada, S., Shimizu, T., Hishikawa, Y., Sasaki, H., Nagamine, H., & Takahashi, K. (1987). Four congenitally blind children with circadian sleep-wake rhythm disorder. *Sleep, 10,* 101–110.

Pelayo, R. P., Thorpy, M. J., & Glovinsky, P. (1988). Prevalence of delayed sleep phase syndrome among adolescents. *Sleep Research, 17,* 391.

Roehrs, T., & Roth, T. (1994). Chronic insomnias associated with circadian rhythm disorders. In M. H. Kryger, T. Roth, & W. C. Dement (Eds.), *Principles and practice of sleep medicine* (2nd ed., pp. 477–482). Philadelphia: Saunders.

Sasaki, M., Kurosaki, Y., Mori, A., & Endo, S. (1986). Patterns of sleep and wakefulness before and after transmeridian flight in commercial airline pilots. *Aviation, Space, and Environmental Medicine, 57*(Suppl.), B29–B42.

Terman, M., Lewy, A. J., Dijk, D. J., Boulos, Z., Eastman, C. I., & Campell, S. (1995). Light treatment for sleep disorders: Consensus report. IV. Sleep phase and duration disturbance. *Journal of Biological Rhythms, 10,* 135–147.

Thorpy, M. J., Korman, E., Speilman, A. J., & Glovinsky, P. B. (1988). Delayed sleep phase syndrome in adolescents. *Journal of Adolescent Health Care, 9,* 22–27.

Wagner, D. R. (1990). Circadian rhythm sleep disorders. In M. J. Thorpy (Ed.), *Handbook of sleep disorders (pp. 493–530).* New York: Marcel Dekker.

Weitzman, E. D., Czeisler, C. A., Coleman, R. M., Dement, W. C., Richardson, G., & Pollak, C. P. (1979). Delayed sleep phase syndrome: A biological rhythm disorder. *Sleep Research, 8,* 221.

Weitzman, E. D., Czeisler, C. A., Coleman, R. M., Speilman, A. J., Zimmerman, J. C., & Dement, W. C. (1981). Delayed sleep phase syndrome: A chronobiological disorder with sleep-onset insomnia. *Archives of General Psychiatry, 38,* 737–746.

Wever, R. (1979). *The circadian system of man: Results of experiments under temporal isolation.* New York: Springer-Verlag.

12

Shift Work

Timothy H. Monk

I t was mentioned in chapter 2 that *Homo sapiens* is a diurnal creature, endowed with biological processes that work under the assumption that the night will be taken up with sleep and the daytime with activity. This temporal orientation is accomplished by the generation of rhythms with a period of about 1 day, which are referred to as *circadian rhythms*. Circadian rhythms are generated by an area of the brain known as the suprachiasmatic nucleus (SCN) and are, to a large extent, endogenous and self-sustaining (Moore, 1982). The timing mechanism of the SCN takes several days to adjust to a new routine (Aschoff, Hoffman, Pohl, & Wever, 1975). Shift workers who are required to work at night or to rotate between morning, evening, and night shifts are therefore fighting against their own biology as well as against a society that expects work during the day, recreation in the evening, and rest at night. There are about 20 million shift workers by the broadest definition; about 22% of the U.S. workforce (16% of full-time and 47% of part-time employees) have at least some experience of regular work outside the "standard" day-work window (Mellor, 1986).

A recent government report (Office of Technology Assessment [OTA], 1991) has emphasized that expert opinion among those who study biological rhythms (chronobiologists) holds the view that shift work is a potentially harmful stressor for the worker. It is surprising, therefore, that protective legislation concerning shift work has been lacking in the United States (see Table 1). A number of recent reviews

Table 1

Regulation of Work, Rest, and Shift Work in Three Countries

Work issue	Germany	Japan	United States
Major source of regulation	Legislation	Legislation	State legislation
Maximum daily hours	10; RC	8	No general regulations; RC
Maximum weekly hours	48; RC	48, averaged over 4 weeks; RC	40
Rest during the day	0.5 hours if work exceeds 6 hours; RWC	45 minutes if work exceeds 6 hours; 1 hour if it exceeds 8	No general regulations
Minimum rest between days or shifts	11 uninterrupted hours; RC	No general regulations	No general regulations
Minimum weekly rest	24 hours, usually on Sunday; RC	1 day	No general regulations
Shift work (except night work)	May work up to 16 hours once every 3 weeks to change shift but must be granted uninterrupted rest of 24 hours at least twice during the 3 weeks; RC	Maximum of 10 hours/day; maximum of 60 hours/week averaged over 4 weeks; RC	No general regulations
Night work only	No general regulations; RW	Extra pay; RWC	No general regulations
Data regulations are valid	1986	1986	1986

Note. RC = restrictions on children; RW = restrictions on women; RWC = restrictions on women and children. From *Biological Rhythms: Implications for the Worker*, by the Office of Technology Assessment, 1991, Washington, DC: U.S. Government Printing Office. Adapted with permission.

have documented the deleterious effects of shift work, particularly risks of gastrointestinal dysfunction (Rutenfranz, Colquhoun, Knauth, & Ghata, 1977) and cardiovascular disease (Knutsson, Akerstedt, Orth-Gomer, Jonsson, 1986). In terms of mental health, rather little evidence has been gathered. Indirectly, Gordon, Cleary, Parker, and Czeisler (1985) showed increases in alcohol and tranquilizer use in rotating-shift workers. Tasto and Colligan (1978) found similar increases in rotating-shift workers and also higher neuroticism scores in shift workers failing to cope, a finding in agreement with several European studies (reviewed by Cole, Loving, & Kripke, 1990). In Austria, Koller et al. (1981) presented a useful review of the literature from several decades ago. Their conclusions were mixed, possibly because of the problem that *existing* shift workers are a "survivor population," reducing the likelihood that a simple comparison of shift workers with day workers would achieve significance. Koller et al. (1981) did find, however, in their own studies, "specific psychosomatic symptoms and disorders significantly more often in shift workers. These symptoms markedly worsened after 20–25 years of shift experience. Furthermore, we found a highly irritated ex-shift worker group with an outstanding high percentage of sleep disturbances, noise sensitivity and psychosomatic complaints" (p. 467).

Various published studies have suggested remedies that might help shift workers in their coping problems. Czeisler et al. (1990), for example, evaluated the use of extremely bright lights at work during the night shift and darkened bedrooms at home in speeding up the realignment of the biological clock, showing the techniques to work well in highly controlled conditions. With the same purpose in mind, Eastman (1987, 1990) has been using "light boxes" (capable of delivering daylight levels of illumination) in the evening at workers' homes, coupled with goggles to limit unwanted daylight exposure during the day. Walsh and colleagues (Walsh, Muehlbach, & Schweitzer, 1984; Walsh, Sugerman, Muehlbach, & Schweitzer, 1988) showed that hypnotics can improve daytime sleep propensity and lessen nighttime sleep propensity in night workers. Harma, Ilmarinen, Knauth, Rutenfranz, and Hanninen (1988) showed the benefits of an exercise program, and Sack and colleagues (personal communication, 1995) found the hormone melatonin to be helpful. Other studies have addressed the speed and direction of shift rotation (see reviews by Folkard, 1992; Monk, 1986; Wilkinson, 1992). There is a need, however, for a structure or framework to encompass the body of information that has been and still needs to be gathered regarding the problems of coping with shift work and the solutions put forward to counter them.

In applying this knowledge for the benefit of shift workers, it is important to recognize that different target audiences require different types of information. Different educational programs need to be provided to the workforce, management, and governmental agencies. It is futile to educate a group in an area in which the members have little influence. For example, the individual shift worker can make changes in his or her lifestyle, bedroom, and diet but can often do little about shift schedules or ambient lighting at work. Equally, the employer can do something about shift schedules, ambient lighting, and canteen facilities but cannot prevent workers from taking a second job or adopting unhelpful behaviors related to sleep or circadian rhythms. Often, employers need governmental regulations to provide an "even playing field" to allow them to remain competitive while adopting procedures more appropriate to their workforce, and they definitely need government funding of the basic and clinical research on which those procedures are based. Thus, information about research needs and possible rational benefits should be provided to governmental agencies.

The study of shift work in Europe and Japan has benefited from government-financed research groups, which have conducted studies that have been reasonably free of interference from special interest groups and have provided "generic" findings that are published in the open literature and are applicable to many different work situations. Unfortunately, in the United States most shift work research is conducted on a consultant basis by moonlighting academic researchers; a lot of U.S. research into shift work has never appeared in the open literature.

The Three-Factor Model

This model of shift work coping ability (taken from Monk, 1988) divides shift work coping determinants into three areas: circadian, sleep, and social–domestic factors (see Figure 1). All three serve to determine the individual's ability to cope with shift work, and all three are interrelated. For example, shift workers' sleep depends on the state of their circadian system and the tranquillity of their household; their circadian system depends on the degree of fragmentation of their sleep and the domestic demands on their daily routine; and their domestic harmony depends on the degree to which they are continually sleep-deprived or

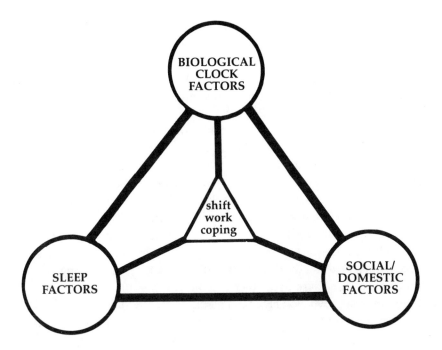

Figure 1. Schematic model of the triad of factors influencing shift work coping ability. From "Coping With the Stress of Shift Work," by T. H. Monk, 1988, *Work & Stress, 2,* 170. Reprinted with permission.

suffering from jet-lag-like symptoms. It is important to note that a failure in any one of the three components of the triad can negate any advances made in the other two. For example, a worker who has plenty of sleep and a perfectly adjusted circadian system fails to cope with shift work if those gains are won at the expense of domestic responsibilities, with possible imminent divorce.

The three components of the triad are considered here in turn, with detailed attention to the various effects. Because the division is arbitrary and the factors interrelated, much of the richness and complexity of the various forces and pressures may be obscured.

Circadian Factors

In discussing circadian factors, we are concerned with the circadian system, or biological clock, whose workings produce the various circadian rhythms that provide the psychological and physiological milieu for the regular cycling of sleep and wakefulness. That cycling presumes a diurnal pattern of restful sleep at night and active wakefulness during the day; in night work and rotating shift situations, therefore, the circadian system has to be realigned to a routine that is more appropriate to the shift worker's schedule. This realignment process is accomplished by the various time cues, or *zeitgebers*, that impinge on the individual (see chapter 2). Zeitgebers can be social, such as meal timing and interpersonal interactions, or physical, such as daylight and darkness (Wever, 1979). Daylight illumination appears to be a particularly potent human circadian zeitgeber (Czeisler et al., 1986; Wever, Poiasek, & Wildgruber, 1983), an unfortunate fact for the hapless night worker trying to obtain a nocturnal circadian orientation. A number of studies both in the laboratory (reviewed by Aschoff et al., 1975; Wever, 1979) and in the field (Knauth & Rutenfranz, 1976) have shown that the adjustment process is a slow one, with many days required. Under normal working conditions, complete phase adjustment to night shifts almost never occurs (Czeisler et al., 1990; Folkard, Monk, & Lobban, 1978).

From the point of view of the work situation, the most important determinant of the status of the circadian system is the particular shift or rotation that the individual is being asked to work. Although most experts agree that the weekly rotating-shift systems are the worst, there is still much controversy about whether very slowly or very rapidly rotating shift systems are the more viable alternatives. The Atlantic Ocean appears to divide those favoring the rapidly rotating systems popular in Europe (Akerstedt, 1985; Wedderburn, 1967) from those promoting the every-3-weeks rotating systems favored by many American authors (Czeisler, Moore-Ede, & Coleman, 1982). Even within Europe, however, there is a lively controversy between those favoring permanent, or fixed, night work and those favoring rapid rotation (Folkard, 1992; Wilkinson, 1992). As discussed by Monk (1986, 1988), the debate rests on the importance that is given to avoiding internal dissociation (a state of disharmony between the various components of the circadian system) as opposed to inappropriate phasing (the need to sleep and work at totally inappropriate points on the circadian curve). Consideration of the type of work to be done may help in resolving this debate. Study of the heterogeneity of circadian performance rhythms has suggested that cognitively loaded tasks may be particularly well suited to rapidly rotating systems, whereas monotonous driving, quality control, and inspection tasks might be better suited to slow rotation (Folkard & Monk, 1979, 1985).

Age is a particularly crucial determinant of circadian adjustment. Studies by Reinberg et al. (1980) and Foret, Bensimon, Benoit, and Vieux (1981) have demonstrated that older people find shift work much harder to deal with than do their younger counterparts. Indeed, there appears to be a certain age—the worker's late 40s or early 50s—when shift work tolerance, which may hitherto have been fairly good, suddenly disappears, leaving the shift worker totally unable to cope. Demographics are changing, with greater proportions of the population over 50; by the late 1990s, when the baby boomers reach a half century in age, there may be a significant crisis in terms of shift work coping ability, particularly in view of sociopolitical trends away from mandatory retirement and other types of age discrimination. The difficulties experienced by elderly shift workers are primarily with the circadian and sleep factors of the triad (social–domestic factors usually *improve*), and at least some of the problems are thought to be due to the fact that circadian rhythms can show a reduced amplitude (flattening) and move to an earlier timing with advancing age (Brock, 1991). Reinberg and colleagues (1984) even showed a complete lack of 24-hour entrainment in intolerant elderly shift workers.

Clearly related to age is the physical and mental health of the shift worker. With regard to physical health, there are some diseases and conditions, such as diabetes, cardiovascular disease, insomnia, epilepsy, and peptic ulcers, that contraindicate shift work (Scott & LaDou, 1990). With regard to mental health, it is distressing how little is known of the incidence of psychopathology in shift work, particularly when the link between psychopathology (particularly depression) and circadian dysfunction has been so well established in the psychiatric literature (Wehr & Goodwin, 1983). At present, there is little evidence concerning whether shift work can induce a major depression. The only information available comes from rather limited symptom reports; there are no definitive studies using established diagnostic criteria (Cole et al., 1990).

Even in psychologically healthy individuals, psychological and chronobiological trait markers can be useful as predictors of shift work tolerance. The circadian trait of "morningness" (Horne & Ostberg, 1976) is the most obvious of these, and a number of authors have shown that extreme morning types suffer more from shift work than their evening-type counterparts (e.g., Hildebrandt & Stratmann, 1979). Reasons for this difference may include the reduced susceptibility to physical time cues evidenced by evening types and the difficulties that morning types have in sleeping during the morning hours. Only one rigorous psychometric study using questionnaires concerning circadian rhythms has been done (Smith, Reilly, & Midkiff, 1978), and much more work in this area needs to be done. One positive development has been the production of a standard shift work index (SSI; Folkard, 1993), which allows a standardization of the questions asked. The SSI is now in use worldwide and has been translated into eight languages. In studies of personality, there remains a need for the application of more sophisticated instruments. Using simple tests, shift work adjustment has been shown to be poorer in persons with the trait of neurotic introversion (Colquhoun & Folkard, 1978) and perhaps to lead to increases in neuroticism (Meers, Maasen, & Verhaegen, 1978).

Sleep Factors

Like circadian factors, the sleep of the shift worker is radically affected by the type of shift system he or she works under. Knauth and coworkers (1980) documented the different lengths of sleep obtained under the various shift systems, showing decrements for night and early-morning shifts. They pointed out that starting times are particularly important in this regard. Although the employer might consider a shift starting at 6:00 a.m. to be a normal day shift, the employees have to wake up at 4:30 a.m. and have some degree of sleep loss. Also important in this regard is overtime, which can make a mockery of everyone's good intentions and severely impact all three factors in the triad.

The importance of age has been discussed previously in relation to circadian factors. For the elderly or even late-middle-aged shift worker, the sleep fragility characteristic of age is compounded with the same characteristic of shift work, often producing a problem that can be solved only by a move to day work. In a study of oil refinery workers, for example, Koller, Kundi, and Cervinka (1978) found that fewer than 20% of the sample expected to continue with shift work until retirement.

The area of sleep need is a complex one. Clearly, those who need less sleep fare better in shift work than those who need more. As Tepas and Mahan (1986) pointed out, this fact may lead shift work researchers to erroneous conclusions. In a large survey study, these researchers showed that night workers who liked night work reported getting less sleep per week than those who disliked it. At least part of the sleep reduction reported for night workers compared with day workers might be explained by a shorter sleep need in this self-selected sample. It certainly remains true, however, that sleep restriction remains a significant problem for many shift workers. In general, shift workers get about 7 hours less sleep per week than their day working counterparts (Akerstedt, 1985).

The problem of the abuse of alcohol, caffeine, nicotine, and other drugs in shift workers is in need of further study. Although some believe such abuse to be rampant in night- and rotating-shift workers, the hard evidence is only preliminary (Gordon et al., 1985; Tasto & Colligan, 1978). It also is unknown whether the abuse comes from the increased opportunities that arise with the lower supervision levels on the night shift or whether it is simply a crutch used by the shift worker to remain awake at work and fall asleep at home.

Related to this issue is the question of sleep hygiene. Sleep hygiene is the label given by sleep disorders practitioners to a series of behavioral measures designed primarily to improve the sleep of persons with insomnia (Hauri & Olmstead, 1986; see also chapter 16, this volume). These measures include limiting the use of drugs, alcohol, and caffeine; imposing regular bedtime rituals; keeping to a regular sleep–wake cycle; and avoiding activities other than sleep and lovemaking in the bedroom. Clearly, such procedures have to be modified in the shift worker's case, but they need to be included in any shift worker education program (Monk & Folkard, 1992).

Some Japanese researchers have shown that sleep "on the job" can represent a useful and workable strategy for improving shift work coping ability (Kogi, 1985). Even when not officially sanctioned, however, sleep on the night shift is extremely common, and researchers would be foolish to ignore it. Many problems with the implementation of new work systems arise because these practices are unrecognized by day working managers who are out of touch with what life is like on the night shift. It is often far better to recognize that such practices exist and to formalize and regulate them than to ignore them.

Social and Domestic Factors

Social and domestic factors probably are the least studied part of the shift-work coping triad, despite being extremely important (Colligan & Rosa, 1990; Walker, 1978, 1985). The reasons are clear: Although it is difficult to obtain sleep and circadian measures from shift workers, it is considerably more difficult to obtain and quantify details of the minutiae of their family life and to be sure that conclusions are drawn from valid data.

An example of such difficulties is provided by the practice of moonlighting, or holding a second job, which is often unreported by the employee for various reasons. Like night-shift sleeping, the practice is ubiquitous and is often the reason some people actively choose to do shift work (Mott, Mann, McLoughlin, & Warwick 1965). Likewise, it often represents a stumbling block to the imposition of new work schedules because such schedules may impede the individual's ability to perform the second job.

The other major social and domestic influence is the need to care for children and manage a household. In present Western cultures, this burden primarily falls to women, and as Gadbois (1981) pointed out, any gender differences in shift-work coping ability are much more likely to be due to societal and domestic demands than to biological differences. Clinicians and educators should be careful not to prescribe shift work coping routines that work well on paper but neglect to take into account the need to take the children to school during the week or to a soccer game on a Saturday morning. Such domestic pressures may make it impossible for shift workers to retain a continuous nocturnal lifestyle, even if their shift schedule is a fixed or slowly rotating one. Domestic responsibilities often require a diurnal orientation during days off, making the rotation in sleep–wake schedule weekly and circadian adjustment therefore incomplete (Monk, 1986; Van Loon, 1963).

Consideration of commuting time is crucially important when 12-hour shifts and overtime are considered. Often, particularly in the United States, commuting involves 90–120 minutes of hard driving per day and should certainly not be regarded as part of the shift worker's recreation time. Indeed, Richardson, Miner, and Czeisler (1990) published data showing that traffic accidents on the way home from work represent a significant risk for rotating-shift workers. One in 5 of this group's sample reported a traffic accident or near miss attributable to sleepiness while driving during the preceding 5 years.

Community support can be a crucial determinant of shift work coping ability. Many shift workers regard themselves as relegated to "marginal" citizenship, forbidden by their work schedule to participate in community recreational and religious activities, which are based on the assumption that evenings and weekends are free for meetings, practice, games, and rehearsals. One could argue that they

are just as excluded as a handicapped person who is denied wheel-
chair access to a museum.

Areas of Application—Three Approaches

Having described the model, I return to the question of how the expertise of psychologists might most effectively be used in improving the
lot of the shift worker. As mentioned previously, different approaches
are called for, depending on the recipient of the advice. The three
approaches considered here are research initiatives, employer counseling, and employee treatment.

Research Initiatives

As in any clinical field, there is a need for research to ensure the best
possible treatment for the patient who is a shift worker. First, there is a
need for rigorous parallel studies using epidemiological techniques to
determine the health risks (mental and physical) of shift work. These
studies should go beyond simple "day worker versus shift worker"
comparisons and move to a sophisticated risk exposure model of the
form employed by Knutsson et al. (1986) in the area of cardiovascular
disease. It is a tragedy that no one can accurately tell shift workers (or
their employers) whether their work schedule is shortening their life
span, irreparably damaging their health, or simply causing transient
difficulties and symptoms.

A second area of research should concentrate on developing a suit-
able animal model of shift work so that the longevity questions can be
addressed. Such models will not, of course, address the psychosocial
stressors of shift work, but limited information from the biological
domain would clearly represent progress. At the moment, the findings coming from the animal literature are mixed and confusing
(OTA, 1991).

Research in the domain of circadian rhythms is also needed to evaluate further the general efficacy of countermeasures such as bright
lights, hypnotics, melatonin, and changes in shift schedule. There is a
strong need for different approaches to be evaluated in parallel,
preferably by a disinterested third party who has no professional or
financial stake in the success of any one intervention. All too often,
studies simply seek to demonstrate an improvement (pre- versus

postintervention) from a single manipulation that the investigators believe will be helpful.

Research is also needed in the domain of sleep. Like the issue of circadian desynchronization, the issues of health and longevity effects from a lifetime of partial sleep deprivation have not been fully addressed. Kripke, Simons, Garfinkel, and Hammond (1979) reported indirect evidence that short sleepers have a reduced life span, but so too do long sleepers (7.5–8 hr per night appears optimal)—the issue is clearly a complex one. Concerning health issues, evidence is now forthcoming about immunological consequences of prolonged sleep loss (Dinges, Douglas, & Zangg, 1993). The sleep deprivation field has the benefit of a working animal model (Rechtschaffen, Gilliland, Bergmann, & Winter, 1983) and some useful work on performance consequences (see review by Dinges & Kribbs, 1991). Although the work is further advanced than in the circadian domain, research in the sleep domain needs to be focused more on the long-term consequences of partial sleep loss rather than on the acute effects of 2 or 3 days without sleep.

With regard to the social domain, the area is wide open for exploration. Does shift work lead to divorce? Do the children of shift workers have poorer school grades? Do shift workers get fewer benefits from the community? How do the social networks of shift workers differ from those of day workers? Would family counseling be a useful tool in helping shift workers to cope? Should shift workers be regarded as a socially disadvantaged group? Current findings are preliminary only (Colligan & Rosa, 1990).

Employer Counseling

The major questions to be answered for most employers relate closely to the "bottom line," or the eventual financial cost, rather than to how long their employees will live or how satisfying their personal relationships will be. The question of cost is not as simple as it may appear, however. First, productivity may be most clearly expressed in terms of absenteeism, poor morale, and job turnover rather than individual performance efficiency in the laboratory sense; therefore, employee well-being becomes a productivity issue. Second, lawsuits have started to appear from employees who were injured in traffic accidents on the drive home or developed disabling illnesses and hold their work schedule, and thus their employer, to blame (OTA, 1991). Such legal claims would undoubtedly benefit from the testimony of experts concerning the reality and ubiquity of shift work problems and the degree to which U.S. legislation lags behind that of much of the rest of the industrialized world (see Table 1).

The development of shift work training and discussion programs and the formation of self-help groups can be a cost-effective solution for the employer, particularly when combined with a change in the shift schedule to remove some of the worst excesses (in a chronobiological sense) of the old system (Czeisler et al., 1982; Orth-Gomer, 1983). Further research is needed to refine what goes into such programs and how they can most effectively be implemented.

Employee Intervention

I use the word *intervention* here in a general sense, rather than restricted to a formal clinician–patient situation. It encompasses all the interactions between the psychologist and the individual shift worker, be they in educational, screening, counseling, or clinical treatment settings.

It is probably unhelpful to the individual shift worker for the psychologist to talk in the global generalities that are more appropriate for employers. Most affected employees are committed to shift work for one reason or another, and the switch to day work may be impossible for them. Rather, they need to hear specifics on how they can use the knowledge gleaned from research to create specific coping strategies that are relevant to their particular circumstance.

Information to be shared regarding circadian rhythms may be suggested by common sense and knowledge of human chronobiology. The eventual aim is to help shift workers to realize the strengths and limitations of their circadian system, to set goals for the system, and to follow behavior patterns that will accomplish those goals. The shift worker should learn which zeitgebers and behaviors are important and which will have positive and which negative effects, given their particular situation (Monk & Folkard, 1992). That approach has the advantage of being flexible should the shift worker's schedule change and a new set of circadian goals become appropriate.

In the sleep field, too, there is much for the shift worker to learn. Many shift workers do not realize the importance of consolidated sleep episodes and other sleep hygiene practices. Like general advice regarding the circadian system, the learning of positive sleep hygiene practices will benefit the individual in many different situations. Here, particularly, the watchword has to be pragmatism. Any advice that appears too dogmatic or unrealistic (e.g., "avoid all caffeine and alcohol") will be rejected out of hand by the shift worker, and the whole purpose of the exercise will be lost. There is so much progress to be made in improving the sleep of shift workers that even modest goals may lead to significant improvements.

As this chapter has repeatedly pointed out, the three factors of the triad are mutually interactive, and social–domestic factors are particularly important agents for facilitating (or wrecking) coping strategies in the circadian and sleep domains. I found out in an intervention study in Connecticut that it was pointless to preach about sleep hygiene and zeitgeber exposure to an individual who had been thrown out of his house and was sleeping in the car. Unfortunately, there is no resource network in place to help shift workers and their families cope with the problem. It would be helpful if "shift worker clinics" could be set up in areas of shift work concentration. Such clinics could be staffed by sleep clinicians, psychologists, and family therapists whose mission would be to provide both clinic-based and community-based support for the population of shift workers they serve.

At present, there are few places that the shift worker can go to for help. The family physician is likely to be the primary contact, but circadian principles still do not figure greatly in many medical school curricula, and a prescription for sleeping pills is often the only outcome. More useful help may come from the sleep disorders clinics that are springing up throughout the United States. However, unless the center is accredited by the American Sleep Disorders Association, the patient is likely to receive only a diagnosis, with little practical help. One major goal regarding shift work should be to provide the medical community with a better understanding of human chronobiology so that the treatment given to shift workers is based on an understanding of the whole circadian system, rather than simply an attempt to treat the symptoms of sleep disruption.

Conclusion

The problem of shift work is not simply a chronobiological problem, a sleep problem, or a social problem. Rather, it is a complex interaction of all three. Only when researchers and clinicians recognize these interactions can satisfactory strategies be developed to ameliorate the difficulties. Developers of these strategies should recognize that the advice and information to be given depends crucially on who is destined to receive it.

REFERENCES

Akerstedt, T. (1985). Adjustment of physiological circadian rhythms and the sleep-wake cycle to shift work. In S. Folkard & T. H. Monk (Eds.), *Hours of work: Temporal factors in work scheduling* (pp. 185–197). New York: Wiley.

Aschoff, J., Hoffman, K., Pohl, H., & Wever, R. A. (1975). Re-entrainment of circadian rhythms after phase-shifts of the zeitgeber. *Chronobiologia, 2,* 23–78.

Cole, R. J., Loving, R. T., & Kripke, D. F. (1990). Psychiatric aspects of shift work. *Occupational Medicine, 5,* 301–314.

Colligan, M. J., & Rosa, R. R. (1990). Shift work effects on social and family life. *Occupational Medicine, 5,* 315–322.

Colquhoun, W. P., & Folkard, S. (1978). Personality differences in body-temperature rhythm and their relation to its adjustment to night work. *Ergonomics, 21,* 811–817.

Czeisler, C. A., Allan, J. S., Strogatz, S. H., Ronda, J. M., Sanchez, R., Rios, C. D., Freitag, W. D., Richardson, G. S., & Kronauer, R. E. (1986). Bright light resets the human circadian pacemaker independent of the timing of the sleep-wake cycle. *Science, 233,* 667–671.

Czeisler, C. A., Johnson, M. P., Duffy, J. F., Brown, E. N., Ronda, J. M., & Kronauer, R. E. (1990). Exposure to bright light and darkness to treat physiologic maladaptation to night work. *New England Journal of Medicine, 322,* 1253–1259.

Czeisler, C. A., Moore-Ede, M. C., & Coleman, R. M. (1982). Rotating shift work schedules that disrupt sleep are improved by applying circadian principles. *Science, 217,* 460–463.

Dinges, D. F., Douglas, S. D., & Zaugg, L. (1993). Human immune function prior to, during, and following recovery from 64 hours without sleep. *Sleep Research, 22,* 329.

Dinges, D. F., & Kribbs, N. B. (1991). Performing while sleepy: Effects of experimentally-induced sleepiness. In T. H. Monk (Ed.), *Sleep, sleepiness and performance* (pp. 97–128). Chichester, England: Wiley.

Eastman, C. I. (1987). Bright light in work-sleep schedules for shift workers: Application of circadian rhythm principles. In L. Rensing, U. an der Heiden, & M. C. Mackey (Eds.), *Temporal disorder in human oscillatory systems* (pp. 176–185). New York: Springer-Verlag.

Eastman, C. I. (1990). Circadian rhythms and bright light: Recommendations for shift work. *Work & Stress, 4,* 245–260.

Folkard, S. (1992). Is there a "best compromise" shift system? *Ergonomics, 35,* 1453–1463.

Folkard, S. (1993). The standard shiftwork index. *Ergonomics, 36,* 313–314.

Folkard, S., & Monk, T. H. (1979). Shift work and performance. *Human Factors, 21,* 483–492.

Folkard, S., & Monk, T. H. (1985). *Hours of work: Temporal factors in work scheduling.* New York: Wiley.

Folkard, S., Monk, T. H., & Lobban, M. C. (1978). Short and long-term adjustment of circadian rhythms in "permanent" night nurses. *Ergonomics, 21,* 785–799.

Foret, J., Bensimon, G., Benoit, O., & Vieux, N. (1981). Quality of sleep as a function of age and shift work. In A. Reinberg, N. Vieux, & P. Andlauer (Eds.), *Night and shift work: Biological and social aspects* (pp. 149–160). Oxford, England: Pergamon Press.

Gadbois, C. (1981). Women on night shift: Interdependence of sleep and off-the-job activities. In A. Reinberg, N. Vieux, & P. Andlauer (Eds.), *Night and shift work: Biological and social aspects* (pp. 223–227). Oxford, England: Pergamon Press.

Gordon, N. P., Cleary, P. D., Parker, C. E., & Czeisler, C. A. (1985). Sleeping pill use, heavy drinking and other unhealthful practices and consequences associated with shift work: A national probability sample study. *Sleep Research, 14,* 94.

Harma, M. I., Ilmarinen, J., Knauth, P., Rutenfranz, J., & Hanninen, O. (1988). Physical training intervention in female shift workers: I. The effects of intervention on fitness, fatigue, sleep and psychosomatic symptoms. *Ergonomics, 31,* 51–63.

Hauri, P. J., & Olmstead, E. (1986). Persistent psychophysiologic (learned) insomnia. *Sleep, 9,* 38–53.

Hildebrandt, G., & Stratmann, I. (1979). Circadian system response to night work in relation to the individual circadian phase position. *International Archives of Occupational and Environmental Health, 43,* 73–83.

Horne, J. A., & Ostberg, O. (1976). A self-assessment questionnaire to determine morningness-eveningness in human circadian rhythms. *International Journal of Chronobiology, 4,* 97–110.

Knauth, P., & Rutenfranz, J. (1976). Experimental shift work studies of permanent night, and rapidly rotating, shift systems: I. Circadian rhythm of body temperature and re-entrainment at shift change. *International Archives of Occupational and Environmental Health, 37,* 125–137.

Knauth, P., Rutenfranz, J., Schulz, H., Bruder, S., Romberg, H. P., Decoster, F., & Kiesswetter, E. (1980). Experimental shift work studies of permanent night, and rapidly rotating, shift systems. II. Behaviour of various characteristics of sleep. *International Archives of Occupational and Environmental Health, 46,* 111–125.

Knutsson, A., Akerstedt, T., Orth-Gomer, K., & Jonsson, B. G. (1986). Increased risk of ischaemic heart disease in shift workers. *Lancet, 2,* 89–92.

Kogi, K. (1985). Introduction to the problems of shift work. In S. Folkard & T. H. Monk (Eds.), *Hours of work: Temporal factors in work scheduling* (pp. 165–184). New York: Wiley.

Koller, M., Haider, M., Kundi, M., Cervinka, R., Katsching, H., & Kufferle, B. (1981). Possible relations of irregular working hours to psychiatric psychosomatic disorders. In A. Reinberg, N. Vieux, & P. Andlauer (Eds.), *Night and shift work: Biological and social aspects* (pp. 465–472). Oxford, England: Pergamon Press.

Koller, M., Kundi, M., & Cervinka, R. (1978). Field studies of shift work at an Austrian oil refinery: I. Health and psychosocial well-being of workers who drop out of shift work. *Ergonomics, 21*, 835–847.

Kripke, D. F., Simons, R. N., Garfinkel, L., & Hammond, E. C. (1979). Short and long sleep and sleeping pills: Is increased mortality associated? *Archives of General Psychiatry, 36*, 103–116.

Meers, A., Maasen, A., & Verhaegen, P. (1978). Subjective health after six months and after four years of shift work. *Ergonomics, 21*, 857–861.

Mellor, E. F. (1986). Shift work and flexitime: How prevalent are they? *Monthly Labor Review, 109*, 14–21.

Monk, T. H. (1986). Advantages and disadvantages of rapidly rotating shift schedules: A circadian viewpoint. *Human Factors, 28*, 553–557.

Monk, T. H. (1988). Coping with the stress of shift work. *Work & Stress, 2*, 169–172.

Monk, T. H., & Folkard, S. (1992). *Making shift work tolerable.* London: Taylor & Francis.

Moore, R. Y. (1982). The suprachiasmatic nucleus and the organization of a circadian system. *Trends in Neurosciences, 5*, 404–407.

Mott, P. E., Mann, F. C., McLoughlin, Q., & Warwick, D. P. (1965). *Shift work: The social, psychological and physical consequences.* Ann Arbor: University of Michigan Press.

Office of Technology Assessment. (1991). *Biological rhythms: Implications for the worker* (OTA-BA-463). Washington, DC: U.S. Government Printing Office.

Orth-Gomer, K. (1983). Intervention on coronary risk factors by adapting a shift work schedule to biologic rhythmicity. *Psychosomatic Medicine, 45*, 407–415.

Rechtschaffen, A., Gilliland, M. A., Bergmann, B. M., & Winter, J. B. (1983). Physiological correlates of prolonged sleep deprivation in rats. *Science, 221*, 182–184.

Reinberg, A., Andlauer, P., DePrins, J., Malbecq, W., Vieux, N., & Bourdeleau, P. (1984). Desynchronization of the oral temperature circadian rhythm and intolerance to shift work. *Nature, 308*, 272–274.

Reinberg, A., Andlauer, P., Guillet, P., Nicolai, A., Vieux, N., & Laporte, A. (1980). Oral temperature, circadian rhythm amplitude, ageing and tolerance to shift work. *Ergonomics, 23*, 55–64.

Richardson, G. S., Miner, J. D., & Czeisler, C. A. (1990). Impaired driving performance in shift workers: The role of the circadian system in a multifactorial model. *Alcohol, Drugs and Driving, 5, 6*, 265–273.

Rutenfranz, J., Colquhoun, W. P., Knauth, P., & Ghata, J. N. (1977). Biomedical and psychosocial aspects of shift work: A review. *Scandinavian Journal of Work, Environment and Health, 3*, 165–182.

Scott, A. J., & LaDou, J. (1990). Shift work: Effects on sleep and health with recommendations for medical surveillance and screening. *Occupational Medicine, 5*, 273–299.

Smith, C. S., Reilly, C., & Midkiff, K. (1978). Evaluations of three circadian rhythm questionnaires with suggestions for an improved measure of morningness. *Journal of Applied Psychology, 74,* 728–738.

Tasto, D. L., & Colligan, M. J. (1978). *Health consequences of shift work* (Project UR11-4426). Menlo Park, CA: Stanford Research Institute.

Tepas, D. I., & Mahan, R. P. (1986). *The many meanings of sleep.* Paper presented at the annual meeting of the American Psychological Association, Washington, DC.

Van Loon, J. H. (1963). Diurnal body temperature curves in shift workers. *Ergonomics, 6,* 267–272.

Walker, J. M. (1978). *The human aspects of shift work.* Bath, England: Pitman Press.

Walker, J. M. (1985). Social problems of shift work. In S. Folkard & T. H. Monk (Eds.), *Hours of work: Temporal factors in work scheduling* (pp. 211–225). New York: Wiley.

Walsh, J. K., Muehlbach, M. J., & Schweitzer, P. K. (1984). Acute administration of triazolam for the daytime sleep of rotating shift workers. *Sleep, 7,* 223–229.

Walsh, J. K., Sugerman, J. L., Muehlbach, M. J., & Schweitzer, P. K. (1988). Physiological sleep tendency on a simulated night shift: Adaptation and effects of triazolam. *Sleep, 11,* 251–264.

Wedderburn, A. A. I. (1967). Social factors in satisfaction with swiftly rotating shifts. *Occupational Psychology, 41,* 85–107.

Wehr, T. A., & Goodwin, F. K. (1983). Biological rhythms in manic-depressive illness. In T. A. Wehr & F. K. Goodwin (Eds.), *Circadian rhythms in psychiatry* (pp. 129–184). Pacific Grove, CA: Boxwood Press.

Wever, R. A. (1979). *The circadian system of man: Results of experiments under temporal isolation.* New York: Springer-Verlag.

Wever, R. A., Poiasek, J., & Wildgruber, C. M. (1983). Bright light affects human circadian rhythms. *Pfulgers Archives European Journal of Physiology, 396,* 85–87.

Wilkinson, R. T. (1992). How fast should the night shift rotate? *Ergonomics, 35,* 1425–1446.

13

Obstructive Sleep Apnea: Natural History and Varieties of the Clinical Presentation

William C. Orr

O bstructive sleep apnea (OSA) syndrome is a complex disorder of neural respiratory control and upper airway dysfunction resulting in repeated complete and partial occlusion of the upper airway during sleep. In itself, this medical phenomenon would not be of particular interest to psychologists. However, there are several aspects of this disorder that bring it quite naturally into the province of experimental or clinical psychology. First, the airway occlusion is a phenomenon that occurs exclusively during sleep, a behavioral state traditionally part of the study of psychology. Second, the most obvious clinical manifestations of this syndrome are alterations in waking behavior, such as excessive daytime sleepiness; personality changes, such as increased irritability and depression; and decreased performance and work productivity (Guilleminault, 1994; Thawley, 1985). In fact, numerous studies have shown an increase in traffic accidents in patients with documented OSA (Findley, 1990). Not uncommonly, a patient will present to the primary care physician or to a psychologist with chief complaints related to one of these behaviors. Thus, it behooves the practicing physician and psychologist to be aware of the many faces and clinical manifestations of the OSA syndrome. This chapter will review a variety of presentations of this common affliction and will emphasize the behavioral symptoms and manifestations.

Historical Perspective

What is now called the OSA syndrome was initially described by Burwell in 1956 (Burwell, Robin, Whaley, & Bikelman, 1956). Burwell described an obese patient who presented with CO_2 retention, somnolence, and polycythemia. The fundamental pathogenesis was attributed to simple hypoventilation, secondary to obesity-related chest wall constriction. Burwell termed this the *Pickwickian syndrome*, after the character "Joe the fat boy" in the Dickens novel *The Pickwick Papers*. Joe the fat boy was a large, somnolent messenger boy who frequently was described as being extremely sleepy under a variety of inappropriate circumstances. It was not until several years later that individuals meeting the criteria of the Pickwickian syndrome as described by Burwell were found to actually have upper airway obstruction during sleep (Gastaut, Tassinari, & Duron, 1965). These authors described repeated episodes of upper airway obstruction in individuals with obesity, snoring, and symptoms of daytime somnolence. This work, and numerous subsequent studies, have inexorably linked symptoms of snoring, obesity, and daytime sleepiness with sleep-related upper airway obstruction, or the OSA syndrome.

Perhaps the sine qua non of this phenomenon is sonorous snoring. Snoring is a phenomenon that is ubiquitous among adult males and is noted in virtually all patients with OSA. Clinically, OSA patients often report a chronic history of loud snoring and a significant exacerbation in snoring within a few years of presentation to a physician.

Snoring as a Medical Phenomenon

Until recently, snoring was regarded as merely an annoyance confined primarily to the snorer's bed partner. It was the source of many jokes and of frustration among spouses but was rarely taken seriously by the medical community. The establishment of a link between snoring and a serious, if not potentially lethal, medical condition (i.e., OSA) has substantially altered the view of this symptom in the medical community. Certainly, snoring under certain circumstances must be taken seriously and regarded as the indication of a potentially serious medical problem. Epidemiologic studies, for example, have shown that chronic snorers have a predisposition to cardiovascular complications such as myocardial infarction and stroke (Lugaresi, Cirignotta, Montagna, & Sforza, 1994). In a prospective study of twins, those identified as habitual snorers were more often affected by angina pectoris and heart or brain ischemia than were nonsnorers (Partinen & Palomaki, 1985).

Epidemiologic studies of snoring have suggested that chronic snoring (i.e., nearly every night) occurs in about 19% of an unselected population. Men snore more frequently than women. The prevalence of snoring increases with age in both sexes up to age 65. It has been estimated that approximately 60% of men and 40% of women between 41 and 64 years of age are habitual snorers (Lugaresi et al., 1994). There is little doubt that obesity favors snoring, as has been noted earlier in terms of the association of obesity, snoring, and OSA. It has been estimated that approximately 60% of overweight men are habitual snorers, whereas just over 30% of nonobese men were so identified (Mondini et al., 1983).

Beyond the nuisance factor associated with chronic loud snoring, the medical complications of snoring relate to increased upper airway resistance. This can vary from trivial increases in airway resistance associated with minimal and benign snoring to increasing levels associated with increasing impairment of airflow and consequent hypoxemia during sleep. The mechanisms of upper airway obstruction will be discussed subsequently, but first let us examine some clinical aspects of snoring that can be helpful in making a decision as to whether or not the possibility of pathological snoring exists. Certainly, the decibel level of snoring is important. Studies have shown that snoring intensity can often exceed 65 dB and often has been noted to be above the noise level considered safe in the workplace by the Occupational Safety and Health Administration (OSHA; Guilleminault, 1994). The decibel level of snoring certainly correlates well with increased upper airway resistance and potential for airway collapse and impaired inspiratory airflow.

Another factor shown to be very predictive of the presence of significant upper airway occlusion is the observation of respiratory pauses during sleep by the sleeping partner (Crocker et al., 1990). Another sign of somewhat more severe snoring is the persistence of snoring in any sleeping position. If snoring occurs predominantly in the supine position, it is much less likely that the upper airway resistance is sufficiently problematic to result in clinical consequences. For example, if snoring occurs habitually when an individual falls asleep sitting in a chair or immediately after sleep onset, it suggests a somewhat more serious elevation in upper airway resistance.

Snoring has been noted to occur immediately after sleep onset and to increase progressively through the nonrapid eye movement (NREM) stages of sleep to reach a peak during Stage 4. It diminishes somewhat during rapid eye movement (REM) sleep. This seems somewhat paradoxical in that apneic episodes are invariably more predominant and longer during REM sleep (Findley, Wilhoit, & Suratt, 1985). Snoring history now is recognized as an important aspect of any medical history and physical exam and can provide very useful predictive information regarding sleep apnea as a possible contributing factor to a variety of behavioral and psychological symptoms.

Natural History

Understanding the natural history of OSA begins with the most obvious manifestation of abnormal airway resistance: snoring. As already noted, the prevalence of snoring in the general population, and the estimated occurrence of OSA in the general population (defined as an apnea index of greater than 5 per hr) is approximately 4% for males and 2% for females (Young et al., 1993). The latter estimates were made using actual home recordings to document the presence of apneas. In a study of heavily snoring but otherwise asymptomatic men, the incidence of upper airway obstruction (apnea-hypopnea index [AHI] of greater than 5) was 13% (Berry, Webb, Block, & Switzer, 1986). In fact, in our laboratory, we have documented the presence of AHIs of greater than 20 in a similar population (Moran, Orr, Fixley, & Wittels, 1984). Given that the natural precursors to clinically significant OSA exist in appreciable numbers in the general population, especially among males, what are the factors that ultimately lead to the development of clinically significant OSA?

There is little doubt that light or occasional snoring represents no medical risk. On the other hand, death rate during sleep is higher among habitually heavy snorers, and there are data to support the notion that an AHI of greater than 20 is associated with an increased risk of mortality (He, Kryger, Zorick, Conway, & Roth, 1988). Perhaps the most important factor in the eventual development of clinically significant OSA is time. The sequence of upper airway obstruction to heavy snoring to eventual OSA with accompanying excessive daytime sleepiness may take as long as 15 to 20 years. Other risk factors that play a role in the eventual manifestation of this disease would certainly be obesity and the condition of upper airway and craniofacial anatomy. For example, if an individual with moderate tonsillar hypertrophy or a slight degree of retrognathia (a slight posterior displacement of the mandible) has mild snoring, as little as 10 lb of weight gain could result in a marked increase in snoring. If weight gain continued or if weight loss were not accomplished over a period of several years, this could result in clinically significant OSA.

Recent work by Lavie and colleagues has shown that the greatest cause of death in patients with OSA is myocardial infarction (personal communication with P. Lavie). The death rate was shown to be several times that which was associated with individuals without OSA; however, the apnea index itself was not a significant predictor. Age, body mass index, and hypertension were in fact significant predictors. This group has suggested that OSA in and of itself will not kill, but rather it is the comorbid factors of obesity and age that account for the mortality. In fact, these are the same factors that have been identified as important in developing significant OSA (AHI > 5) over time (Young et al., 1993). As alluded to earlier, these studies noted that habitual snorers had a sixfold risk of developing an AHI index of greater than 5. Once manifest, OSA may progress quite rapidly in terms of the severity of its clinical manifestations. Svanborg and colleagues have shown that individuals with OSA in whom repeat sleep studies have been conducted at varying intervals from 6 to 32 months had a rather remarkable exacerbation of apneic episodes as well as the desaturation index (Svanborg & Larsson, 1993).

It appears from this discussion on natural history that the occurrence of repeated episodes of upper airway obstruction during sleep is a necessary but not sufficient condition to produce potentially lethal cardiopulmonary complications such as hypertension and increased risk for cardiovascular complications. However, it should be noted that the clinically significant OSA (AHI > 10) produces a significant hypoxemia and sleep fragmentation. Both of these events have been implicated in the pathogenesis of the profound excessive daytime sleepiness that is seen in the vast majority of these patients (Orr, Imes, Martin, Rogers, & Stahl, 1979). This cannot be ignored as a prominent feature in the issue of morbidity and mortality in patients with OSA because it has been shown in numerous studies by Findley and colleagues that OSA patients have a greater incidence of fatal and nonfatal traffic accidents (Findley, 1990).

Pathogenesis of Upper Airway Obstruction

In understanding how the upper airway remains patent or becomes progressively diminished in circumference, eventually leading to complete occlusion, it is necessary to understand those factors that naturally occur to keep the airway open. In healthy individuals, each inspiratory effort is associated with a collapsing negative pressure and a simultaneous burst of activity from a variety of upper airway muscles that serve to prevent collapse. Perhaps the best example of this comes from work by Harper and Sauerland in which they demonstrated that inspiratory efforts are associated with a concomitant phasic burst of activity from the genioglossus muscle (Harper & Sauerland, 1978). This muscle controls the protrusion and stability of the tongue, and phasic inspiratory activity of this muscle would prevent collapse of the tongue against the posterior pharyngeal wall during inspiration. Studies from our laboratory and others have demonstrated that there are many dilating muscles of the upper airway that act in concert to maintain airway patency and stability during inspiration (Sauerland, Orr, & Hairston, 1981).

The interaction of the dynamic collapsing and dilating forces of the upper airway have been nicely consolidated into a model of upper airway obstruction by Remmers and colleagues (Remmers, deGroot, & Sauerland, 1978). In this model, they integrate their research data showing that upper airway patency or relative patency is maintained if the dilating forces of the upper airway overcome the tendency for the airway to collapse via increased airway resistance and inspiratory effort. It is clear that reflexes exist to ensure increasing inspiratory effort associated with increased resistance to airflow into the lungs. It is also clear that a relatively small-diameter upper airway is more susceptible to collapse than is a normally patent airway (Kuna & Sant'Ambrogio, 1991). Thus, anatomical factors that decrease the cross-sectional area of the upper airway will render it more susceptible to collapse with inspiratory effort.

Extrapolating from this, one can postulate a variety of factors that would lead to airway occlusion by means of either decreasing the dilating forces of the upper airway or increasing the tendency of the upper airway to collapse with inspiratory effort. For example, studies have shown that the timing of the onset of the dilating activation of the upper airway muscles must be precisely timed with diaphragmatic contraction (Strohl, Hensley, Hallett, Saunders, & Ingram, 1980). Obviously, the dilating forces must occur prior to diaphragmatic contraction, and if the onset of upper airway dilation is a fraction of a second too late, the collapsing forces of inspiratory effort (i.e., diaphragmatic contraction) will result in airway collapse. On the other hand, decreasing the cross-sectional diameter of the upper airway by means of a variety of anatomical abnormalities will create a tendency for airway collapse in spite of normal upper airway dilation with inspiration. In fact, it has now been well documented that the vast majority of individuals with OSA do have compromised upper airway diameter (Hoffstein & Slutsky, 1987). This can manifest itself in terms of adenotonsillar hypertrophy, retrognathia, macroglossia (enlarged tongue), or simple obesity with fat deposition in the upper airway, thereby constricting its cross-sectional diameter.

There are considerable data to suggest that the onset of upper airway obstruction results from diminished central drive to breathe. For example, studies in our laboratory have shown that prior to the onset of airway occlusion, there is a progressive decrease in the central drive to breathe that is associated with a concomitant increase in upper airway resistance, resulting in total airway occlusion (Martin, Pennock, Orr, Sanders, & Rogers, 1981). Obviously, during sleep there is an absence of the waking drive to breathe, and it is clear that individuals with OSA manifest their breathing disorder only during sleep. It would appear that sleep does induce a risk that any one of several complex mechanisms may malfunction, thereby predisposing one to upper airway obstruction. Certainly, the complex interaction of these various neurophysiologic mechanisms with sleep is not well understood, but it is clear that the full manifestation of this medical syndrome represents a complex array of neurophysiological and psychophysiological phenomena.

Varieties of the Clinical Presentation

As alluded to earlier, the psychophysiological complexity of the OSA syndrome often results in the manifestation of symptoms that can masquerade as a variety of other conditions. Perhaps the most frequent and obvious misdiagnosis is narcolepsy (Dement, 1976). The confusion here is easy to understand because both conditions have excessive daytime sleepiness as a primary symptom manifestation.

The term *narcolepsy* has frequently been used as synonymous with excessive daytime sleepiness. Not uncommonly, physicians refer to patients with loud snoring and evidence of airway obstruction as having narcolepsy. This simply refers to the fact that such patients may actually present to the referring physician with a primary complaint of excessive daytime sleepiness. It is not understood or appreciated that narcolepsy represents a completely separate and distinct medical entity whose primary presenting symptom is also excessive and uncontrollable daytime sleepiness. There are, however, numerous factors that differentiate these conditions that can be easily obtained from the patients' medical histories.

For example, most narcoleptics have an onset of symptoms in their early teenage years, and the sleepiness has been generally unrelenting since that time. Many patients report being concerned about their sleepiness but are unaware that it represents the manifestation of an actual medical disorder. Many patients report that they do not necessarily feel that there is anything different about them in that they believe that everyone has the same problem with sleepiness. Such patients will often report difficulties in high school or college classes in keeping awake, reprimands in the military for falling asleep on a watch or on duty, or reprimands from work supervisors who have noticed them sleeping on the job. In essence, excessive sleepiness is a long-standing problem in patients with narcolepsy.

On the other hand, the development of sleepiness in the patient with OSA syndrome is much more insidious, but symptoms are usually evident only well into the patient's adult years. The average age of onset of symptoms in OSA syndrome is in the mid-40s. Most commonly, symptoms have been present for as few as 1 to 2 years or as long as 5 to 10 years. Manifestations of excessive sleepiness in patients with OSA and with narcolepsy are similar in many ways; there are some subtle differences between the two patient groups. Most obvious is the response to napping. Most narcoleptic patients will report a history of considerable refreshment and invigoration from a relatively short nap of perhaps 15 to 20 minutes. On the other hand, patients with OSA will rarely report feeling refreshed from a nap, and in fact, they usually state that they feel worse after a nap than before. In addition, narcoleptic patients will frequently experience a vivid dream accompanying a short nap. This is a fairly common ancillary symptom of narcolepsy called *hypnogogic hallucinations*. Although most people will experience this phenomenon on occasion, it is quite common and frequent in narcoleptic patients.

The hypnogogic hallucination is a manifestation of a sleep pattern that can differentiate the narcoleptic patient from the patient with OSA: the sleep onset REM period (SOREM). A definitive diagnosis of narcolepsy can be made by documenting the presence of the onset of REM sleep immediately after sleep onset (usually within 15 to 20 min). The behavioral manifestation of this is the report of an usually intense and vivid dream shortly after the onset of sleep. This is common in narcoleptics but rarely encountered in patients with OSA. The actual documentation of the SOREM is made in the sleep laboratory and is discussed in chapter 10

The behavioral manifestations of this syndrome produce symptoms that may result in consultation with psychologists. Most notable would be the appearance of excessive daytime sleepiness, which may be seen as a purely psychological symptom. In addition, depression and other commonly encountered personality changes in this patient group may also result in referrals to a psychologist. The perspicacious psychologist should be aware of not only the behavioral manifestations of OSA but also its attendant and rather significant medical complications. An awareness of the presenting symptoms of OSA, particularly those that differentiate it from other medical conditions, can provide information that strongly suggests the presence of OSA to the psychological consultant and indicates a possible referral to a sleep specialist.

The psychophysiological complexity of OSA emphasizes the importance of an interdisciplinary medical team in appropriately diagnosing and treating this condition. Ideally, the behavioral scientist and the internist will work closely together in the optimal management of this common and complicated condition, and the routine presence of the psychologist as part of the management team will optimize patient care delivery and satisfaction.

REFERENCES

Berry, D. T. R., Webb, W. B., Block, A. J., & Switzer, D. A. (1986). Sleep-disordered breathing and its concomitants in a subclinical population. *Sleep, 9*(4), 478–483.

Burwell, C., Robin, E., Whaley, R., & Bikelman, A. (1956). Extreme obesity associated with alveolar hypoventilation: A Pickwickian syndrome. *American Journal of Medicine, 21*, 811–818.

Crocker, B. D., Olson, L. G., Saunders, N. A., Hensley, M. J., McKeon, J. L., Allen, K. M., & Gyulay, S. G. (1990). Estimation of the probability of disturbed breathing during sleep before a sleep study. *American Review of Respiratory Disease, 142*, 14–18.

Dement, W. C. (1976). Daytime sleepiness and sleep "attacks." In C. Guilleminault, W. C. Dement, & P. Passouant (Eds.), *Narcolepsy* (pp. 17–42). New York: Spectrum Publications.

Findley, L. J. (1990). Automobile driving in sleep apnea. In F. G. Issa, P. M. Suratt, & J. E. Remmers (Eds.), *Sleep and respiration: Proceedings of the First International Symposium on Sleep and Respiration* (pp. 337–345). New York: Wiley-Liss.

Findley, L. J., Wilhoit, S. C., & Suratt, P. M. (1985). Apnea duration and hypoxemia during REM sleep in patients with obstructive sleep apnea. *Chest, 87*(4), 432–436.

Fletcher, E. C., DeBehnke, R. D., Lovoi, M. S., & Gorin, A. B. (1985). Undiagnosed sleep apnea in patients with essential hypertention. *Annals of Internal Medicine, 103*, 190–195.

Gastaut, H., Tassinari, C. A., & Duron, B. (1965). Polygraphic study of the episodic diurnal and nocturnal (hypnic and respiratory) manifestations of the Pickwick syndrome. *Brain Research, 2*, 167–186.

Guilleminault, C. (1994). Clinical features and evaluation of obstructive sleep apnea. In M. H. Kryger, T. Roth, & W. C. Dement (Eds.), *Principles and practice of sleep medicine* (2nd ed., pp. 667–677). Philadelphia: W. B. Saunders.

Harper, R. M., & Sauerland, E. K. (1978). The role of the tongue in sleep apnea. In C. Guilleminault & W. C. Dement (Eds.), *Sleep apnea syndromes* (pp. 219–234). New York: Alan R. Liss.

He, J., Kryger, M. H., Zorick, F. J., Conway, W., & Roth, T. (1988). Mortality and apnea index in obstructive sleep apnea. *Chest, 94*, 9–14.

Hoffstein, V., & Slutsky, A. S. (1987). Pharyngeal structure and function as a determinant of sleep-related breathing disorders: A unifying hypothesis. *Medical Hypothesis, 24*, 191–199.

Imes, N. K., Orr, W. C., Smith, R. O., & Rogers, R. M. (1977). Retrognathia and sleep apnea: A life threatening condition masquerading as narcolepsy. *Journal of the American Medical Association, 237*, 1596–1598.

Kuna, S. T., & Sant' Ambrogio, G. (1991). Pathophysiology of upper airway closure during sleep. *Journal of the American Medical Association, 266*(10), 1384–1389.

Lugaresi, E., Cirignotta, F., Montagna, P., & Sforza, E. (1994). Snoring: Pathogenic, clinical, and therapeutic aspects. In M. H. Kryger, T. Roth, & W. C. Dement (Eds.), *Principles and practice of sleep medicine* (2nd ed., pp. 621–629). Philadelphia: W. B. Saunders.

Martin, R. J., Pennock, B. E., Orr, W. C., Sanders, M. H., & Rogers, R. M. (1981). Respiratory function during sleep in obstructive sleep apnea. *Journal of Applied Physiology, 84*, 432–437.

Mondini, S., Zucconi, M., Cirignotta, F., Aguglia, U., Lenzi, P. L., Zauli, C., & Lugaresi, E. (1983). Snoring as a risk factor for cardiac and circulatory problems: An epidemiological study. In C. Guilleminault & E. Lugaresi (Eds.), *Sleep/wake disorders: Natural history, epidemiology, and long-term evolution.* New York: Raven Press.

Moran, W. B., Orr, W. C., Fixley M. S., & Wittels, E. (1984). Nonhypersomnolent patient with obstructive sleep apnea. *Transactions of Otolaryngology, Head and Neck Surgery, 92*, 608.

Orr, W. C., Imes, N. K., Martin, R. J., Rogers, R. M., & Stahl, M. L. (1979). Hypersomnolent and nonhypersomnolent patients with upper airway obstruction during sleep. *Chest, 75*, 418–422.

Orr, W. C., Levine, N. S., & Buchanan, R. T. (1987). The effect of cleft palate repair and pharyngeal flap surgery on upper airway obstruction during sleep. *Journal of Plastic & Reconstructive Surgery, 80*(20), 226–232.

Orr, W. C., Males, J. L., & Imes, N. K. (1981). Myxedema and obstructive sleep apnea. *American Journal of Medicine 70*, 1061–1066.

Orr, W. C., & Martin, R. (1981). Obstructive sleep apnea associated with tonsillar hypertrophy in adults. *Archives of Internal Medicine, 141*, 990–992.

Partinen, M., & Palomaki, H. (1985). Snoring and cerebral infarction. *Lancet, 2*, 1325–1326.

Rauscher, H., Popp, W., & Zwick, H. (1992). Systemic hypertension in snorers with and without sleep apnea. *Chest, 102*, 367–371.

Remmers, J. E., deGroot, W. J., & Sauerland, E. K. (1978). Pathogenesis of upper airway occlusion during sleep. *Journal of Applied Physiology, 44*, 931–938.

Sauerland, E. K., Orr, W. C., & Hairston, L. E. (1981). EMG patterns of oropharyngeal muscles during respiration in wakefulness and sleep. *Electromyography & Clinical Neurophysiology, 21*, 307–316.

Shepard, J. W. (1985). Gas exchange and hemodynamics during sleep. *Medical Clinics of North America, 69*, 1243–1269.

Strohl, K. P., Hensley, M. J., Hallett, M., Saunders, N. A., & Ingram, R. H., Jr. (1980). Activation of upper airway muscles before onset of inspiration in normal subjects. *Journal of Applied Physiology, 49*, 638–642.

Svanborg, E., & Larsson, H. (1993). Natural evolution of obstructive sleep apnea syndrome. *Sleep, 16*(Suppl. 8), 124–125.

Thawley, S. E. (1985). *The medical clinics of North America: Symposium on sleep apnea disorders* (Vol. 69, No. 6). Philadelphia: W. B. Saunders.

Young, T., Palta, M., Dempsey, J., Skatrud, J., Weber, S., & Badr, S. (1993). The occurrence of sleep-disordered breathing among middle-aged adults. *New England Journal of Medicine, 328*(17), 1230–1235.

14

Obstructive Sleep Apnea: Treatment Options, Efficacy, and Effects

Paul Saskin

S leep apnea is a condition in which people stop breathing during sleep. The most common type, obstructive sleep apnea (OSA), occurs primarily as a result of the collapse of upper airway tissues during sleep. It is most often associated with loud snoring and episodes of gasping witnessed by a bed partner. The management of (OSA) encompasses a variety of decisions, many of which can involve the skills of behavioral assessment and change that are unique to psychology. It is important to remember that OSA is not a disease but a final common pathway of many diseases (Kryger, 1994). In determining an appropriate course of treatment, the clinician must be sensitive to the multidimensional nature of sleep apnea syndrome (SAS) and the types of anatomic obstruction that can predispose to the occlusion of the airway during sleep. The selection of a therapy for OSA depends, therefore, on many factors.

Weight Loss

The majority of patients with sleep apnea syndrome are overweight, and weight reduction can lead to improvement of the obstructive apnea (Browman et al., 1982). Patients with sleep apnea often become trapped in a cycle of despair concerning their inability to sustain even short-term weight loss, however. As their syndrome progresses, the accompanying daytime sleepiness and fatigue affects their ability to initiate exercise. With the ensuing lethargy, patients succumb to an increasingly sedentary lifestyle that is further exacerbated by lack of motivation and frustration over increased weight.

Weight loss is complex and difficult to manage in patients with morbid obesity, yet it must be considered a first step in the treatment of sleep apnea. An effective combination of dietary control and increased exercise can often be achieved through the application of a team approach. The team, composed of the physician, nurse, dietitian, and perhaps most important, peer group, can be markedly helpful in allowing a patient to make appropriate psychological and lifestyle adjustments that will permit long-lasting weight control.

Pharmacological Impediments

Although it is not considered treatment for sleep apnea syndrome, the elimination of various pharmacological elements may play a crucial role in the initial management of sleep-disordered breathing. Along with weight loss, avoidance of respiratory suppressant products may greatly enhance the patient's underlying physiological state while appropriate, required intervention is arranged.

Alcohol

Alcohol has been identified as the most readily available substance that can adversely affect sleep apnea. Alcohol increases the frequency of upper airway obstructive events by selectively reducing the motor activity of upper airway dilator muscles, promoting airway collapse. This results in a propensity toward closure of the airway during sleep (Remmers, DeGroot, Sauerland, & Anch, 1978). In addition to increasing the frequency of sleep-disordered breathing events, alcohol may decrease the arousal response to apnea and decrease the oxygen supply to the brain, both of which are essential to the eventual termination of a prolonged episode of apnea.

Avoidance of alcohol may help prevent the progression of the apnea syndrome. Recommending the elimination of alcohol alone, like encouraging weight loss alone, may simply be a "band-aid" measure, insufficient to prevent the eventual worsening of sleep-disordered breathing.

Sedative Medications

Many patients with sleep apnea are inadvertently or intentionally given prescriptions for sedative–hypnotic medications, in part for their anxiolytic effect and in part to alleviate some of the underlying sleep-maintenance difficulties. Barbiturates are not widely used in this regard, although their continued use for reduction of anxiety or for sleep induction may remain a concern for some patients. Like alcohol, these agents may reduce the neural activity of upper airway muscles, predisposing to occlusion during sleep and precipitating apnea (Simmons & Hill, 1974).

Although they have not been widely studied as a group, the benzodiazepines represent the largest pharmacological family used for the treatment of anxiety or sleep problems. Flurazepam (e.g., Dalmane) is a widely used hypnotic agent that has been studied extensively with regard to sleep-disordered breathing. Use of flurazepam before sleep may worsen apnea in some patients with preexisting disease and precipitate sleep-disordered breathing in some individuals who otherwise do not have it (Dolly & Block, 1982; Mendelson, Garnett, & Gillin, 1981). Additionally, flurazepam may adversely affect some elderly patients, substantially increasing the severity of otherwise asymptomatic sleep-disordered breathing (Guilleminault, Eldridge, Tilkian, Simmons, & Dement, 1977) and prolonging the arousal response to lowered brain oxygen in a similar manner to alcohol (Gothe, Cherniak, & Williams, 1986; Hedemark & Kronenberg, 1985).

It is probable that benzodiazepines, like alcohol, increase the likelihood of upper airway collapse during sleep. Under these circumstances, patients with a history of loud snoring and a possible diagnosis of sleep apnea who require sedative–hypnotic assistance should be encouraged to explore alternative medications or aggressive behavioral strategies.

Narcotics

There have been no systematic studies of the effects of narcotic medications on sleep apnea. Anecdotal reports, however, have suggested that upper airway obstruction may develop following administration of narcotics (Rafferty, Ruskis, Sasaki, & Gee, 1980). With these concerns, it may be prudent to minimize the use of narcotic medications both in the management of pain-related complaints and in the preparation for or treatment with operative procedures in patients apparently predisposed to sleep apnea.

Hypothyroidism

There appears to be a relatively high prevalence of sleep-disordered breathing in patients with hypothyroidism. (Rajagopal et al., 1984). The concomitant obesity often evident in hypothyroidism confounds to a certain extent the explanations of underlying pathophysiology of sleep-disordered breathing. It has been demonstrated that administration of thyroid replacement significantly reduces the number of episodes of sleep-disordered breathing without any significant weight loss (Grunstein & Sullivan, 1988; Rajagopal et al., 1984).

Pharmacological Treatments

Efforts at the management of sleep apnea with the use of medication alone have employed protriptyline, a nonsedating tricyclic medication typically used in the treatment of depression. In a small population of patients with sleep apnea, it was noted that protriptyline taken at bedtime reduced nocturnal deoxygenation and apnea frequency (Brownell, West, Sweatman, Acres, & Kryger, 1982). This was apparently associated with the reduced amount of time spent in rapid eye movement (REM) sleep relative to total sleep time, the reduction of REM time being an initial effect of administration of tricyclic medications. Because more frequent episodes of apnea and prolonged oxygen desaturation are seen in REM sleep, the improvement in sleep-disordered breathing evident with protriptyline may reflect the sleep-stage-specific effect of this medication.

Other investigators have explored the use of agents designed to augment progesterone, a strategy derived from early observations of a relative absence of obstructive apnea in premenopausal women. Although several limited studies concluded that medroxyprogesterone acetate might be beneficial in selected individuals (Hensley, Saunders, & Strohl, 1981; Orr, Imes, & Martin, 1979; Strohl et al., 1981), placebo-controlled studies have shown no reduction in apnea frequency or duration (Cook, Benich, & Wooten, 1989; Rajagopal, Abbrecht, & Jabbari, 1986).

Theophylline and similar respiratory stimulant medications have long been a mainstay in the management of asthma and other disorders of breathing. It has therefore been a tantalizing prospect that such medications might have some beneficial effect on sleep-disordered breathing. Although they are potentially useful in the management of associated central apnea conditions or other problems of diminished ventilatory effort (e.g., Cheyne–Stokes periodic breathing), no systematic benefit has been evident from the use of these medications in the treatment of obstructive sleep apnea (Espinoza, Antic, Thornton, & McEvoy, 1987).

Several studies emerged in the early 1980s to suggest a beneficial role of L-tryptophan, an essential amino acid involved in the regulation of the brain neurotransmitter serotonin. Schmidt (1983, 1985) demonstrated a reduction of apnea in patients with relatively mild disease (a disturbance index of less than 20 events per hour of sleep). A recently identified risk associated with L-tryptophan use has been the development of the eosinophilia-myalgia syndrome (Hertzman et al., 1990). This disorder, characterized by generalized fatigue and muscle weakness, evidence of hepatic inflammation, pulmonary infiltrates, and other lung diseases, has occurred in some patients given L-tryptophan for a variety of conditions (e.g., insomnia, anxiety) as well as in patients who obtained this product through commercial sources (health food and nutrition stores). Although the beneficial effect of L-tryptophan in patients with mild sleep apnea may be evident, the risks associated with its use may outweigh any therapeutic advantage.

Sleeping Position

Sleep clinicians will often learn of a positional component to sleep apnea through the caricature of the snoring husband with bruised ribs. The spouse, aware of her husband's tendency to snore while on his back and subsequently have episodes of apnea, will describe a brief arousal from her own sleep to nudge him gently (or not so gently!) in order to readjust his sleeping posture. This reflects perhaps the earliest and most widely used initial therapy for sleep apnea. The documentation of a higher frequency of sleep-disordered breathing events in the supine position has been confirmed, at least anecdotally, by virtually every sleep laboratory. Cartwright (1984) reported an apnea–hypopnea index of 24 unselected patients with sleep apnea to be twice as high during the time spent sleeping in the supine position as in the time spent in the lateral position. It was noted, however, that the degree of body position dependency was inversely related to the degree of obesity, with a greater probability of sleep apnea evident in all sleep positions among patients who were more obese.

For position-dependent sleep apnea, particularly in patients without obesity or significant consequences of sleep apnea (e.g., changes in arterial oxygen saturation, overt cardiac dysrhythmias, excessive daytime sleepiness), it is not unreasonable to offer suggestions for "positional re-training." This technique, which has been demonstrated to be effective, uses a gravity-activated position alarm that sounds if the patient remains in the supine position for more than 15 seconds (Cartwright, Lloyd, Lilie, & Kravitz, 1985).

Alternative commercially available products can be purchased, usually consisting of positional sensors that attach to an electrode delivering a minimal shock, awakening the patient briefly and, one hopes, ensuring that he or she rolls over while sleeping. Similar results can be achieved at less cost by having patients sew pockets onto the back of a sleep T-shirt, allowing them to sleep with one or several tennis balls on their back to prevent them from remaining asleep in the supine position.

Dental Appliances

A variety of dental orthotic devices have been employed in the management of sleep apnea. Most are insertion devices with the purpose of mandibular advancement—shifting the lower jaw forward to increase the posterior airway space. Although many brief reports on these devices have described improvement in sleep apnea parameters, few have been subject to the close scrutiny of physiological sleep investigations.

Schmidt-Nowara, Meade, and Hays (1991) evaluated the sleep and symptoms of 68 patients for whom a dental orthotic was employed. The study included assessment of sleep apnea, subjective evaluation of snoring by bed partners, compliance, and side effects. Snoring was improved or eliminated in most patients, and indices of sleep apnea were decreased by at least 50%, with concomitant improvement in brain oxygenation and sleep stage parameters. They advocated the use of a dental orthotic appliance for patients with primary snoring or with minimal to moderate sleep apnea.

Evaluation of the effect of treatment for sleep apnea must be based on an individual assessment of patient need. Although factors of compliance with a device that must be inserted in the mouth nightly need to be addressed, this relatively noninvasive means of management remains a useful option.

Surgical Interventions

The surgical treatment of obstructive sleep apnea, more than any other treatment, requires a comprehensive understanding of and sensitivity to the dynamics of the upper airway in sleep. For many patients, the site of collapse remains consistent—within the pharynx (upper airway)—although the region of the pharynx that collapses and the mechanism of collapse may vary (Sher, 1980). The upper airway of patients with obstructive sleep apnea may be more predisposed to collapse as a result of diminished cross-sectional area (Haponik et al., 1983; Rivlin et al., 1984; Suratt, Dee, Atkinson, Armstrong, & Wilhoit, 1983). This observation appears to correlate quite well with the negative pressure required to sustain pharyngeal collapse (Issa & Sullivan, 1984).

Treatment of the upper airway obstruction, therefore, requires careful consideration of anatomic factors in the selection of eventual surgical intervention. For example, removal of tonsils and adenoids may be sufficient, particularly in children, to alleviate the focus of obstruction by increasing the upper airway cross-sectional area. For others, the focus of obstruction may be deeper within the area (hypopharynx), so that consideration of the site of collapse is much more important.

Early surgical interventions were almost exclusively confined to tracheostomy, an opening in the windpipe. In bypassing the level of obstruction, this procedure allows patients to sleep with an open hole in their throat, which is closed off during the day. Apart from the relative lack of acceptance of the procedure by many individuals, the increased medical complications (e.g., risk of infection, need for localized skin care) necessitated the development of alternative surgical techniques.

Current procedures focus on the pattern of collapse of the pharynx in sleep, classified according to the location, relative to the base of the tongue and its location within the palate. In 1964, Ikematsu and his colleagues described a treatment for snoring, the uvulopalatopharyngoplasty (UPPP). This technique, adapted by Fujita (1984), allowed a surgical means of correcting snoring and sleep apnea. The technique typically involves a resectioning of the uvula and a portion of the edge of the soft palate as well as tonsillar pillars. It creates a wider pharyngeal cross-section and removes potential sites of obstruction. Although it is markedly effective in the elimination of snoring, there is a lack of practical methods for predicting which patients will achieve a surgical cure. Recently Larsson, Carlsson-Nordlander, and Svanborg (1994) showed that 50% of initial responders to UPPP had relapsed according to follow-up 4 years after surgery. Subsequent treatment was required in 63% of nonresponders, who remained clinically symptomatic. A variety of factors may have contributed, the most important of which was increased weight. Additionally, no subjective or objective differences could be discerned between responders and nonresponders to surgery; fully 73% reported complete or partial improvement in sleepiness despite polysomnographic evidence of residual disease.

Recent attempts have been made to use a carbon dioxide (CO_2) laser in the treatment of snoring. The laser-assisted UPPP (LAUP) is noteworthy in that it can be performed in the office setting, under local anesthesia, with reportedly minor discomfort (American Sleep Disorders Association, 1994). The method has been used clinically in France, but no objective evaluations of patients with obstructive sleep apnea have been published. Recent report's (Krespi et al., 1994) have no appreciable difference in snoring or in objective measurement of sleep apnea among patients undergoing laser-assisted surgery (Kamami, 1983). Of major concern has been the identification of large numbers of snoring patients by physicians trained in LAUP, who may be successful in the ablation of snoring without paying careful attention to the underlying possibility of sleep apnea. The American Sleep Disorders Association, in a Practice Parameters Report, stated that because "adequate peer-reviewed objective data do not exist regarding the effectiveness of LAUP for the treatment of sleep-related breathing disorders, including OSA, LAUP is not recommended for the treatment of these disorders." (American Sleep Disorders Association, 1994)

Surgical alternatives also include maxillomandibular advancement with hyoid suspension (Riley, Powell, & Guilleminault, 1986). This complex and aggressive procedure, developed at Stanford University, offers an almost 95% cure rate for sleep apnea; typically, it is performed in conjunction with UPPP. Although it is effective in treating nonresponders to traditional airway surgery, the cost and complexity of this operation may prevent widespread application.

Nasal Continuous Positive Airway Pressure (CPAP)

Nasal CPAP therapy was introduced by Sullivan in 1981 and has since become the most popular therapy for obstructive sleep apnea (Sanders, Moore, & Eveslage, 1983; Sullivan, Berthon-Jones, Issa, & Eves, 1981). Nasal CPAP consists of a high-flow blower that delivers a continuous stream of room air into a sealed mask that the patient wears over the nose during sleep (see Figures 1 and 2).

This infusion of positive air pressure creates a pneumatic splint, maintaining upper airway patency during sleep and preventing its

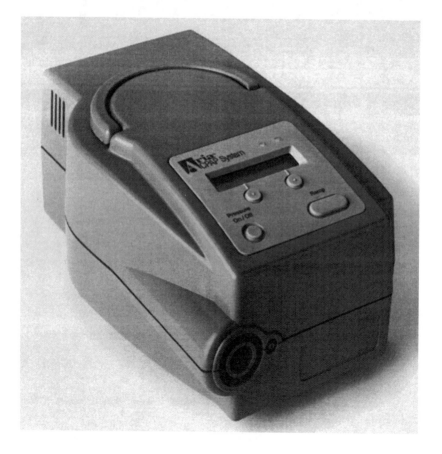

Figure 1. Nasal CPAP machine. The compact machine is designed to rest on the patient's bedside table. The blower hose connection attaches to a flexible silicone mask, which sits over the nose. CPAP = continuous positive airway pressure. Photo courtesy Respironics, Inc.

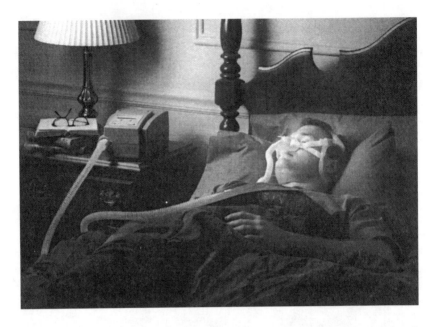

Figure 2. CPAP mask and headgear. The CPAP mask is held in place with soft headgear. With proper mask fitting, patients can sleep comfortably with minimal interruption. Photo courtesy Respironics, Inc.

collapse. The success of nasal CPAP has been associated with its demonstrated ability to abolish most episodes of apnea, eliminate associated oxygen desaturation, and allow for the consolidation of sleep state architecture. All of these benefits result in an improvement in daytime function.

Patients must be observed in the sleep laboratory for nasal CPAP to be implemented. Although the majority of patients require pressure settings in the range of 5–15 cm water pressure, the individual variability of nasal airway size, upper airway factors, and patient tolerance significantly affects the success of this mechanical device in the treatment of sleep apnea.

Typically, patients with sleep apnea return to the sleep laboratory for a second night of sleep recording following their initial diagnostic evaluation. In the facility that I direct, patients view a commercial videotape that describes CPAP treatment and answers some of the most common questions asked have about its viability. The technician spends a great deal of time ensuring that the mask used is comfortable for the patient; the mask represents the most important interface between the sleeping patient and the CPAP blower. A variety of different masks may be tried, some of which completely cover the nose in sleep. Alternative mask devices include nasal pillows or prongs that sit under the nasal orifices, creating a seal that approximates that available with the use of the complete nasal mask.

During this introductory phase, the sleep technician allows the patient to sit quietly with the CPAP mask in place and the blower set on a low pressure. This accommodation period is particularly helpful for patients with some underlying discomfort or more evident claustrophobia.

For patients who require markedly elevated CPAP pressure settings, a variety of options are available. The impact of high CPAP pressure (>13 cm water pressure) may be akin to an attempt to breathe in or out against a flow of air equivalent to having one's head out the car window at 80-plus miles per hour! Although the inspiratory pressure may be more easily accepted, the effort required to exhale against such a flow is formidable.

To ease adaptation to higher inspiratory pressure, many current CPAP devices offer a "ramping" feature. This control allows the individual to initiate sleep with the CPAP mask in place while the blower generates a relatively low pressure. Over a 15- to 30-minute period, the pressure gradually increases to the prescribed setting, allowing the patient to fall asleep with greater comfort. Awakenings during the night can be managed in a similar manner.

For patients for whom the pressure is unmanageable, particularly in terms of the effort required for exhalation, there is a variation of CPAP known as *nasal bilevel pressure*. In this method, the inspiratory pressure (IPAP) is generally set higher than the pressure required for expiration (EPAP). This modification can increase patients' comfort by reducing the force of pressure against which they must exhale. This treatment option is equally effective to standard CPAP in the management of obstructive sleep apnea, although the higher cost associated with the bilevel pressure machine can be prohibitive for some patients.

Mechanical treatment of sleep apnea with continuous or bilevel airway pressure is effective for most patients. Ongoing research and development of new products appear to offer sleep clinicians a greater range of options in the use of nasal CPAP. These options include automated setting systems, such as a demand positive airway pressure device (DPAP). This experimental self-adjusting positive airway pressure system detects changes in inspiratory flow (breathing in), compensating by increasing the pressure through the system to allow for airway maintenance. By monitoring and adjusting on a breath-by-breath basis, the DPAP system appears to avoid some of the difficulties associated with very high starting pressures. With ongoing research in this method, it is hoped that systems such as this will improve patient compliance, an area to be addressed in the next chapter.

Conclusion

Sleep apnea syndrome is a common medical disorder, characterized by pauses in breathing during sleep. With the growth of sleep medicine in the past 20 years, the identification of sleep apnea has become more prevalent, as have the options for the management of this potentially life-threatening condition. With features of obesity, loud snoring, and the adverse effects of substances (e.g. sleeping pills, alcohol) on sleep-related breathing, the role of the psychologist in the management of sleep apnea syndrome becomes more important.

An understanding of the underlying mechanisms of sleep apnea and its most common effective treatment modalities can be helpful to the clinician in working with this complex problem. Weight management interventions, both through behavioral means and as an adjunct for pharmacologic support, can facilitate improvement of the patient's overall state. Early identification of the use or abuse of substances (alcohol, tobacco, street drugs) and an understanding of their role in sleep-disordered breathing can be essential in helping the patient make appropriate lifestyle changes. An appreciation of the process through which mechanical ventilatory devices, such as nasal CPAP (continuous positive airway pressure), can eliminate episodes of apnea in sleep will help both the clinician and patient with long term compliance in treatment. This will ultimately result in improvement in daytime function and a reduction of symptoms that may be attributable to the daytime sleepiness and fatigue caused by the sleep apnea itself. Finally, an understanding of surgical outcomes along with some knowledge of alternative therapies (oral appliances, positional retraining) will allow the psychologist involved in management of this condition to provide appropriate feedback and support for the individual facing significant lifestyle changes.

As sleep medicine emerges from the research settings into the mainstream of clinical medicine, the psychologist as health care provider must become equipped to offer both a supportive role in treatment as well as guidelines for the facilitation of behavioral change.

REFERENCES

American Sleep Disorders Association. (1994). Practice parameters for the use of laser-assisted uvulopalatoplasty. *Sleep, 17,* 744–748.

Browman, C. P., Sampson, M. G., Yolles, S. F., Gujavarty, K. S., Weiler, S. J., Walsleben, J. A., Hahn, P. M., & Mitler, M. M. (1984). Obstructive sleep apnea and body weight. *Chest, 1982,* 291–294.

Brownell, L. G., West, P., Sweatman, P., Acres, J. C., & Kryger, M. H. (1982). Protriptyline in obstructive sleep apnea. *New England Journal of Medicine, 307,* 1037–1042.

Cartwright, R. D. (1994). Effect of sleep position on sleep apnea severity. *Sleep, 7,* 110–114.

Cartwright, R. D., Lloyd, S., Lilie, J., & Kravitz, H. (1985). Sleep position training as treatment for sleep apnea syndrome: A preliminary study. *Sleep, 8,* 87–94.

Cook, W. R., Benich, J. J., & Wooten, S. A. (1989). Indices of severity of obstructive sleep apnea syndrome do not change during medroxyprogesterone acetate therapy. *Chest, 96,* 262–266.

Dolly, F. R., & Block, A. J. (1982). Effect of flurazepam on sleep-disordered breathing and nocturnal desaturation in asymptomatic subjects. *American Journal of Medicine, 73,* 239–243.

Espinoza, H., Antic, R., Thornton, A. T., & McEvoy, R. D. (1987). The effects of aminophylline on sleep and sleep-disordered breathing with obstructive sleep apnea syndrome. *American Review of Respiratory Disease, 136,* 80–84.

Fujita, S. (1984). U.P.P.P. for sleep apnea and snoring. *Ear, Nose and Throat Journal, 63,* 227–235.

Gothe, B., Cherniak, N. S., & Williams L. (1986). Effect of hypoxia on ventilatory and arousal response to CO_2 during n-REM sleep with and without flurazepam in young adults. *Sleep, 9,* 24–37.

Grunstein, R. R., & Sullivan, C. E. (1988). Sleep apnea and hypothyroidism: Mechanisms and management. *American Journal of Medicine, 85,* 775–779.

Guilleminault, C., Eldridge, F. L., Tilkian, A., Simmons, F. B., & Dement, W.C. (1977). Sleep apnea syndrome due to upper airway obstruction: A review of 25 cases. *Archives of Internal Medicine, 137,* 296–300.

Haponik, E. F., Smith, P. L., Bohlman, M. E., Allen, R. P., Goldman, S. M., & Bleecker, E. R. (1983). Computerized tomography in obstructive sleep apnea. *American Review of Respiratory Disease, 127,* 221–226.

Hedemark, L. L., & Kronenberg, R. S. (1985). Flurazepam attenuates the arousal response to sleep in normal subjects. *American Review of Respiratory Disease, 131,* 41–45.

Hensley, M. J., Saunders, N. A., & Strohl, K. P. (1981). Medroxyprogesterone treatment of obstructive sleep apnea. *Sleep, 3,* 441–446.

Herzman, P. A., Blevins, W. L., Mayer, J., Greenfield, B., Ting, M., & Gleich, G. J. (1990). Association of the eosinophilia-myalgia syndrome with the ingestion of tryptophan. *New England Journal of Medicine, 322,* 869–873.

Issa, F. G., & Sullivan, C. E. (1984). Upper airway closing pressure in snorers. *Journal of Applied Physiology (Respiratory, Environmental and Exercise Physiology), 57,* 528–535.

Kamami, Y (1993). Ambulant treatment of sleep apnea syndrome with CO2 laser. In *Proceedings of the XV World Congress of Otorhinolaryngology, Head and Neck Surgery* (pp. 953–957). Istanbul, June 20–25.

Kryger, M. H. (1994). Management of obstructive sleep apnea: Overview. In M. Kryger, T. Roth, & W.C. Dement (Eds.), *Principles and practice of sleep medicine* (pp. 736–747). Philadelphia: Saunders.

Larsson, L. H., Carlsson-Nordlander, B., & Svanborg, E. (1994). Four year follow-up after uvulopalatopharyngoplasty in 50 unselected patients with obstructive sleep apnea syndrome. *Laryngoscope, 104,* 1362–1368.

Mendelson, W. B., Garnett, D., & Gillin, J. C. (1981). Flurazepam-induced sleep apnea syndrome in a patient with insomnia and mild sleep-related respiratory changes. *Journal of Nervous and Mental Disease, 160,* 261–264.

Orr, W. C., Imes, N. K., & Martin, R. J. (1979). Progesterone therapy in obese patients with sleep apnea. *Archives of Internal Medicine, 139,* 109–111.

Rafferty, T. D., Ruskis, A., Sasaki, C., & Gee, J. B. (1980). Perioperative considerations in the management of tracheostomy for the obstructive sleep apnea patient. *British Journal of Anaesthesia, 52,* 619–621.

Rajagopal, K. R., Abbrecht, P. H., Derderian, S. S., Picket, C., Hofeldt, F., Tellis, C., & Zwillich, C. W. (1984). Obstructive sleep apnea in hypothyroidism. *Annals of Internal Medicine, 101,* 491–494.

Rajagopal, K. R., Abbrecht, P. H., & Jabbari, B. (1986). Effects of medroxyprogesterone acetate in obstructive sleep apnea. *Chest, 90,* 815–821.

Remmers, J. E., DeGroot, W. J., Sauerland, E. K., & Anch, A. M. (1978). Pathogenesis of upper airway occlusion in sleep. *Journal of Applied Physiology, 44,* 931–938.

Riley, R. W., Powell, N. P., & Guilleminault, C. (1986). Inferior sagittal osteotomy of the mandible with hyoid myotomy-suspension: A new procedure for obstructive sleep apnea. *Otolaryngology Head and Neck Surgery, 94,* 589–593.

Rivlin, J., Hoffstein, V., Kalbfleish, J., McNicholas, W., Zamel, N., & Bryan, A. C. (1984). Upper airway morphology in patients with idiopathic obstructive sleep apnea. *American Review of Respiratory Disease, 129,* 355–360.

Sanders, M. H., Moore, S. E., & Eveslage, J. (1983). CPAP via nasal mask: A treatment for occlusive sleep apnea. *Chest, 83,* 144–145.

Schmidt, H. S. (1983). L-tryptophan in the treatment of impaired respiration during sleep. *Bulletin of European Physiopathology and Respiration, 19,* 625–629.

Schmidt, H. S. (1985). Combined L-tryptophan and protryptiline in the treatment of obstructive sleep apnea. *Sleep Research, 14,* 209.

Schmidt-Nowara, W. W., Meade, T. E., & Hays, M. B. (1991). Treatment of snoring and obstructive sleep apnea with a dental orthosis. *Chest, 99,* 1378–1385.

Sher, A. (1980). Obstructive sleep apnea syndrome: A complex disorder of the upper airway. *Otolaryngologic Clinics of North America, 23,* 593–608.

Simmons, F. B., & Hill, M. W. (1974). Hypersomnia caused by upper airway obstructions: A new syndrome in otolaryngology. *Annals of Otolaryngology, 83,* 670–673.

Strohl, K. P., Hensley, M. J., Saunders, N. A., Scharf, S. M., Brown, R., & Ingram, R. H., Jr. (1981). Progesterone administration and progressive sleep apneas. *Journal of the American Medical Association, 245,* 1230–1232.

Sullivan, C. E., Berthon-Jones, M., Issa, F. G., & Eves, L. (1981). Reversal of obstructive sleep apnoea by continuous positive airway pressure applied through the nares. *Lancet, 1,* 862–865.

Suratt, P. M., Dee, P., Atkinson, R. L., Armstrong, P., & Wilhoit, S. C. (1983). Fluoroscopic and computed tomographic features of the pharyngeal airway in obstructive sleep apnea. *American Review of Respiratory Disease, 127,* 487–492.

15

Methods and Problems of Treatment Compliance in Obstructive Sleep Apnea

Nancy Barone Kribbs

Q uestions regarding the successful administration of therapy for obstructive sleep apnea syndrome (OSAS) are overwhelmingly behavioral. Therefore, sleep psychologists have quite naturally filled a unique and important role in treating, measuring, and evaluating the quality of care provided to patients with sleep apnea. This chapter focuses on the therapeutic problems faced by the OSAS patient, the issues that must be considered when evaluating the success of continuous positive airway pressure (CPAP) therapy, and how these issues have been informed by behavioral science.

Obstructive sleep apnea is the periodic occlusion of the upper airway during sleep, caused by a loss of rigidity in the oropharyngeal musculature that allows soft tissue to collapse inward and block airflow. This blockage results in numerous arousals from sleep throughout the night for the patient to breathe and reduced oxyhemoglobin levels during apneic events. In turn, these events lead to extreme daytime sleepiness, deteriorated performance due to lack of sleep, and chronic cardiovascular consequences.

Pharmacological treatments for sleep-disordered breathing are theoretically possible, but they have been disappointing to date. There have also been attempts to stimulate the neuromuscular input to the airway electrically, but it is a tricky business to accomplish this without causing arousals from sleep, which are already an integral problem of the syndrome. Such modes of treatment are still in development, are not yet well documented, and have not met with universal acceptance as treatment for OSAS.

Obstructive sleep apnea is often associated with obesity, and weight loss is one of the best, although not a guaranteed successful, means of alleviating the condition. However, the field of weight loss research, which has a prolific and controversial body of literature, points to the difficulty in achieving and maintaining success. Therefore, weight loss is not usually viewed as an immediate, viable option, although it can be suggested for long-term benefit. Typically, other treatments for sleep apnea are used while a patient embarks on a weight loss program.

The best of the remaining treatment options are those that attempt to keep the upper airway open through physical means (see chapter 20). This can be accomplished temporarily with a tracheostomy or permanently with surgery that clears and scrapes the redundant soft tissue of the oropharynx. Surgical procedures have been refined, and greater precision is possible than in the past. However, surgery is still a risky option that patients and clinicians are often unwilling to attempt, especially because it is not always successful in permanently eliminating sleep apnea.

Other means of keeping the airway open include use of a variety of dental appliances, worn at night, that bring the jaw or tongue forward and thereby prevent airway obstruction. Also, a side sleep position, rather than a supine sleep position, can eliminate apnea in patients with mild, position-dependent OSAS. Mechanical devices or position changes are usually successful only when the illness is mild.

These treatment options have not been thoroughly evaluated or given full credit in this brief review, but they are mentioned to explain why CPAP is the current treatment of choice for sleep apnea. CPAP forces the airway to remain open with a constant stream of air blown through the nose via a mask or nasal prongs. It was first developed in 1981 (Sullivan, Berthon-Jones, Issa, & Eves, 1981), has become the most accepted treatment for sleep apnea, and is widely regarded as the most effective therapeutic option.

What is CPAP?

A CPAP machine is an air blower housed in a plastic box, about the size of a toaster oven, that can be placed on a bedside nightstand or floor. The outward appearance of these devices varies with the particular manufacturer, but most are portable, with minimal, patient-accessible controls. Air pressure is adjustable by a technician and measurable with a pressure transducer so that the prescribed pressure (measured in cm H_2O) is administered to the patient. The more sophisticated of these devices automatically adjust airflow to increase and compensate when leaks occur at the mask, thereby always providing the appropriate pressure levels. Flexible plastic tubing is attached to a port on the device, with a soft plastic mask or nasal prongs at the patient end of the tubing. The mask is held in place by bands that are strapped around the patient's head and attached by hook-and-loop closures. Often a humidifier, which is a plastic container filled with water, is connected between the CPAP machine and the patient tubing to moisten the air, which increases comfort in patients suffering from nasal dryness and nosebleeds. When in operation, CPAP machines produce a constant mild, "shushing" air sound. Newer devices, developed in the last 5 years, are quieter than the original machines, but they are still clearly audible to the user.

Much of the existing literature on general treatment compliance for illnesses involves the determination of the reliable use of medications. The findings and suppositions of these pharmaceutical investigations are, in part, applicable to the study of compliance with CPAP therapy. However, CPAP therapy is unique in several respects: The machine must be turned on and "worn" during sleep. CPAP is almost always prescribed to patients for use *every night* during sleep, for the *entire night's* sleep period, and often for an indefinite period of time, possibly for the rest of the patient's life. Therefore, the successful and continued use of this therapy requires dedication and persistence on the part of patients, who become physically involved in the management of their own condition. This level of patient involvement in treatment is rivaled perhaps only by diabetes in terms of physical demands and vigilant maintenance of treatment administration in the home environment, without the routine intervention of a health care provider.

For approximately the first 10 years of CPAP use in sleep centers, most studies of adherence to CPAP therapy were conducted through patient interviews. Patients were consulted during follow-up visits and over the telephone regarding their level of CPAP use (e.g., Anand, Ferguson, & Schoen, 1991; Katsantonis, Schweitzer, Branham, Chambers, & Walsh, 1988; Nino-Murcia, McCann, Bliwise, Guilleminault, & Dement, 1989; Rauscher, Popp, Wanke, & Zwick, 1991). Some more detailed studies were also conducted, which used a cumulative time counter that indicated the total amount of time the CPAP machine had been operated

(Krieger, & Kurtz, 1988). To analyze data from these counters, the time readout was divided by the number of days CPAP was available for patient use, resulting in a crude but useful measure of mean daily use. The general conclusions of these studies were that CPAP enjoyed up to a 90% acceptance rate by patients and was used every day by up to 75% of all patients. However, one must be cautious in the interpretation of and reliance on patients' subjective reports that are not supplemented with objective data, because they usually overestimate the adherence rate (Rand & Wise, 1994), as I show later.

It is difficult to determine exactly when CPAP is used if only a cumulative time counter of total power use is engaged. This method gives no indication of the daily pattern of use, which results in an underestimation of regular daily use if CPAP is occasionally skipped for an entire night. Also, if a patient used CPAP for 8 hours per night for the first half of the measurement period and then stopped using it altogether in the second half, the mean use across the measurement period (4 hr) would qualify that patient as compliant according to the adherence criteria set in previous research. Additionally, for all but a few of the previous studies, there were no means of determining whether CPAP was used appropriately, that is, whether there was any mask pressure applied. Using a verification procedure that does not include pressure measurements can result in the appearance of compliance even if the mask has a serious leak, falls off, or is never worn at all.

Monitoring Compliance

In 1993 my colleagues and I at the University of Pennsylvania and Johns Hopkins University reported a collaborative study in which we objectively measured day-to-day CPAP treatment compliance using a microcomputer monitoring device that we developed for this purpose (Kribbs, Pack, Kline, Smith, et al., 1993). This monitor covertly measured precise use by assessing both power to the machine and pressure levels with a pressure transducer. A time and date marker was stored for each of four events: power on, power off, mask on, and mask off. Thus, we could determine exactly when a patient used CPAP and when it was used at the correct pressure. Precedent for a study of this kind can be found in asthma inhaler studies using a microprocessor in the medication canister (Tashkin et al., 1991). We supplemented our objective monitoring with an initial enrollment questionnaire that requested

detailed demographic information and subjective answers about pre-
treatment symptomatology (e.g., sleepiness). We also obtained subjective information about posttreatment symptom recovery, side
effects, and satisfaction with treatment through the use of follow-up
questionnaires.

Ethical Considerations

Because patient use of CPAP was not previously reported using objective criteria, we conducted this study without full patient knowledge of
the sophistication of our monitoring procedures. We thought that even
the knowledge of our monitoring might be sufficient motivation for
patients to increase what otherwise would be their "natural" home use
of the device, and we wanted to avoid interference with their usual
clinical care. Patients underwent informed consent procedures in
which they agreed to participate in a study of their CPAP use, but they
did not know the precise capability of our monitoring device. We
developed our protocol with the guidance of the institutional review
boards at our respective universities to ensure ethical conduct, including participant debriefing. The issue of patient monitoring has
increased in importance as current medical research needs, combined
with advanced technological capability, have presented new challenges for the health research field in terms of ethical conduct of studies. The psychology profession has a distinguished history of
sensitivity to ethical issues in research, and health psychologists are in
a position to provide a leadership role in the medical community in this
respect. For a more detailed review of the ethical considerations in this
and similar research studies, the reader is directed to a series of editori-
als in which we and other investigators discussed the implications of
these issues for medical research (Dinges, Kribbs, Schwartz, Smith, &
Pack, 1994; Klocke, 1994; Levine, 1994; Rand, 1994).

Patterns of CPAP Use

A detailed picture of patient CPAP use emerged from the data gathered
on the 35 patients in our study who initially accepted and received
CPAP as a treatment for their OSAS. The CPAP monitor provided a
"window" into therapy use on a daily basis, from which we created
profiles of individual patient use across several weeks of treatment. A
representation of daily use in four different patients across a 14-week

period is displayed in Figure 1. The patient represented in the upper left quadrant of this figure used CPAP every day (100% of days), for a mean of 7.1 hours per day (calculated only for days CPAP was used). This patient was undoubtedly compliant with CPAP therapy in that he used CPAP every night for a period of time that permitted adequate sleep. The periodic increases in duration of use (extensions of the lines to the right in the figure) that are observed about every 7 days represent weekends, when the patient "slept in" on Saturday and Sunday mornings. There is also one Sunday afternoon CPAP nap that can be observed in this patient's profile.

The lower left panel shows a patient who was also a consistent user (100%), but his mean use per night was only 4.6 hours. This patient was considered compliant with CPAP therapy—he used it virtually every night—but his use time per night was low. We do not know from our

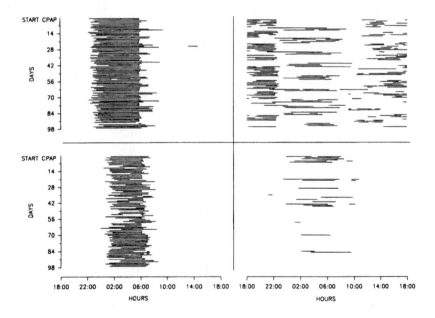

Figure 1. Profiles of patterns of use of continuous positive airway pressure (CPAP) for 14 weeks in four patients. The horizontal black lines indicate the times when the CPAP machine was in operation, with the first day of therapy starting at the top. Each quadrant of the figure represents one patient. From "Objective Measurement of Patterns of Nasal CPAP Use by Patients With Obstructive Sleep Apnea," by N. B. Kribbs, A. I. Pack, L. R. Kline, P. L. Smith, et al., 1993, *American Review of Respiratory Disease, 147,* 893. Reprinted with permission.

results exactly when he slept; it is possible that he turned his CPAP device off and remained in bed (we are currently investigating the incidence of this practice in a separate study). Nonetheless, we can presume the amount of undisturbed, or treated, sleep available to him. We know from sleep deprivation research that at least 4 hours of sleep per night are required to avoid serious performance decrements; therefore, this person's daytime sleepiness has probably not been adequately treated. The problem may be one of poor sleep hygiene practice (see chapter 16 of this volume concerning insomnia treatment). The point is, however, that a patient can be compliant with use of CPAP therapy and still require education to enhance sleep hygiene through clinical support services.

The patient displayed in the upper right quadrant of Figure 1, a rotating-shift worker, provides another example of the need for careful clinical assessment and advisement. This patient used CPAP regularly (95% of days; mean use = 5.8 hr per day), but he kept an unusual and constantly varying sleep–wake schedule. Such a schedule could have a negative impact on his ability to work and perform, in addition to the problems associated with his sleep-disordered breathing (see chapter 14).

The lower right panel shows a patient who attempted some CPAP use (20% of days; mean use = 5 hr per day) but would be considered noncompliant by any clinician's standards. This patient reported that he used CPAP every night in his subjective follow-up questionnaire.

Frequency and Duration of Use

Although the level of adherence to CPAP treatment by a patient can be objectively monitored, there is no satisfactory consensus on what constitutes a "compliant" patient. This stems, in part, from the variability in recommended treatment regimens prescribed to patients, that is, how much emphasis is placed on regular nightly use and duration of use each night by the health care provider. Our overall findings indicated that CPAP use was attempted (i.e., used for at least 20 min) an average of 66.3% of days ($SD = 37.6$), with a mean duration of 4.88 hours per night ($SD = 1.97$). Although 60% of patients reported using CPAP every day on the follow-up questionnaire, only 43% actually did so, as shown in the monitor data. Patients also overestimated their subjective duration of use per night by a mean of approximately 1 hour (69 min, $SD = 110$).

The 66% compliance rate is comparable to that found in asthma inhaler studies, which have demonstrated compliance rates in the range of 30–70% (Rand & Wise, 1994). However, this rate does not take into consideration the duration of time CPAP is used, and the results are markedly different when the threshold for duration of use per night is varied. For example, in Figure 2, the nightly CPAP use for all the patients in our study across a 60-day period is displayed first with a 4-hour use criterion shown in the top half (mean days = 51.1%, SD = 37.7). This figure is compared with one for the same patients using a stricter 7-hour use criterion, shown in the bottom half of the figure. Our original 20-minute compliance rate of 66.3% dropped to a mean of 16.6% (SD = 21.6) of days at the 7-hour criterion level. Clearly, a different picture of patient compliance emerges depending on the standard of adequate use set by the clinician. We considered an average of 7 hours of CPAP use per night (i.e., quality sleep) to be "optimal" for an individual patient, yet only two of the patients in our group achieved this level on average! Less than 5 hours of "treated," undisturbed sleep per night is low and begs the question of the adequacy of CPAP treatment for the constellation of symptoms presented in sleep apnea, with an emphasis on the associated level of sleepiness.

Also of importance is the fact that initial patient compliance with therapy, measured in the first month, correlated highly (r = .94, p < .0001) with later compliance, measured during the third month of treatment. This finding is consistent with studies of patient adherence to therapy in other disciplines (Sherbourne, Hays, Ordway, DiMatteo, & Kravitz, 1992) and is a clear argument for actively engaging patients "up front" in their own treatment.

Regularity of Use

For the next step in my group's research, we divided our CPAP monitor population retrospectively into "regular" and "irregular" treatment groups (somewhat sidestepping the issue of defining compliance!) so that comparisons could be made of related factors. These divisions were based on a liberal approximation of the amount of nondisrupted sleep we believed was required to avoid serious daytime performance decrements according to previous research. Regular CPAP users (45.7%) used their CPAP device for at least 4 hours per night (duration) on at least 70% of all nights (frequency), whereas irregular users (54.3%) failed to meet either the frequency or duration criteria. Further analyses tried to probe the various subjective and objective variables in an attempt to discern a distinction between regular and irregular users.

Adequate treatment should begin with an understanding of how these symptoms may be related to the interaction of disease state and sleep. All too often, patients and clinicians assume that the primary disease is the cause of all symptoms and overlook the impact of sleep. A better understanding on the part of the patient may help to improve compliance with the prescribed treatment regimen.

REFERENCES

Bye, P. T., Issa, F., Berthon-Jones, M., & Sullivan, C. F. (1984). Studies of oxygenation during sleep in patients with interstitial lung disease. *American Review of Respiratory Disease, 129,* 27–32.

Douglas, N. J. (1994a). Asthma. In M. Kryger, T. Roth, & W. Dement (Eds.), *Principles and practice of sleep medicine* (pp. 748–756). Philadelphia: Saunders.

Douglas, N. J. (1994b). Breathing during sleep in patients with chronic obstructive pulmonary disease. In T. Roth & W. Dement (Eds.), *Principles and practice of sleep medicine* (pp. 758–768). Philadelphia: Saunders.

Koella, W. P. (1985). CNS side effects of β-blockers with special reference to mechanisms of action. *European Journal of Clinical Pharmacology, 28* (suppl.), 55–63.

Levine, S., Henson, D., & Levy, S. (1988). Respiratory muscle rest therapy. *Clinics in Chest Medicine, 9,* 297–309.

Mitler, M. M., Poceta, S., Menn, S. J., & Erman, M. K., (1991). Insomnia in the chronically ill. In P. Hauri (Ed.), *Case studies in insomnia* (pp. 223–236). New York: Plenum Press.

Verrier, R. L., & Kirby, D. A. (1988). Sleep and cardiac arrhythmias. *Annals of the New York Academy of Science, 533,* 238–251.

19

Sleep and Sleep Disorders in Noncardiopulmonary Medical Disorders

Mark R. Pressman, Stephen Gollomp, Robert L. Benz, and Donald D. Peterson

S leep disruption is a common symptom of many medical disorders, and sleep disorders are diagnosable in almost all medical subspecialties. Sometimes sleep disorders are a consequence of medical pathophysiology, and sometimes they are a cause or precursor of that pathophysiology. This chapter reviews the relationship between sleep disorders and a variety of relatively common neurological and medical disorders that are not directly related to cardiopulmonary function.

End-Stage Renal Disease

Chronic kidney failure, or end-stage renal disease (ESRD), has long been associated with sleep complaints, especially in patients undergoing dialysis. Patient sleep complaints focus on problems with both sleep maintenance (frequent awakenings) and daytime alertness. Early reports described patients whose night and day were reversed and who suffered from restless legs (Papper, 1978; Karacan, Salia, & Williams, 1973). More recent surveys of patients undergoing dialysis have found a sleep complaint in 41–52% (Holley, Nespor, & Rault, 1991; Millman, Kimmel, Shore, & Wasserstein, 1985). Presenting complaints run the gamut from sleep onset and sleep-maintenance problems to difficulty breathing and involuntary movements of the legs.

Excessive daytime sleepiness is a frequent complaint, and it is common to enter a dialysis unit during the daytime and find almost all patients fast asleep while being dialyzed.

One of the most common complaints among patients with ESRD is restless legs (Montplaisir & Godbout, 1989). This is a subjective complaint in which patients describe an irritating "creepy, crawling" feeling deep in the muscles of the lower leg, typically in the calf muscle. This sensation can be relieved only by movement of the leg and foot, including stamping of the feet and walking. The sensation typically appears when patients are at rest, most frequently in the hours before the usual bedtime. The irritating sensation coupled with frequent voluntary movements of the legs interferes with normal sleep onset and may delay sleep by hours.

Polysomnographic studies of patients with ESRD have demonstrated a high incidence of both sleep apnea and periodic leg movements in sleep (PLMS; Kimmel, Miller, & Mendelson, 1989; Millman et al., 1985; Pressman, Benz, & Peterson, 1995). In patients undergoing dialysis who have a complaint of a sleep disorder, recent studies have found sleep apnea in 53–75% (Kimmel et al., 1989; Mendelson, Wadhwa, Greenberg, Gujavarty, & Bergofsky, 1990; Millman et al., 1985). In our own case series of 45 dialysis patients with sleep complaints, significant sleep apnea was found in 43, or 94% (Pressman, Benz, & Peterson, 1995). In a recent study of randomly selected patients undergoing dialysis, sleep apnea was found to be present in 72.5%, suggesting that sleep apnea may be present in many patients who are unaware of the problem (Hallett, Burden, Stewart, & Farrell, 1995). The sleep apnea found in the majority of patients with ESRD is generally not of the obstructive variety found in most patients who have sleep apnea. Rather, central and mixed sleep apnea, suggesting a malfunction in the respiratory centers of the brain, is most common. Patients with ESRD are among the few groups of patients in whom repetitive central apnea has been identified.

PLMS also occurs in much higher numbers in patients with ESRD when compared with other patients with PLMS. In our case series of 45 patients, 32 patients, or 71%, had significant PLMS (Pressman, Benz, & Peterson, 1995). Several patients had more than 1,500 leg movements in a single night. These patients represent the worst cases of PLMS ever seen in our sleep laboratory. These leg movements were frequently associated with arousals from sleep, resulting in severe sleep fragmentation and daytime fatigue.

Patients undergoing dialysis have a high rate of mortality. On average, 24% of all such patients die each year (Owen, Lew, Yan Liu, Lowrie, & Lazarus, 1993). There have been numerous attempts to determine risk factors or predictors of this mortality. Among the leading predictors of mortality is poor nutrition, as measured by albumin levels, and less than adequate dialysis, as measured by the urea reduction ratio (URR; Owen et al., 1993). In reviewing patients with ESRD in our case series whom we had studied in the sleep laboratory during the last 4 years, we were surprised to note that 10 of the 45 patients had subsequently died. On close examination, we found that all of the patients who had died had very high levels of periodic leg movements and relatively low levels of sleep apnea (Benz, Pressman, & Peterson, 1994). Usually, the number of movements exceeded 35 per hour of sleep. Patients with high levels of sleep apnea, generally thought to be a disorder with significant cardiopulmonary risks, had survived. A review of albumin and URR levels for these patients found that they did not predict the patient mortality and did not distinguish the surviving patients from the deceased. Only the presence of PLMS predicted mortality in these patients. A Fisher exact probability test showed that a PLMS index (number of leg movements per hour) of 35 per hour or greater predicted mortality at $p = .0009$. The PLMS index and the index of arousing PLMS (leg movements found to cause arousals from sleep) were also the only factors found to be significantly different between surviving and deceased groups of patients undergoing dialysis. Generally, PLMS produces symptoms by causing sleep fragmentation, and these patients did have severely fragmented sleep. It is possible that the sleep deprivation that resulted from this sleep fragmentation exacerbated underlying medical disorders, of which patients on dialysis have many. An alternative explanation is that the presence of high numbers of PLMS is a result of inadequate removal of toxins by dialysis, resulting in some type of cerebral dysfunction that is not easily seen in any other way. In this sense, the PLMS would represent a novel marker of decline in medical status that precedes the more commonly accepted predictors of death.

PLMS and RLS have been reported to respond well to treatment with medication. L-dopa, in particular, has been shown to reduce the number and severity of both disorders (Montpleisir & Godbout, 1989). Sleep apnea in ESRD is often more difficult to treat than in the usual patient with obstructive sleep apnea. Many of the apnea episodes found in ESRD patients are central in nature. However, administration of nasal continuous positive air pressure (NCPAP) has been shown to produce significant reductions in the frequency and severity of sleep apnea episodes (Pressman, Benz, Schleifer, & Peterson, 1993). Unfortunately, as in the general population, compliance with this method of treatment can be difficult, and only 40–60% of patients are able to use the apparatus as prescribed (Kribbs et al., 1993). Hemodialysis does not have an effect on the frequency or severity of sleep apnea in this group (Mendelson et al., 1990).

Patients with ESRD have a high incidence of major sleep disorders, whose main effects are the fragmentation of sleep and decrease in daytime alertness. These disorders are likely to result from both the initial kidney failure and failure of dialysis to normalize the levels of toxins in the blood. Sleep disorders of ESRD are easily diagnosable and often treatable. Complete cures have also been reported following kidney transplant (Langevin, Fouque, Leger, & Robert, 1993; Yasuda, Nishimura, Katsuki, & Tusji, 1986).

Stroke (Cerebrovascular Accident)

Strokes have a circadian pattern similar to that of cardiovascular events, with a peak in the early morning. However, 13–44% of all strokes are known to occur during sleep, being discovered only on awakening (Argentino et al., 1990; Marler et al., 1989; Marsh et al., 1990; Marshall, 1977; Wroe et al., 1992). There is a growing body of evidence that sleep-disordered breathing—snoring, apnea–hypopnea, and their consequences—are predictors, and perhaps the trigger, of strokes during sleep. Snoring has been shown to be an independent risk factor for stroke resulting in an increased odds ratio of 2.13–3.2 (Palomaki, 1991; Palomaki, Partinen, Juvela, & Kaste, 1989; Partinen & Palomaki, 1985). Snorers are more likely to be admitted to the hospital for stroke, and the risk of mortality in the 6 months following discharge from the hospital for stroke was found to be positively correlated with the severity of snoring (Spriggs et al., 1992). Level of consciousness on admission to the hospital was also found to be significantly reduced in snorers. When, in addition to snoring, apnea, daytime sleepiness, and obesity are present, the statistical risk of stroke is increased by 8 times (Palomaki, 1991).

Obstructive sleep apnea syndrome includes many of the signs and symptoms reported to be independent risk factors for stroke. These include hypertension, hypoxemia, obesity, and sudden changes in cerebral perfusion and intracranial pressure during sleep (Shepard, 1990). Reviews have found that 48–96% of all patients with diagnosed sleep apnea have hypertension (Levinson & Millman, 1991). Individual apnea episodes are associated with transient increases in blood pressure that may be extremely high. Cardiac arrhythmias are also common during sleep in patients with sleep apnea and may not be present during daytime electrocardiography (Guilleminault, Connolly, & Winkle, 1983). Sleep apnea is also reported to be associated with sudden increases in intracranial pressure and decreases in cerebral perfusion, with resultant changes in cerebral blood flow (Jennum & Borgeson, 1990). Balfours and Franklin (1994) recently reported that changes in blood pressure are so sudden with apnea and hypopnea that the autoregulatory mechanism that protects the brain from changes in arterial blood pressure may be insufficient, resulting in a cerebrovascular event.

Hypoxemia is also a risk factor for stroke and is a common consequence of sleep apnea. When the upper airway becomes obstructed, oxygen saturation declines, sometimes precipitously, and returns to normal only when the patient awakens briefly at the termination of the apnea. The severity of the hypoxemia is related to its duration, the patient's obesity, and the patient's lung volumes (Shepard, 1990). Obesity, alcohol, and age are all independent risk factors for stroke and also are known to cause significant worsening of sleep apnea (Ancoli-Israel et al., 1991; Issa & Sullivan, 1992). The presence of untreated sleep apnea has been shown to be significantly related not only to increased morbidity but also to increased mortality (He, Kryger, Zorick, Conway, & Roth, 1988; Partinen, Jamieson, & Guilleminault, 1988).

Although sleep researchers strongly believe that there is a real link between sleep apnea and stroke, there is limited published clinical and polysomnographic material available confirming the epidemiological studies. There is only a single report in which the signs of a stroke were observed directly during a sleep study. Rivest and Reiher (1987) reported observing a transient ischemic attack (TIA) immediately following polysomnographically documented sleep apnea. There are several recent studies of sleep apnea in patients presenting with stroke. Pressman, Schetman, et al. (1995) recently reported two cases of older women who awakened from sleep with the signs of a TIA or minor stroke. In both, the symptoms had completely or largely resolved. When these two patients were studied in the sleep laboratory, both were found to have severe sleep apnea associated with severe drops in oxygen saturation to below 50% (see Figure 1). Both were successfully treated with NCPAP and have had no recurrence of symptoms in the 2 years since they were studied. Kapen, Goldberg, and Wynter (1991) found significant sleep apnea in 72% of 47 patients presenting with a stroke. In a study of 10 patients within 1 year of their stroke, Mohsenin and Valor (1995) found that the patients with stroke averaged 51 episodes of apnea–hypopnea per hour, consistent with severe sleep apnea, compared with a group of normal controls who averaged 3 episodes of apnea–hypopnea per hour. Good, Henkle, Gelber, Welsh, and Verhulst (1996) recently reported that 95% of 19 patients with stroke undergoing full polysomnography were found to have severe sleep apnea. Additionally, they reported that patients with stroke and proven sleep apnea had higher rates of mortality at 1 year and that these patients' functional abilities were lower at discharge and at 3 and 12 months after discharge. They proposed that sleep apnea may be an independent predictor of poor functional outcome in patients with stroke. Most of the patients included in this study had a history of snoring that predated the stroke, suggesting that sleep apnea may have played a role in the onset of the stroke. However, most patients also had significant physical and functional deficits after the stroke that may have contributed to the presence or exacerbation of sleep apnea. The most recent study of sleep apnea and stroke found significant sleep apnea in 10 of 13 (77%) men and 7 of 11 (64%) women. In normal controls, the figures were 23% and 14%, respectively (Dyken, Somers, Yamada, Ren, & Zimmerman, 1996). A total of 13 of the 24 patients had their strokes during sleep. A 4-year follow-up study of these patients found a mortality rate of 20.8%. All patients who died had been previously diagnosed with sleep apnea.

It is uncertain from the research whether the sleep apnea caused the stroke or the stroke caused the sleep apnea in the patients studied. Clearly, sleep apnea is a common finding in patients who have had stroke, and it appears to influence both patients' functional state and their survival. It is clear as well that sleep apnea is a significant risk factor and could be the trigger of strokes during sleep. Successful treatment of sleep apnea has been reported to reduce both morbidity and mortality from cardiovascular causes (Motta, Guilleminault, Schroeder, & Dement, 1978; Partinen & Guilleminault, 1990). However, there are no large studies showing the same effect with stroke. Nevertheless, the presence of sleep apnea should always be considered in patients with stroke and treated when appropriate.

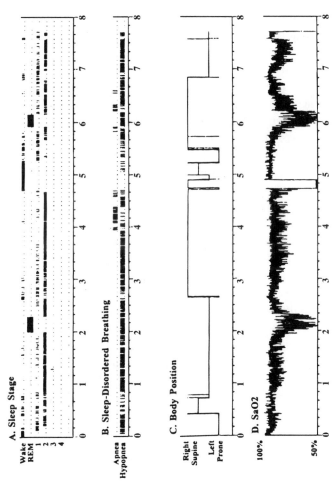

Figure 1.   Histograms displaying results of diagnostic polysomnogram for patient who awakened from sleep with signs of a minor stroke. Histogram A shows frequent fragmentation of sleep. Histogram B shows repetitive apnea and hypopnea episodes that occurred whenever sleep was present. Histogram C shows that apnea and hypopnea occurred in all body positions. Histogram D shows that oxygen saturation level (SaO$_2$) declined abnormally with each apnea and hypopnea episode, reaching 50% for episodes occurring during rapid eye movement (REM) sleep.

Parkinsonism

Parkinson's disease is one of the most common chronic neurological disorders of the aging population. Sleep disturbances are quite common among these patients, with as many as 75% making complaints (Aldrich, 1993; Ashkenasy, 1993). Sleep is typically fragmented in parkinsonism, with longer sleep latencies and decreased sleep efficiency (percentage of time in bed asleep). Specifically, light Stage 1 sleep is significantly increased, whereas both REM sleep and deep sleep are reduced. Careful polysomnographic studies have also demonstrated reduced K-complex and sleep spindle formation, which are common electroencephalographic (EEG) signs of intermediate Stage 2 sleep. Rapid eye movements (REMs) may occur during NREM sleep, and muscle tone may be present during REM sleep. This sleep alteration appears to be predominantly the result of increased motor activity through the night, although the dopamine depletion at the heart of parkinsonism also may result in disruption of basic neurophysiological sleep–wake controls (Rubio, Buruera, Sobrino, Ameabe, & Fenollosa, 1995; Van Hilten et al., 1994). The typical tremors of parkinsonism are generally reduced or absent during sleep, but they may appear during arousals, longer awakenings, and sleep stage changes. The presence of these tremors during the night may make return to sleep difficult. Periodic leg movements in sleep may occur in as many as one-third of all patients, and irregular respiration, characterized by both obstructive and central apnea, may be present. Many patients with parkinsonism also demonstrate frequent motor activation and behaviors during REM sleep, consistent with REM behavior disorder (Commella, Tanner, & Ristoanovoic, 1993; Menza & Rosen, 1995). REM behavior disorder can be precipitated in these patients by treatment with selegiline at normal therapeutic doses (Louden, Morehead, & Schmidt, 1995). Disruptive nocturnal behavior is more common in patients with Parkinson's disease and dementia than in patients with Alzheimer's disease, possibly reflective of the depletion of monoamines in the brain stem in parkinsonism (Bliwise et al., 1995).

Epilepsy

Epilepsy is one of the most common neurological disorders encountered in clinical practice and has been well recognized since antiquity.

There is a complex relationship between sleep and epilepsy. It has long been recognized that sleep deprivation can provoke seizures, particularly in patients with poorly controlled epilepsy, but oversleep does not appear to have any significant effects on frequency of seizures. Patients, particularly children with benign childhood epilepsy with centrotemporal spikes and whose seizures are confined to sleep, generally experience a higher remission rate of their seizure disorder than patients with waking disorders. Sleep efficiency can be significantly reduced in this population, further complicating the individual's quality of life on a daily basis. Slow wave sleep is frequently reduced or absent in these patients, contributing to the overall reduced quality of sleep. REM sleep disturbances are common in unmedicated epilepsy, although it is well known that anticonvulsants can have a substantial impact on this portion of sleep. Some patients have exaggerated periodic leg movements of sleep with arousals, possibly related to epileptiform discharges and exacerbated by medication but seemingly unrelated to nocturnal seizures. Sleep apnea does not appear to be more common in this population. However, the presence of sleep apnea appears to worsen seizure frequency. Treatment of the sleep apnea can be quite beneficial in helping reduce seizure frequency (Devinsky, Ehrenberg, Barthlen, Abramson, & Luciano, 1994; Miyajima, Kurihara, Mizanu, Tamagawa, & Komiya, 1993; Newell & Drake, 1994; Rajna & Veres, 1993).

Multiple Sclerosis

Multiple sclerosis is another common disorder of the nervous system with a progressive but variable clinical course. Fatigue is a common complaint among these patients, although only some have alterations of sleep (Taphoorn et al., 1993). These patients have reduced sleep efficiency and more awakenings during sleep, typically secondary to leg spasms, pain, immobility, nocturia, or medication. Sleep apnea does not appear to be more common than in controls (Tachibana et al., 1994). Sleep architecture is not different from that of controls, but the frequency of periodic leg movements is significantly higher (Ferini-Stambi et al., 1994). It is interesting that morning dream recall may be impaired in multiple sclerosis, possibly reflective of underlying acute disease activity affecting brain areas concerned with REM sleep control (Sandyk, 1995).

Headaches

Another ubiquitous neurological disorder that has a complex, poorly understood interaction with sleep is migraine (Inamorato, Minatti-Hannuch, & Zukerman, 1993). On the basis of clinical experience and questionnaire studies, it has been recognized for many years that migraine can be precipitated by sleep deprivation and, to a lesser degree, by sleep excess. Sleep itself is one of the most effective means of relieving migraine. Morning or nocturnal headaches are frequent indicators of underlying sleep disturbance, particularly sleep apnea. Headaches in patients with substance abuse problems may be associated with insomnia (Pavia, Batista, Martins, & Martins, 1993).

Summary

Sleep disorders are a common feature of many medical disorders. The relationship is often complex, with sleep disorders sometimes serving as the triggers or precursors of medical disease and sometimes occurring as a consequence of medical disorders. Often, sleep disorders can be diagnosed and treated separately from the medical disorder that brought the patient to medical attention. Patients with medical disorders who present with sleep complaints should be evaluated fully for the presence of underlying sleep disorders, and the underlying cause of the sleep disturbance should be treated whenever possible.

REFERENCES

Aldrich, M. S. (1993). Parkinsonism. In M. H. Kryger, T. Roth, & W. C. Dement (Eds.), *Principles and practice of sleep medicine* (pp. 351–357). Philadelphia: Saunders.

Ancoli-Israel, S., Kripke, D. F., Klauber, M. R., Mason, W. J., Fell, R., & Kaplan, O. (1991). Sleep disordered breathing in community dwelling elderly. *Sleep, 14,* 486–495.

Argentino, C., Toni, D., Rasura, M., Violi, R., Sacchetti, M. L., Allegretta, A., Balsano, F., & Fieschi, P. (1990). Circadian variation in the frequency of ischemic stroke. *Stroke, 21,* 387–389.

Ashkenasy, J. J. (1993). Sleep in Parkinson's disease. *Acta Neurologica Scandinavia, 87*(3), 167–170.

Balfours, E. M., & Franklin, K. A. (1994). Impairment of cerebral perfusion during obstructive sleep apneas. *American Journal of Respiratory and Critical Care Medicine, 150,* 1588–1591.

Benz, R. L., Pressman, M. R., & Peterson, D. D. (1994). Periodic Leg Movements of Sleep Index (PLMSI): A sensitive predictor of mortality in dialysis patients. *Journal of the American Society of Nephrology, 5,* 433.

Bliwise, D. L., Watts, R. L., Watts, N., Rye, D. B., Irbe, D., & Hughes, M. (1995). Disruptive nocturnal behavior in Parkinsons disease. *Journal of Geriatric Psychiatry and Neurology, 8*(2), 107–110.

Commella, C. L., Tanner, C. M., & Ristoanovic, R. K. (1993). Polysomnographic measures in Parkinson's disease patients with treatment-induced hallucinations. *Annals of Neurology, 34,* 710–714.

Devinsky, O., Ehrenberg, B., Barthlen, G. M., Abramson, H. S., & Luciano, D. (1994). Epilepsy and sleep apnea syndrome. *Neurology, 44,* 2060–2064.

Dyken, M. E., Somers, V. K., Yamada, T., Ren, Z., & Zimmerman, M. B. (1996). Investigating the relationship between stroke and obstructive sleep apnea. *Stroke, 27,* 401–407.

Ferini-Stambi, L., Filippi, M., Martinelli, V., Oldani, A., Rovaris, M., Zucconi, M., Comi, G., & Smirne, S. (1994). Nocturnal sleep study in multiple sclerosis: Correlations with clinical and brain magnetic resonance imaging findings. *Journal of Neurological Science, 125*(2), 194–197.

Good, D. C., Henkle, J. Q., Gelber, D., Welsh, J., & Verhulst, S. (1996). Sleep-disordered breathing and poor functional outcome after stroke. *Stroke, 27,* 252–259.

Guilleminault, C., Connolly, S. J., & Winkle, R. A. (1983). Cardiac arrhythmia and conduction disturbances during sleep in 400 patients with sleep apnea syndrome. *American Journal of Cardiology, 52,* 490–494.

Hallett, M., Burden, S., Stewart, D., & Farrell, P. (1995). Sleep apnea and end stage renal disease. *ASAIO Journal, 41*(1), S54.

He, J., Kryger, M. H., Zorick, F. J., Conway, W., & Roth, T. (1988). Mortality and apnea index in obstructive sleep apnea. *Chest, 94,* 9–14.

Holley, J. L., Nespor, S., & Rault, R. (1991). Characterizing sleep disorders in chronic hemodialysis patients. *Transactions of the American Society of Artificial Internal Organs, 38,* M456–457.

Inamorato, E., Minatti-Hannuch, S. N., & Zukerman, E. (1993). The role of sleep in migraine attacks. *Neuropsiquiatry 51,* 429–432.

Issa, F. G., & Sullivan, C. E. (1992). Alcohol, snoring and sleep apnea. *Journal of Neurology, Neurosurgery and Psychiatry, 45,* 353–359.

Jennum, P., & Borgeson, S. E. (1990). Intracranial pressure and obstructive sleep apnea. *Chest, 95,* 279–283.

Kapen, S., Goldberg, J., & Wynter, J. (1991). The incidence and severity of obstructive sleep apnea in ischemic cerebrovascular disease. *Neurology, 41* (suppl.), 121.

Karacan, I., Salia, P. J., & Williams, R. (1973). Clinical disorders of sleep. *Psychosomatics, 14,* 77–88.

Kimmel, P. L., Miller, G., & Mendelson, W. B. (1989). Sleep apnea syndrome in chronic renal disease. *American Journal of Medicine, 86,* 308–314.

Kribbs, N. B., Pack, A. I., Kline, L. R., Smith, P. L., Schwartz, A. R., Schubert, N. M., Redline, S., Henry, J. N., Getsy, J. E., & Dinges, D. (1993). Objective measurement of patterns of NCPAP use by patients with obstructive sleep apnea. *American Review of Respiratory Diseases, 147*, 887–895

Langevin, B., Fouque, D., Leger, P., & Robert, D. (1993). Sleep apnea syndrome and end state renal disease: Cure after renal transplantation. *Chest, 103*, 1330–1335.

Levinson, P. D., & Millman, R. P. (1991). Causes and consequences of blood pressure alterations in obstructive sleep apnea. *Archives of Internal Medicine, 151*, 455–462.

Louden, M. B., Morehead, M. A., & Schmidt, H. S. (1995). Activation by selegiline (Eldepryl) of REM sleep behavior in parkinsonism. *West Virginia Medical Journal, 91*(3), 101.

Marler, J. R., Price, T. R., Clark, G. L., Muller, J. E., Roberston, T., Mohr, J. P., Hier, D. B., Wolf, P. A., Caplan, L. R., & Foulkes, M. A. (1989). Morning increase in onset of ischemic stroke. *Stroke, 20*, 473–476.

Marsh, E. E., Biller, J., Adams, H. P., Marler, J. R., Hulbert, J. R., Love, B. B., & Gordon, D. L. (1990). Circadian variation in onset of acute ischemic stroke. *Archives of Neurology, 47*, 1178–1180.

Marshall, J. (1977). Diurnal variation in occurrence of strokes. *Stroke, 8*, 230–231.

Mendelson, W. B., Wadhwa, N. K., Greenberg, H. E., Gujavarty, K., & Bergofsky, E. (1990). Effects of hemodialysis of sleep apnea syndrome in end-stage renal disease. *Clinical Nephrology, 33*, 247–251.

Menza, M. A., & Rosen, R. C. (1995). Sleep in Parkinson's disease. The role of depression and anxiety. *Psychosomatics, 36*, 262–266.

Millman, R. P., Kimmel, P. L., Shore, E. T., & Wasserstein, A. G. (1985). Sleep apnea in hemodialysis patients: The lack of testosterone effect on its pathogenesis. *Nephron, 40*, 407–410.

Miyajima, T., Kurihara, E., Mizanu, Y., Tamagawa, K., & Komiya, K. (1993). Prognosis of epilepsy in psychoneurologically normal children. *No To Hattatsu, 25*(1), 59–64.

Mohsenin, V., & Valor, R. (1995). Sleep apnea in patients with hemispheric stroke. *Archives of Physical Medicine and Rehabilitation, 76*, 71–76.

Montplaisir, J., & Godbout, R. (1989). Restless legs syndrome and periodic leg movements in sleep. In M. H. Kryger, T. Roth, & W. C. Dement (Eds.), *Principles and practice of sleep medicine* (pp. 402–409). Philadelphia: Saunders.

Motta, H., Guilleminault, C., Schroeder, J. S., & Dement, W. C. (1978). Tracheostomy and hemodynamic changes in sleep induced apnea. *Annals of Internal Medicine, 89*, 454–458.

Newell, S. A., & Drake, M. E. (1994). Sleep apnea and periodic movements in epilepsy. *Clinical Electroencephalography, 25*(4), 153–155.

Owen, W. F., Lew, N. L., Yan Liu, S. M., Lowrie, E. G., & Lazarus, J. M. (1993). The urea reduction ratio and serum albumin concentrations as predictors of mortality in patients undergoing dialysis. *New England Journal of Medicine, 329*, 1001–1006.

Palomaki, H. (1991). Snoring and the risk of ischemic brain infarction. *Stroke, 22*, 21–25.

Palomaki, H., Partinen, M., Juvela, S., & Kaste, M. (1989). Snoring as a risk factor for sleep-related brain infarction. *Stroke, 20*, 1311–1315.

Papper, S. (1978). *Clinical nephrology*. Boston: Little, Brown.

Partinen, M., & Guilleminault, C. (1990). Daytime sleepiness and vascular morbidity at seven-year follow-up in obstructive sleep apnea patients. *Chest, 97*, 27–32.

Partinen, M., Jamieson, A., & Guilleminault, C. (1988). Long-term outcome for obstructive sleep apnea syndrome patients: Mortality. *Chest, 94*, 1200–1204.

Partinen, M., & Palomaki, H. (1985). Snoring and cerebral infarction. *Lancet, 2*, 1325–1326.

Pavia, T., Batista, A., Martins, P., & Martins, A. (1993). The relationship between headaches and sleep disturbances. *Headache, 35*, 590–596.

Pressman, M. R., Benz, R. L., & Peterson, D. D. (1995). High incidence of sleep disorders in end stage renal disease patients. *Sleep Research, 25*, 321.

Pressman, M. R., Benz, R. L., Schleifer, C. R., & Peterson, D. D. (1993). Sleep disordered breathing in ESRD: Acute beneficial effects of treatment with nasal continuous positive airway pressure. *Kidney International, 43*, 1134–1139.

Pressman, M. R., Schetman, W. R., Figueroa, W. G., Van Uitert, B., Caplan, H. J., & Peterson, D. D. (1995). Transient ischemic attacks and minor stroke during sleep: Relationship to obstructive sleep apnea syndrome. *Stroke, 26*, 2361–2365.

Rajna, P., & Veres, J. (1993). Correlations between night sleep duration and seizure frequency in temporal lobe epilepsy. *Epilepsia, 34*, 574–579.

Rivest, R., & Reiher, J. (1987). Transient ischemic attacks triggered by symptomatic sleep apneas. *Stroke, 18*, 293.

Rubio, P., Buruera, J. A., Sobrino, R., Ameabe, Y., & Fenollosa, B. (1995). Sleep disorders and Parkinson disease. *Revue Neurologue, 23(120)*, 265–268.

Sandyk, R. (1995). Weak electromagnetic fields restore dream recall in patients with multiple sclerosis. *International Journal of Neuroscience, 82(1–2)*, 113–125.

Shepard, J. W. (1990). Cardiopulmonary consequences of obstructive sleep apnea. *Mayo Clinic Proceedings, 65*, 1250–1259.

Spriggs, D. A., French, J. M., Murdy, J. M., Curless, R. H., Bates, D., & James, O. F. (1992). Snoring increases the risk of stroke and adversely affects prognosis. *Quarterly Journal of Medicine, 83*, 555–662.

Tachibana, N., Howard, R. S., Hirsch, N. P., Miller, D. H., Mosley, I. F., & Fish, D. (1994). Sleep problems in multiple sclerosis. *European Journal of Neurology, 34*, 320–323.

Taphoorn, M. J., van Someren, E., Snoek, F. J., Strijers, R. L., Swaab, D. F., Visscher, F., de Wall, L. P., & Polman, C. H. (1993). Fatigue, sleep disturbances and circadian rhythm in multiple sclerosis. *Journal of Neurology, 240*, 446–448.

Van Hilten, B., Hoff, J. I., Middelkoop, H. A., van der Velde, E. A., Kerkhof, G. A., Wauquier, A., Kamphuisen, H. A., & Roos, R. A. (1994). Sleep disruption in Parkinson's disease. Assessment by continuous activity monitoring. *Archives of Neurology, 51*, 922–928.

Wroe, S. J., Sandercock, P., Bamford, J., Dennis, M., Slattery, J., & Warlow, C. (1992). Diurnal variation in incidence of stroke: Oxfordshire community stroke project. *British Medical Journal, 304(6820)*, 155–157.

Yasuda, T., Nishimura, A., Katsuki, Y., & Tusji, Y. (1986). Restless legs syndrome treated successfully by kidney transplantation: A case report. *Clinical Transplants*, 138.

20

Effects of Hospitalization, Surgery, and Anesthesia on Sleep and Biological Rhythms

Mark R. Pressman, Thomas J. Meyer, Donald D. Peterson, Lee W. Greenspon, and William G. Figueroa

The first hospital in the United States, Pennsylvania Hospital in Philadelphia, was opened in 1752 with 20 beds (Williams, 1976). In 1753 there was a total of 64 hospital admissions. Even in colonial times, there were definite expectations about the purpose and experience of hospital care. Hospitals were expected to be places of not only healing but also rest and recuperation. On August 15, 1751, Benjamin Franklin described his views of the advantages of hospital care in the *Philadelphia Gazette*. The concept of a hospital was new in the colonies, and he wanted to convince the residents of Philadelphia and Pennsylvania of the need for a hospital and to solicit funds for the hospital's construction and operation.

> In an hospital his case will be treated according to the best rules of art, by men of experience and known abilities in their profession. His lodging will be commodious, clean and neat, in a healthy and open situation, his diet will be well chosen, and properly administered: He will have many other necessary conveniences for his relief, such as hot and cold baths, sweating rooms, chirurgic machines, bandage &c. which can rarely be procured in the best private lodgings, much less in those miserable loathsome holes, which are the common receptacles of the diseas'd poor that are brought to the city.—In short a beggar in a well regulated hospital, stands an equal chance with a prince in his palace for a comfortable subsistence, and an expeditious and effectual cure of his diseases. (*Franklin Writings*, 1987, pp. 366–367)

Benjamin Franklin could never have imagined the growth in hospital numbers and in the complexity of their services, much less the inequities of the modern health care system in the United States. In 1992, the American Hospital Association's annual survey of hospitals identified 6,539 registered hospitals in the United States (American Hospital Association, 1993). These hospitals operated with 1,178,000 beds. In 1992, there were 33,536,000 inpatient admissions, for a total of 295,103,000 patient days in the hospital. Patient "days" also include nights, and therefore sleep, in the hospital for this large group of patients. Patients who sleep in the hospital are expected to have all the usual sleep disorders found in the general population. In many cases, the expected incidences of sleep disorders may be higher than in the general population owing to the patients' admitting diagnoses. Additionally, the hospital environment, medications, surgery, and procedures provide many additional opportunities for sleep and biological rhythm disruptions that are unique to the hospital and important to consider when evaluating inpatients in all types of hospital settings.

Sleep Quantity and Quality

Intensive Care Units

Both sleep quantity and sleep quality in the intensive care unit (ICU) following surgery or admission for medical reasons have been found to be extremely poor. Aurell and Elmqvist (1985) reported that patients averaged 2 hours per day of sleep over the first 48 hours following major noncardiac surgery. Deep sleep and rapid eye movement (REM) sleep were either severely or completely suppressed. Five of the patients studied did not sleep at all during the first 24 hours after surgery. Of interest, the sleep EEG findings differed significantly from the nursing staff estimates over the same period, with the nursing staff estimates significantly higher than the objective measurements. All studies of sleep in the ICU have reported significant sleep disruptions (Broughton & Baron, 1978; Dohno, Paskewitz, Lynch, Gimbel, & Thomas, 1979; Hilton, 1976; Johns, Egan, Gay, & Masterton, 1970; Johns, Large, Masterton, & Dudley, 1974; Orr & Stahl, 1977; Wood, 1993). Lesser amounts of sleep disruption are reported to occur with patients undergoing less serious types of surgery, although deep sleep and REM sleep are often suppressed during the first 1–2 days after surgery. It is uncertain whether the sleep changes are due to the shock, pain, or discomfort of the surgery or to the effects of anesthesia or other medications.

Changes in sleep may extend for several weeks following surgery. Orr and Stahl (1977) reported that some patients still showed REM sleep abnormalities 2–4 weeks after open heart surgery. When deep sleep and REM sleep are suppressed by experimental techniques or by medication and then are allowed to return to normal, quantities of REM sleep may initially be higher than expected. This phenomenon, termed *rebound sleep*, may also occur in hospitalized patients. Krill, Moote, Skinner, and Rose (1990) reported that following abdominal surgery, the REM sleep of 12 patients was severely suppressed for 2 days. On the third day, the REM sleep percentage returned to normal limits, but on the fourth day increased above normal limits and was associated with an increase in the number of rapid eye movements (REM, density). REM sleep is known to be associated with rapid changes in cardiovascular function. It has been suggested that REM-sleep-related cardiac arrhythmias, ischemia, and sudden changes in blood pressure may be related to myocardial infarctions and stroke. Krill and colleagues pointed out that many of the worst complications of surgery, including myocardial infarction, stroke, and delirium, occur between the second and fifth postoperative days. They suggested that REM sleep rebound and its associated physiological changes have a similar timing and may contribute to the appearance of these complications.

Patients admitted to ICU units also have recently been found to have a high incidence of sleep apnea. Recent research has shown that 31 of 41 (76%) consecutive patients admitted to an ICU for cardiovascular diseases had significant sleep apnea (Nahmias, Singh, & Karetsky, 1995). Additionally, 17 of 29 (59%) consecutive patients admitted to the ICU for noncardiovascular diseases had significant sleep apnea. This is a surprisingly high percentage for a group of patients with medical diagnoses who did not have a prior diagnosis of sleep apnea. The presence of undiagnosed sleep apnea in an ICU population is of concern because sleep apnea may be associated with cardiac arrhythmias, hypertension, hypoxia, fragmented sleep, daytime fatigue, and decreased cognitive functioning, all of which may be unexplained in terms of the patient's admitting diagnosis. Failure to identify sleep apnea in the ICU may lead to improper diagnosis and treatment.

Non-ICU Hospital Rooms

Few studies of sleep have been performed in areas of the hospital other than the ICU. Yinnon, Ilan, Tadmor, Altaescu, and Hershko (1992) studied sleep on general medical services at two Israeli hospitals using rating scales. Sleep EEG was not measured. Overall they found that 51% of all patients reported sleeping significantly worse in the hospital when compared with their home. Most cited an increased number of awakenings, lesser quantity of sleep, and less restorative sleep. Of patients who did not use sedative–hypnotic medication at home, 26% reported using such medication at the hospital. Patients pointed to noise made by other patients and hospital staff as the main reason for their sleeping difficulties, with pain and discomfort from their illnesses secondary. These findings may differ slightly from findings in American hospitals because the Israeli hospitals studied typically had three to five patients per room. Of interest is that 18% of the patients surveyed reported that they slept better in the hospital than at home. This finding was attributed to successful treatment of their admitting complaints.

Sources of Sleep Disruption in the Hospital

Environmental

Staff. Exhibit 1 lists the many possible sources of sleep disruption in the hospital. Normal procedures in the ICU often prevent patients from getting sufficient uninterrupted sleep. Meyer et al. (1994) found sleep to be interrupted on an hourly basis throughout the night in the ICU, with no uninterrupted period of sleep exceeding 4 hours. Interruptions may be even more frequent in the first 48 hours after major surgery (Hilton, 1976). Even seemingly minor interactions that do not require direct contact with the patient, such as adjusting an intravenous line, are reported to result in patient arousal (Orr & Stahl, 1977).

Light. Meyer et al. (1994) also examined lighting levels in the ICU. They found there was indeed a distinct difference between day and night lighting. However, during the night, medical ICU rooms still averaged 190 lux, whereas a respiratory ICU averaged 1445 lux. The researchers believe this difference was a result of frequent but brief bursts of high intensity light. Under all conditions, lighting was certainly higher than most patients experience in their home environment;

Exhibit 1

Possible Sources of Sleep Disruption in the Hospital

Anticipatory anxiety
Anxiety and depression
Change of sleep environment
Pain and discomfort from admitting medical disorder
Pain, discomfort, and shock following surgery
Effects of medical illness
Effects of medication
Effects of withdrawal from medication
Effects of typical nursing procedures
Biological rhythm disorders resulting from absence of usual time
    cues (zeitgebers)
Noise
Light (too much or too little)
Effects of preexisting sleep disorders such as sleep apnea

---

however, it was not generally high enough to cause shifts in biological rhythms.

Noise. Several studies have found sound levels in the ICU to be much higher than recommended (Bentley, Murphy, & Dudley, 1977; Hansell, 1984; Meyer et al., 1994; Topf & Davis, 1993). The Environmental Protection Agency recommends that sound levels in hospitals not exceed 45 dB during the day and 35 dB during the night (U.S. Environmental Protection Agency, 1974). However, sound levels exceeding 70–80 dB have been frequently noted. Meyer et al. (1994) noted that sounds did display a day–night pattern, with less sound at night, but that over 150 sounds of 80 dB or higher were detected from midnight to 6:00 am. A sound of 80 dB is similar to that of traffic noise on a busy street. Bentley et al. (1977) noted that most noise during the night originated from staff conversations or from equipment. When numerous locations in the ICU were studied, rooms nearest nursing stations were found to be the noisiest. ICU noise has been found to result directly in arousal from sleep (Aaron, Carskadon, Meyer, Hill, & Millman, 1995), and peak sound levels greater than 80 dB were found to be positively and significantly related to arousal from sleep.

Patients receiving the very close monitoring required in intensive care units are attached to a variety of sophisticated electronic medical equipment. Changes in patient status monitored by this equipment are signaled to ICU staff by alarms. Cropp, Woods, Raney, and Bredle (1994) counted 33 different audio signals in their ICU, 10 of which they considered critical alarms. They reported that during a typical day shift, 50 audio alarms sounded every hour. Nighttime rates were not reported. Paradoxically, when alarm sounds were tape recorded and presented to ICU staff, staff were able to identify only 50% of the critical alarms and 40% of the noncritical alarms. This finding suggested to the authors that much of the noise originating from equipment may not be essential, although they also suggested that staff may have needed additional training. Because ICU care is around-the-clock, it seems likely that similar levels of alarm noise are present at night, representing a significant source of sleep-disrupting noise.

Biological Rhythm Disturbances

When patients enter the hospital, they leave behind the usual external time cues that organize their 24-hour rhythms of sleep and wakefulness. Family, job, light–darkness, and other cues are no longer present during the hospital stay. These may or may not be replaced by other cues. Farr, Gaspar, and Munn (1984) studied seven physiological variables in 12 female inpatients (mean age = 30.7 yr) during their hospitalization for minor surgery. They found that all patients experienced desynchronization of at least one variable from its usual position related to the sleep–wake rhythm. Most of the patients experienced a phase delay in the timing of measured variables. Patients who were able to maintain normal circadian synchrony of the most variables were also reported to return to normal activities faster after discharge than patients who were more desynchronized. In other studies by the same group, 23 patients who had undergone various types of surgery experienced phase delays of 2–12 hours (Farr, Keene, Samson, & Michael-Jacoby, 1984). Patients with the most severe phase delays took the longest time to reestablish normal circadian patterns of sleep and wakefulness following discharge. Similar findings have been associated with surgery in animals. Farr, Campell-Grossman, and Mack (1988) studied rats before and after surgery. After surgery, they found initially a total loss of circadian rhythmicity followed by a delay in circadian timing that lasted for 2–5 days, with rats with the most severe phase delay taking the longest to return to normal patterns of activity. Baskett, Cockrem, and Todd (1991) also reported changes in the timing of melatonin secretion in elderly medical patients who were hospitalized when compared with healthy elderly persons living in the community. Under normal circumstances, bright light (2500 lux or more) suppresses the secretion of melatonin during daylight hours. The hospitalized patients showed a daytime peak of melatonin secretion that was not present at all in the community-living elderly participants as well as an earlier rise in the typical nocturnal peak of melatonin. This earlier rise may represent a phase advance in the hospitalized patients' 24-hour rhythms. Although most people in settings without time cues experience phase delay (go to sleep later), some elderly people may experience phase advance (go to sleep earlier). The changes in melatonin secretion are attributed to the lack of sufficiently bright light in the hospital setting. As noted previously, hospital lighting rarely approaches the 2500 lux necessary to suppress melatonin and have other circadian-rhythm entraining effects.

Patients admitted to hospitals may experience biological rhythm disturbances owing to the absence of the usual time cues or the effects of surgery, medication, or illness. This may leave the patient in a state comparable to severe jet lag. Circadian rhythm disturbances may in turn cause the patient to become sleep-deprived. If a phase delay in the patient's usual sleep–wake rhythms shifts the patient's biologically best time for sleep from 4:00 a.m. to noon, doctors arriving for morning rounds at 7:00 a.m. will awaken patients in the middle of their sleep period. Once the patient is awakened, he or she may not have the opportunity to return to sleep until much later. Phase delays in the timing of sleep and wakefulness may affect the delivery of medication at bedtime. If medication is given at a socially acceptable bedtime, perhaps 11:00 p.m., but the patient's biologically best bedtime is 4:00 a.m., is that medication being administered properly?

Anesthesia

Administration of anesthesia may have a variety of effects on patients' sleep and wakefulness. As noted earlier, anesthesia may be partially responsible for desynchronization of circadian rhythms. However, when certain types of anesthesia were given experimentally without surgery, shifts in circadian rhythms were not found (Sessler, Lee, & McGuire, 1991). Thus, the shock, pain, and discomfort of surgery may be necessary for the phase delay to occur. A more serious complication of anesthesia related to sleep and sleep disorders is the possible exacerbation or induction of obstructive sleep apnea (Connolly, 1991).

Obstructive sleep apnea is a potentially life-threatening disorder characterized by repetitive closures of the upper airway. Apnea is associated with hypoxemia, cardiac arrhythmias, hypertension, and changes in cerebral blood flow and perfusion (Guilleminault, Connolly, & Winkle, 1983; Jennum & Borgeson, 1990; Levinson & Millman, 1991). The presence of untreated obstructive sleep apnea is associated with increased mortality (He, Kryger, Zorick, Conway, & Roth, 1988). Epidemiological studies have shown that snoring and other symptoms of sleep apnea increase the risk of stroke by 8 times (Palomaki, 1991). Successful treatment of sleep apnea has been reported to decrease cardiovascular morbidity (Partinen & Guilleminault, 1990).

Any depression of central nervous system activity is likely to result in worsening of existing sleep apnea and may induce significant sleep apnea when none was previously present (Connolly, 1991). Central nervous system depressants, including anesthetics, sedative–hypnotic medications, narcotics, and alcohol, are well known to increase the severity of sleep apnea by delaying the arousal response that terminates apnea episodes as well as by reducing the tone of upper airway muscles, decreasing the pressure necessary for causing the apnea (Bonora, St. John, & Bledsoe, 1985; Connolly, 1991). Almost all types of anesthesia have a similar effect. There are numerous reports in the medical literature describing a finding of sleep apnea in patients under anesthesia who had no prior history of this disorder and even in patients who had just undergone surgery for treatment of sleep apnea (Hanning, 1989; Keamy, Cadieux, Kofke, & Kales, 1987; Reeder et al., 1991; Rennotte, Baele, Aubert, & Rodenstein, 1995; Rosenberg & Kehlet, 1991; Tierney, Pollard, & Doran, 1989). In patients receiving general anesthesia with intubation during surgery, previously undiagnosed sleep apnea has been discovered in the recovery room following surgery or, in some cases, following preoperative sedation. Serious complications and death have been attributed to the effects of undetected or untreated sleep apnea caused by anesthesia (Rennotte et al., 1995; Rosenberg & Kehlet, 1991; Tierney et al., 1989). Rosenberg, Pedersen, Ramsing, and Kehlet (1992) investigated the unexpected deaths of 18 hospitalized patients following abdominal surgery. They found that 13 of these patients had died during the night, presumably during sleep. Cardiac arrhythmias were thought to be the most likely cause of most deaths, with undiagnosed sleep apnea a possible contributing factor. Reports of complications following anesthesia caused by sleep apnea indicated that a history of sleep apnea was generally not taken by medical personnel prior to the surgery. In many cases, it was fortunate that postsurgical monitoring included the use of an oximeter capable of detecting changes in oxygen saturation associated with apnea. Current guidelines recommend taking a thorough sleep history and, if necessary, keeping the patient intubated until anesthesia wears off (Connolly, 1991; Rennotte et al., 1995). Use of nasal continuous positive airway pressure (NCPAP) equipment, the outpatient treatment of choice for sleep apnea, is also recommended before and after surgery (Rennotte et al., 1995).

Exacerbation or induction of sleep apnea is also possible with use of presurgical sedatives, postsurgical pain killers, and medications for conscious sedation for outpatient procedures. These medications can induce life-threatening episodes of sleep apnea in undiagnosed patients (VanDecar, Martinez, & DeLisser, 1991). Any suppression of cental nervous system activity is likely to induce sleep apnea in patients who have undiagnosed and unrecognized sleep apnea. These findings have led some hospitals to require continuous monitoring of oxygen levels during outpatient procedures using conscious sedation.

Anesthesia and other medications used before, during, and after surgery may also have direct effects on the quality and quantity of sleep. Morphine, for instance, is a potent suppresser of REM sleep, and benzodiazepines reduce slow wave sleep activity (Kay, Eisenstein, & Jasinski, 1969).

Hypnotic Medication

The days of routine prescription of hypnotic medication for all patients in the hospital are generally thought to be over. However, prn (as needed) prescription of hypnotic medications remains common (Berlin, 1984). A recent Dutch study of hypnotic prescribing patterns in three hospitals found that 47% of all patients on both medical and surgical services had a prescription for a sleep medication, although only 34% had taken sleep medication that night (Halfens, Cox, & Kuppen–Van Merwijk, 1994).

This pattern is similar to those noted in the United States in the early 1980s. A 1984 study found 46% of patients on medical services had been prescribed hypnotic medication, although only 31% actually used this medication during their hospitalization. On surgical services, 96% of all patients were prescribed hypnotic medications, whereas 88% used this medication during their hospitalization (Perry & Wu, 1984).

In most cases hypnotics were prescribed prn, but nursing staff made the final decision about whether or not the patient received the sleep medication. A review of the nursing notes found no correlation between the decision to give sleeping medication and the patient's quantity and quality of sleep.

The hospital may be the place where patients are first exposed to the use of sleep medication. In the Dutch study described earlier, 53% of patients who had never used sleep medication at home took it for the first time in the hospital (Halfens et al., 1994). Of those who had never taken sleeping medication before and who took it five or more times in the hospital, almost 15% continued to take sleeping medication at home following discharge. In a survey of hypnotic drug use in general medical practice, 21.6% of all patients taking hypnotic medication were found to have started taking this medication while hospitalized (Clift, 1975).

Effects of Sleep Deprivation on Hospitalized Patients

As noted in chapter 3, this volume, sleep deprivation has a variety of effects on physiology and reflexes that may worsen existing medical conditions and interfere with medical procedures. Sleep deprivation has been reported to depress ventilatory responses to hypercapnia (increased carbon dioxide) and hypoxia (decreased oxygen) in otherwise normal persons, suggesting that it could contribute to hypoventilation in hospitalized patients (White, Douglas, Pickett, Zwillich, & Weil, 1983; Schiffman, Trontell, Mazar, & Edelman, 1983). Sleep-deprived dogs also showed delayed or depressed arousal responses to hypoxia, hypercapnia, and stimulation of the upper airway (Bowes, Woolf, Sullivan, & Phillipson, 1980). Respiratory muscle endurance has been shown to be affected after sleep deprivation (Chen & Tank, 1989). Specifically, inspiratory muscle activity endurance is significantly decreased, whereas end tidal carbon dioxide is increased. Genioglossus muscle activity (related to movement of the tongue) was also decreased with sleep deprivation in older research participants (Leiter, Knuth, & Bartlett, 1985). The effects of sleep deprivation on cardiopulmonary functioning may be much greater in patients with existing disease such as chronic obstructive pulmonary disease (Phillips, Cooper, & Burke, 1987). However, almost all studies of sleep deprivation have been performed on young, normal persons deprived of sleep for 60 hours or less. Extrapolation of these findings to hospitalized patients should be done with caution.

Sleep deprivation may affect immune function (for a complete review, see chapter 21, this volume). Complete sleep deprivation of rats for several weeks results in death (Rechtschaffen, Bergmann, Everson, Kushida, & Gilliland, 1989). More recent research has suggested that the cause of death in these rats is a total breakdown of host defenses caused by immunosuppression, permitting the pathogens that are normally present in the blood but well controlled by the immune system to flourish, producing severe septicemia, or blood poisoning (Everson, 1993). Brown, Pang, Husband, and King (1989) reported that sleep deprivation interfered with immune responses to respiratory viruses administered nasally in rats even though the rats had been previously inoculated against that respiratory virus.

Sleep deprivation has also been shown to worsen sleep apnea, with an effect similar to that of medication that depresses the central nervous system. Both acute total sleep deprivation and partial, cumulative sleep deprivation have been shown to increase the volume of snoring as well as increase the frequency and severity of sleep apnea episodes. Daytime sleepiness also increases out of proportion to the sleep loss (Pearson & Svanborg, 1996; Stoohs & Dement, 1994).

The most commonly accepted theory of sleep is that it serves the purpose of tissue restoration, with peak activities in protein synthesis and cell division occurring during sleep (Horne, 1988). Sleep deprivation may thus disrupt restorative activities of the body. Most researchers of immune function and sleep deprivation have studied healthy persons who underwent total sleep deprivation for 24–80 hours. This acute form of sleep deprivation may not appropriately mimic the sleep deprivation of hospitalized patients, who may already be sleep-deprived owing to the pain and discomfort of their medical disorder and are more likely to suffer from partial, cumulative sleep deprivation over a long period of time. Additionally, hospitalized patients may already have impaired immune function that could be more easily affected by sleep deprivation.

ICU Psychosis

Patients admitted to the ICU sometimes develop acute changes in their mental status and cognitive function. ICU psychosis, or ICU syndrome, typically develops after 3 to 7 days in the ICU (Blachy & Starr,

1964; Hansell, 1984; Helton, Gordon, & Nunnery, 1980; Johns et al., 1974; Krachman , D'Alonzo, & Criner, 1995; Lazarus & Hagen, 1968). Symptoms may include agitation, combativeness, delirium, disorientation, irritability, delusions, hallucinations, and paranoia. The patient's age, type and severity of illness, and psychological and drug history, as well as the use of a cardiopulmonary bypass pump, are thought to be contributing factors.

Although there is no consensus on the matter, ICU syndrome has more recently been reported to be associated with both severe sleep deprivation and circadian rhythm desynchronization. A study of 62 ICU patients who exhibited ICU syndrome found that 24% of these patients experienced 50% or more sleep loss, whereas another 16% had more moderate sleep deprivation (Helton et al., 1980). A significant correlation was found between the degree of sleep deprivation and the severity of the ICU syndrome. Another researcher found ICU syndrome in 24% of 100 patients after cardiothoracic surgery; 27% of those patients were thought by nursing staff to be severely sleep-deprived (Heller et al., 1970).

ICU syndrome has been reported to resolve within 1–2 days after transfer from the ICU (Helton et al., 1980). Of course, the transfer may have indicated that the medical or surgical problems that had led to the admission of the patient to the ICU originally were no longer present, suggesting that the patient was healthier and using fewer medications.

Conclusion

Sleep disorders are a common consequence of hospitalization, surgery, anesthesia, and medical disorders that result in significant sleep deprivation. Sleep deprivation appears to be maximized in patients following major surgical procedures during stays in the ICU, but it may occur anywhere in the hospital. Recovery of normal sleep patterns may take weeks. The hospital environment is often not conducive to normal sleeping. Staff interruptions, noise, and light in addition to pain and discomfort may cause significant reductions in both the quantity and quality of sleep. Biological rhythms may also become disrupted, leaving the patient in a state similar to severe jet lag after only a few days in the hospital. Anesthesia and other medications that depress the central nervous system can cause sleep apnea to appear in patients who have not been previously diagnosed as well as suppression of both REM sleep and deep sleep. Sleep deprivation and circadian rhythm disorders are likely to be important factors in the development of the ICU syndrome. Assessment of changes in the quantity and quality of sleep, as well as of the presence of sleep disorders, should be part of all evaluations of patients in the hospital. Sleep deprivation and circadian rhythm disorders may affect not only mental status and cognitive functioning but also the course, treatment, and recovery from medical disorders and surgery.

REFERENCES

Aaron, J., Carskadon, M., Meyer, T., Hill, T., & Millman, R. (1995). Environmental noise is a cause of sleep disruption in a respiratory care unit. *American Journal of Respiratory and Critical Care Medicine, 151,* 4, A495.

American Hospital Association. (1993). *AHA hospital statistics.* Chicago: Author.

Aurell, J., & Elmqvist, D. (1985). Sleep in the surgical intensive care unit: Continuous polysomnographic recording of sleep in nine patients receiving postoperative care. *British Medical Journal, 290,* 1029–1032.

Baskett, J. J., Cockrem, J. F., & Todd, M. A. (1991). Melatonin levels in hospitalized elderly patients: A comparison with community based volunteers. *Age & Ageing 20,* 430–434.

Bentley, S., Murphy, F., & Dudley, H. (1977). Perceived noise in surgical wards and an intensive care area: An objective analysis. *British Medical Journal, 2,* 1503–1506.

Berlin, R. M. (1984). Management of insomnia in hospitalized patients. *Annals of Internal Medicine, 100,* 398–404.

Blachy, P. H., & Starr, A. (1964). Post-cardiotomy delirium. *American Journal of Psychiatry, 121,* 371–375.

Bonora, M., St. John, W. M., & Bledsoe, T. A. (1985). Differential elevation of protriptyline and depression by diazepam of upper airway respiratory motor activity. *American Review of Respiratory Diseases, 131,* 41–45.

Bowes, G., Woolf, G. M., Sullivan, C. E., & Phillipson, E. A. (1980). Effect of sleep fragmentation on ventilatory and arousal response of sleeping dogs to respiratory stimuli. *American Review of Respiratory Diseases, 125,* 286–289.

Broughton, R., & Baron, R. (1978). Sleep patterns in the intensive care unit and on the ward after acute myocardial infarction. *Electroencephalography and Clinical Neurophysiology, 45,* 348–360.

Brown, R., Pang, G., Husband, A. J., & King, M. G. (1989). Suppression of immunity to influenza virus infection in the respiratory tract following sleep disturbance. *Regional Immunity, 2,* 321–325.

Chen, H., & Tank, Y. (1989). Sleep loss impairs inspiratory muscle endurance. *American Review of Respiratory Diseases, 140,* 907–909.

Clift, A. D. (1975). Dependence on hypnotic drugs in general practice. In A. D. Clift (Ed.), *Sleep disturbance and hypnotic dependence* (pp. 71–95). Amsterdam: Excerpta Medica.

Connolly, L. A. (1991). Anesthetic management of obstructive sleep apnea patients. *Journal of Clinical Anesthesia 3*, 461–469.

Cropp, A. J., Woods, L. A., Raney, D., & Bredle, D. L. (1994). Name that tone: The proliferation of alarms in the intensive care unit. *Chest, 105*, 1217–1220.

Dohno, S., Paskewitz, D. A., Lynch, J. J., Gimbel, K. S., & Thomas, S. A. (1979). Some aspects of sleep disturbance in coronary patients. *Perceptual and Motor Skills, 48*, 199–205.

Everson, C. A. (1993). Sustained sleep deprivation impairs host defense. *American Journal of Physiology, 265*, R1148–R1154.

Farr, L. A., Campell-Grossman C., & Mack, J. M. (1988). Circadian disruption and surgical recovery. *Nursing Research, 37*, 170–175.

Farr, L. A., Gaspar, T., & Munn, D. (1984). Desynchronization with surgery. In E. Haus & H. F. Kabat (Eds.), *Chronobiology* (pp. 544–547). New York: Karger.

Farr, L. A., Keene, A., Samson, D., & Michael-Jacoby, A. (1984). Alterations in circadian excretion of urinary variables and physiological indicators of stress following surgery. *Nursing Research, 33*, 140–146.

Farr, L. A., Keene, A., Samson, D., & Michael-Jacoby, A. (1986). Relationship between disruption of rhythmicity and reentrainment in surgical patients. *Chronobiologia, 13*, 105–113.

Franklin Writings. (1987). New York: Library of America.

Guilleminault, C., Connolly, S. J., & Winkle, R. A. (1983). Cardiac arrhythmias and conduction disturbances during sleep in 400 patients with sleep apnea syndrome. *American Journal of Cardiology, 52*, 490–494.

Halfens, R., Cox, K., & Kuppen–Van Merwijk, A. (1994). Effect of use of sleep medication in Dutch hospitals on the use of sleep medication at home. *Journal of Advanced Nursing, 19*(1), 66–70.

Hanning, C. D. (1989). Obstructive sleep apnoea. *British Journal of Anaesthesia, 63*, 477–488.

Hansell, H. N. (1984). The behavioral effects of noise on man: The patient with "intensive care unit psychosis." *Heart & Lung, 13*(1), 59–65.

He, J., Kryger, M. H., Zorick, F. J., Conway, W., & Roth, T. (1988). Mortality and apnea index in obstructive sleep apnea. *Chest, 94*, 9–14.

Heller, S. S., Frank, K. A., Malm, J. R., Bowman, T. O., Harris, P. D., Charlton, P. D., & Kornfeld, D. S. (1970). Psychiatric complications of open-heart surgery. *New England Journal of Medicine, 283*, 1015–1020.

Helton, M. C., Gordon S. H., & Nunnery, S. L. (1980). The correlation between sleep deprivation and the intensive care unit syndrome. *Heart & Lung, 9*, 464–468.

Hilton, B. A. (1976). Quantity and quality of sleep and sleep disturbing factors in a respiratory care unit. *Journal of Advances in Nursing, 1*, 453–468.

Horne, J. A. (1988). *Why we sleep: The function of sleep in humans and other mammals.* New York: Oxford University Press.

Jennum, P., & Borgeson, S. E. (1990). Intracranial pressure and obstructive sleep apnea. *Chest, 95*, 279–283

Johns, M. W., Egan, P., Gay, T. J. A., & Masterton, J. P. (1970). Sleep habits and symptoms in male medical and surgical patients. *British Medical Journal, 2,* 509–512.

Johns, M. W., Large, A. A., Masterton, J. P., & Dudley, H. A. F. (1974). Sleep and delirium after open heart surgery. *British Journal of Surgery, 61,* 377–381.

Kay, D. C., Eisenstein, R. B., & Jasinski, D. R. (1969). Morphine effects on human REM state, waking state and NREM sleep. *Psychopharmacologia (Berlin), 14,* 404–416.

Keamy, M. F., Cadieux, R. J., Kofke, W. A., & Kales, A. (1987). The occurrence of obstructive sleep apnea in a recovery room patient. *Anesthesiology, 66,* 232–234.

Krachman, S. L., D'Alonzo, G. E. & Criner, G. J. (1995). Sleep in the intensive care unit. *Chest, 107,* 1713–1720.

Krill, R. L., Moote, C. A., Skinner, M. I., & Rose, E. A. (1990). Anesthesia with abdominal surgery leads to intense REM sleep during first postoperative week. *Anesthesiology 73,* 52–61.

Lazarus, H. R., & Hagen, J. H. (1968). Prevention of psychosis following open-heart surgery. *American Journal of Psychiatry, 124,* 1190–1195.

Leiter, J. C., Knuth, S. L., & Bartlett, D. (1985). The effect of sleep deprivation on activity of the genioglossus muscle. *American Review of Respiratory Diseases, 132,* 1242–1245.

Levinson, P. D., & Millman, R. P. (1991). Causes and consequences of blood pressure alterations in obstructive sleep apnea. *Archives of Internal Medicine, 151,* 455–462.

Meyer, T. J., Eveloff, S. E., Bauer, M. S., Schwartz, W. A., Hill, N. S., & Millman, R. P. (1994). Adverse environmental conditions in the respiratory and medical ICU settings. *Chest, 105,* 1211–1216.

Nahmias, J., Singh, J., & Karetsky, M. (1995). Prevalence of sleep apnea in an intensive care population admitted with cardiovascular events. *Chest, 105*(3), 164S.

Orr, W. C., & Stahl, M. L. (1977). Sleep disturbances after open heart surgery. *American Journal of Cardiology, 39,* 196–201.

Palomaki, H. (1991). Snoring and the risk of ischemic brain infarction. *Stroke, 22,* 1021–1025.

Partinen, M., & Guilleminault, C. (1990). Daytime sleepiness and vascular morbidity at seven year follow-up in obstructive sleep apnea patients. *Chest, 97,* 27–32.

Pearson, H. E., & Svanborg, E. (1996). Sleep deprivation worsens obstructive sleep apnea. *Chest, 109,* 645–650.

Perry, S. W., & Wu, A. (1984). Rationale for the use of hypnotic agents in a general hospital. *Annals of Internal Medicine, 100,* 441–446.

Phillips, B. A., Cooper, K. R., & Burke, T. V. (1987). The effect of sleep loss on breathing in chronic obstructive pulmonary disease. *Chest, 91,* 29–32.

Rechtschaffen, A., Bergmann, B. M., Everson, C. A., Kushida, C. A., & Gilliland, M. A. (1989). Sleep deprivation in the rat: X. Integration and discussion of findings. *Sleep, 12,* 68–87.

Reeder, M. K., Goldman, M. D., Loh, L., Muir, K. R., Casey, K. R., & Gitlin, D. A. (1991). Postoperative obstructive sleep apnoea: Hemodynamic effects of treatment with nasal CPAP. *Anaesthesia, 46,* 849–853.

Rennotte, M., Baele, P., Aubert, G., & Rodenstein, D. O. (1995). Nasal continuous positive airway pressure in perioperative management of patients with obstructive sleep apnea submitted to surgery. *Chest, 107,* 367–374.

Rosenberg, J., & Kehlet, H. (1991). Postoperative episodic oxygen desaturation in the sleep apnoea syndrome. *Acta Anaesthesiology Scandinavia, 35,* 368–369.

Rosenberg, J., Pedersen, M. H., Ramsing, T., & Kehlet, H. (1992). Circadian variation in unexpected postoperative death. *British Journal of Surgery, 79,* 1300–1302.

Schiffman, P. L., Trontell, M. C., Mazar, M. E., & Edelman, N. H. (1983). Sleep deprivation decreases ventilatory response to CO_2 but not load compensation. *Chest, 84,* 695–698.

Sessler, D. I., Lee, K. A., & McGuire, J. (1991). Isoflurane anesthesia and circadian temperature cycles in humans. *Anesthesiology, 75,* 985–989.

Stoohs, A., & Dement, W. C. (1994). Snoring and sleep-related breathing abnormality during partial sleep deprivation. *New England Journal of Medicine, 328,* 1279.

Tierney, N. M., Pollard, B. J., & Doran, B. R. H. (1989). Obstructive sleep apnoea. *Anaesthesia, 44,* 235–237.

Topf, M., & Davis J. E. (1993). Critical care unit noise and rapid eye movement (REM) sleep. *Heart & Lung, 22,* 252–258.

U.S. Environmental Protection Agency. (1974). Information on levels of environmental noise requisite to protect public health and welfare with an adequate margin of safety. Washington, DC: Government Printing Office.

Van Decar, D. H., Martinez, A. P., & DeLisser, E. A. (1991). Sleep apnea syndromes: A potential contraindication for patient controlled analgesia. *Anesthesiology, 74,* 623–624.

White, D. P., Douglas, N. J., Pickett, C. K., Zwillich, C. W., & Weil, J. V. (1983). Sleep deprivation and control of ventilation. *American Review of Respiratory Diseases, 128,* 984–986.

Williams, W. H. (1976). *America's first hospital: The Pennsylvania Hospital 1751–1841.* Wayne, PA: Haverford House.

Wood, A. M. (1993). A review of literature relating to sleep in hospital with emphasis on the sleep of the ICU patient. *Intensive & Critical Care Nursing* 9(2), 129–136.

Yinnon, A. M., Ilan, Y., Tadmor, B., Altaescu, G., & Hershko, C. (1992). Quality of sleep in the medical department. *British Journal of Clinical Practice, 46(2),* 88–91.

Sleep Deprivation
and the Immune System

Carol A. Everson

Although common sense warns that sleep deprivation can predispose to illness, particularly infections, experimental investigations of sleep-deprivation-induced changes in the immune system are few and, therefore, the evidence is sparse. The purpose of this chapter is to review the evidence that exists linking sleep deprivation with alterations in host defense and the immune system. Six general findings indicate that sleep and the immune system are intricately and functionally related: (a) Sleep deprivation in humans results in activation of the first line of host defense; (b) bacterial products and immunomodulators are potent somnogenic agents; (c) changes in plasma levels of immunomodulators covary with sleep; (d) antitumor factors and antibody production appear to be altered by sleep deprivation in laboratory animals; (e) host defense fails during prolonged sleep deprivation in laboratory rats; and (f) changes in sleep parameters are associated with infectious disease in humans and laboratory animals.

Perspectives on Human Sleep Deprivation Studies

Short-term sleep deprivation in normal young adults studied under carefully controlled experimental and environmental conditions without added exertion has not produced illness, and most markers of the integrity of the immune response remain within or near normal limits. Consequently, a dysfunction has not yet been found in humans resulting from sleep deprivation that would attach clinical significance to the mild changes that have been found in some immune-related parameters. Still, to avoid concluding prematurely that sleep deprivation has no role in host defense and immune function, it is important to consider two points: (a) Human participants generally have been young, and all have been in excellent health; and (b) most sleep deprivation studies have consisted of only 1 or 2 nights of sleeplessness. In the first case, the relatively young and healthy are remarkably resistant to many biological insults in the short term. Studies in the laboratory rat have shown that sleep-deprivation-induced pathologies evolve slowly over a 3-week period and eventuate in a life-threatening state (discussed later). This slowly developing pattern also occurs during deprivation of other basic requirements such as food and water. It might be expected, therefore, that the initial physiological changes in healthy human persons deprived of sleep for one or two nights would be subtle.

The duration of the sleep deprivation period employed in most studies of humans in which immune-related parameters have been measured is 48 hours (i.e., 2 days and 1 night) or 64 hours (3 days and 2 nights), preceded by a baseline period and followed by a recovery period. Sleep-deprivation-induced symptoms that are known to occur in humans include a decrease in oral temperature; an increased sensitivity to painful stimuli, changes in mood (e.g., irritability); and most striking, a marked deterioration in cognitive performance (Horne, 1988; Kleitman, 1963). After 68–76 hours of sleep deprivation, the deterioration in cognitive performance cannot be overcome by increased incentives and mustering of willpower (Horne, 1988). This suggests that, at least for brain function, a more fundamental biological impairment occurs after three days and three nights of sleeplessness, which is beyond the time frame of observation in most studies. All changes in mood and cognitive performance are quickly reversed after subsequent rebound sleep, indicating that the physiological changes induced by sleep deprivation are quickly reversible by sleep (Horne, 1988).

Sleep-Deprivation-Induced Changes in Immune-Related Parameters in Humans

During sleep deprivation, the number of circulating white blood cells (WBCs) commonly increases. In 1925, investigators at Georgetown University kept participants awake for up to three nights. The only remarkable physiological finding was that the leukocyte count increased gradually to levels well above normal in 6 of 8 participants (cited in Kleitman, 1963). Much later, in 1969, Kuhn, Brodan, Brodanová, and Ryšánek reported a gradual increase in WBCs in participants who were sleep-deprived for 72–126 hours. Recently, Dinges and colleagues (1994) also reported a gradual increase in circulating WBC numbers in individuals who were sleep-deprived for 64 hours.

The majority of leukocytes (60–80%) are granulocytes, composed of polymorphonuclear neutrophils, eosinophils, and basophils, which have the principal protective function of phagocytosis. Granulocytes lack two attributes typically associated with immunity: antigenic specificity and memory. Neutrophils are usually the first cells to respond to a challenge to the host, arriving at a site of injury where they release antibacterial substances and digestive enzymes. Increased levels of neutrophils are expected with infection, inflammation, trauma, poisoning, and ketoacidosis, whereas increases in eosinophils are generally associated with parasitic infestation. Both eosinophils and basophils are associated with allergic reactions and asthma. The increase in leukocytes during sleep deprivation has been attributed to neutrophils (Kuhn et al., 1969) and to both granulocytes (excluding eosinophils) and monocytes (Dinges et al., 1994).

Monocytes, which make up 2–10% of leukocytes, differentiate mostly into mononuclear phagocytes, or macrophages. Macrophages are second to the neutrophils in responding quickly after stimulation. Within 24 hours, they leave the blood and arrive at the sites of reaction or injury. Along with granulocytes, macrophages serve as surveillance cells in antitumor defense. Macrophages not only help to eliminate invading microorganisms but also remove old and damaged serum proteins and cellular debris from the circulation. As phagocytes, macrophages release a number of powerful chemicals, enzymes, complement proteins, and regulatory factors. One of these secreted products is an antigen-nonspecific soluble factor (i.e., cytokine), interleukin-1, which has been found to increase during sleep deprivation (Moldofsky, Lue, Davidson, & Gorczynski, 1989). This substance is also known as a somnogen (Krueger, Walter, Dinarello, Wolff, & Chedid, 1984).

The third type of leukocyte is the lymphocyte, which accounts for 20–40 percent of the leukocytes. Lymphocytes have the immune response attributes of memory and specificity and therefore serve the major recognition and reaction functions of the immune response. In a study of sleep-deprived persons, Dinges and colleagues (1994) reported no changes in total lymphocyte number during 64 hours; Kuhn and colleagues (1969) reported a decrease throughout most of 72–126 hours. Hertz, who in 1923 deprived himself of sleep for 80 hours, also reported a decrease in lymphocytes, along with an increase in neutrophils (cited in Kleitman, 1963). Because there are many subtypes of lymphocytes with different traffic patterns among the blood and organs, the total lymphocyte count contains little information.

Of the lymphocytes, 70–80% are T lymphocytes, which are responsible for cell-mediated immunity. B lymphocytes, a second category, are responsible for antibody production and humoral immunity. When activated, lymphocytes emerge from a resting state and begin to proliferate. Among the T lymphocytes are effector cells, such as cytotoxic T cells, which directly attack the membrane of a transformed or infected cell and release toxic chemicals. Others are regulatory, such as helper T cells, which act on B lymphocytes and other cells in the immune system. Lymphocytes express different markers on their cell surface, denoted as "cluster designations" (CD), which indicate their reactivity with different types of cells. Analysis of the lymphocyte CD subsets in participants sleep-deprived for 64 hours (Dinges et al., 1994) revealed no changes in numbers of B cells (CD20), cytotoxic T cells (CD8), inducer–helper cells (CD29), and inactivated (CD45RA) or activated (HLA-DR receptor) T cells. However, there was a linear decline of the regulatory cell, helper T (CD4), and an increase over basal levels after the second sleep deprivation night in the number of natural killer cells (CD16, CD56, and CD57).

To test the function of lymphocyte cells, one stimulates them in vitro with various mitogens that interact with B and T lymphocytes in different ways to trigger proliferation and differentiation. Lipopolysaccharides (endotoxin) from the cell wall of gram-negative bacteria are T–independent antigens because they stimulate B cells directly. Responses to pokeweed mitogen (PWM) require B- and T-cell interactions (i.e., T-dependent antigen). Two plant lectins, concanavalin A (Con A) and phytohemagglutinin (PHA), are particularly potent mitogens for T cells. The mitogen effect is assessed by measuring the rate of incorporation of a radioactive substance (tritiated thymidine) into deoxyribonucleic acid (DNA) as the lymphocyte cells become mitotic. Sleep deprivation has not produced a consistent and unambiguous effect on lymphocyte proliferation. PHA reactivity of lymphocytes was depressed in one study of persons who were sleep-deprived for 48 hours (Palmblad, Petrini, Wasserman, & Åkerstedt, 1979) and unchanged in two studies of persons sleep-deprived for 40 (Moldofsky et al., 1989) and 64 hours (Dinges et al., 1994). PWM stimulation of proliferation, which normally shows a night-time increase over wakefulness during sleep (Moldofsky, Lue, Eisen, Keystone, & Gorczynski, 1986), was suppressed by one night of sleep deprivation until the early-morning hours, suggesting an alteration of the timing of the response (Moldofsky et al., 1989). In the most recent study by Dinges et al. (1994), lymphocyte proliferation responses to PHA, Con A, and PWM were not found to vary substantially, but blood was drawn only once daily during 64 hours of sleep deprivation.

Although no clear changes in the end point of lymphocyte proliferation have been found, there are indications that activation of lymphocytes has occurred, which might be expected to eventuate in proliferation. This induction is indicated by the results of measurements of the phases of DNA synthesis before cell mitosis. As sleep deprivation progressed, lymphocytes incubated in vitro with PHA showed a significant and linear increase in the number of cells in the DNA synthesis phase, compared with the pre-DNA and post-DNA synthesis phases (Dinges et al., 1994). By 64 hours of sleep deprivation, a shift had occurred with increased proportions of cells in the DNA synthesis and post-DNA synthesis phases. Moreover, after 70 hours of incubation without PHA stimulation, the proportion of cells in the DNA-synthesis phase increased across the period of sleep deprivation, which suggests an induction within the host that was independent of PHA (i.e., T-independent). During the recovery period after sleep deprivation, the proportion of cells in the DNA-synthesis phase remained high if incubated with PHA but dropped if not incubated with PHA. The shift in DNA synthesis phases, in the absence of changes in total lymphocyte number, resembled most closely the changes found in numbers of CD56 and CD57. Although CD56 and CD57 antigens may be attributed to activated T lymphocytes, they are most commonly assigned to a third type of lymphocyte, natural killer cells.

Natural killer cells are large granular lymphoid cells that participate in cell-mediated immunity by killing antigen without prior sensitization to it. Natural killer cells lack memory, and their behavior is therefore consistent with an innate, rather than acquired, immunity—hence the term *natural*. The killing of target cells by natural killer cells occurs before cell-mediated effector T cells have been sensitized, and it is directed at viral infected cells, neoplastic cells, and foreign tissues. Unlike granulocytes and macrophages, natural killer cells are not phagocytotic; rather, they release cytotoxic substances after binding to the target. Natural killer cell activity exhibits a normal nighttime increase that is part of a diurnal, biphasic pattern. Although 40 hours of sleep deprivation suppressed this nighttime increase (Moldofsky et al., 1989), prolonging the sleep deprivation through a second night resulted in an increase above predeprivation levels in both natural killer cell number ($\cong$20%) and cytotoxicity (13.9%) (Dinges et al., 1994). In addition to the control of tumor cell growth and of the spread of microbes (especially viruses), the major functions reported for natural killer cells include a role in the regulation of cell-mediated immunity and antibody responses, the control of stem cell growth and differentiation, involvement in allograft rejections, and the production of cytokines.

One primary stimulus of natural killer cells is the cytokine interferon. Interferon has several functions, but its name resulted from an initial recognition of its ability to "interfere" with viral entry and replication and to serve a protective role. Interferon production is increased by cells throughout the body during most challenges to host defense, including those of rickettsiae, mycoplasma, protozoa, fungi, bacterial endotoxins, and nucleic acids, and they increase in response to other immunomodulators. Leukocytes produce interferon-α in relatively large quantities. Fibroblasts, macrophages, and epithelial cells produce interferon-β, which share several characteristics of structure and function with interferon-α. T lymphocytes produce interferon-γ. During a 77-hour vigil that combined sleep deprivation with various stressors experienced by military personnel, such as loud noise and battle simulation, the interferon-producing ability of leukocytes, both overall and per leukocyte, was found to increase progressively and dramatically (Palmblad et al., 1976). The sleep deprivation and stimulus bombardment regimen was associated with an increased plasma concentration of cortisol, which is not otherwise found during sleep deprivation alone (Åkerstedt, Palmblad, de la Torre, Marana, & Gillberg, 1980; Dinges et al., 1994; Moldofsky et al., 1989). Increases in cortisol and catecholamines associated with stress were likely mediators of a suppression of phagocytic activity and a tendency toward decreased lymphocyte numbers that were found in this study (Palmblad et al., 1976); these hormones became dissociated from the interferon production. This is because their levels fell during the recovery period, whereas interferon production continued to rise. If it were known what type of interferon increased during the 77-hour sleep deprivation and stressor study, it might provide clues to the leukocyte type that is the source of the production. Nevertheless, increased interferon production ability would be expected to induce, as its consequence, the activity and increased effectiveness of other cells. For one thing, interferon has synergistic relationships with other cytokines, such as interleukin-1 and interleukin-2, the latter of which is secreted by activated T cells.

Cytokines are generally rapidly secreted in response to a stimulus. Among them, the interleukins serve communicative functions among leukocytes ("inter-leukin"). Moldofsky and colleagues (1989) reported that sleep deprivation of only 40 hours' duration enhanced nocturnal plasma interleukin-1-like and interleukin-2-like activities over basal levels and that the interleukin-1-like enhancement continued into the post-sleep-deprivation phase. Interleukin-1 is produced not only by monocytes and macrophages but also by many other different cells including dendritic cells, Langerhans cells, epithelial cells, endothelial cells, astrocytes, and microglia in the brain. Interleukin-1 augments the immune response by activating phagocytes, promoting prostaglandin production, and inducing fever. Interleukin-1 stimulates the production of interleukin-2 by helper–inducer T cells (CD4) and also the synthesis of other cytokines. Interleukin-1 induces expression of T-cell receptors for interleukin-2, and the latter is a cytotoxic T-cell differentiation factor. Both interleukin-1 and interleukin-2 influence B-cell activation and activate natural killer cells. Increases in the interleukin-1 and interleukin-2 cytokines in sleep-deprived persons therefore suggest that macrophages and other cells that produce them are functionally activated and that there is increased communication among macrophages, natural killer cells, and lymphocytes.

In summary, sleep deprivation in humans evokes the first line of host defense. Taken together, the overall indications are such that throughout three days and two nights of sleep deprivation, the number of circulating phagocytes and monocytes is increased, followed by an increase in natural killer cell numbers and their cytotoxicity. Furthermore, there are indications of immune system activation by increased concentrations of interferon and the interleukins. The increases in these nonantibody proteins imply that there is increased communication among and activation of other cells. Besides the increase in interferon production, the increase in interleukin-2 concentration suggests the presence of activated T lymphocytes. However, in vitro measurement of lymphocyte proliferation responses to antigens has not revealed an unambiguous change in either T or B lymphocytes. As such, none of the changes are considered part of the adaptive apparatus of the immune system per se, because there are no strong indications of changes in cell-mediated and humoral immunity. The sleep-deprivation-induced changes are therefore considered nonspecific, not because they are inconsequential but because of the diverse stimuli and the many cell types that can produce them and the several functions they can serve.

The functional consequences of the observed changes are unknown, and there are many possibilities. On the one hand, activation of phagocytes, macrophages, and natural killer cells might be maladaptive because of, for example, the release of cytotoxic chemicals. On the other hand, the observed changes might be adaptive and regulatory. For example, natural killer cells might attack neoplastic and other abnormal cells that sleep deprivation might produce, or they might kill immature cells that are released in excess and thereby regulate their number. Accordingly, it is not yet possible to determine whether increases in leukocytes and natural killer cells during sleep deprivation are adaptive responses that provide surveillance and protection or whether their release has benign or even maladaptive consequences.

The products of an increase in the activity of nonspecific immune-related factors would be expected, in turn, to stimulate cell-mediated and humoral immunity (i.e., the components of the immune response itself). Changes in other immune-related parameters are unknown, such as immunoglobulins and complement, because they have not yet been evaluated. In this regard, the findings of sleep deprivation are yet equivocal for activation versus suppression of immune system, owing to the many complexities in both the system and its measurement. For example, findings from in vitro studies might not reflect the manner in which the same cells would respond within the in vivo neuroendocrine milieu of the host. As a second example, even many immune-related diseases and lethal septicemia are not associated with reliable responses by lymphocytes. Yet another consideration is the likelihood that sleep deprivation, as a challenge to host defense, is qualitatively different from, for example, a sudden injection of endotoxin. That is, there may be differences in immunogenicity whereby the effects of sleep deprivation are less "foreign" to the host than endotoxin, which can produce rapid proliferation of T lymphocytes. Finally, under many conditions the DNA synthesis and cell division of lymphocytes can take time. For instance, it can take 48 hours for a T cell to respond to antigen and, subsequently, 7 days for the antibody production by B cells to be detectable in the serum. Added to that, characteristics of the immune response vary depending on whether the stimuli that elicit immune responses become modified and whether they are persistent. Therefore, the degree of the responsiveness of the immune system does not necessarily reflect the severity of the offending stimulus. By way of further illustration, treatment after exposure to hepatitis B requires an immediate injection of antibody because the host does not mount a response soon enough to avoid infection that can turn deadly. The lack of a specific immune response notwithstanding, it seems remarkable that sleep deprivation, without other encumbrance (e.g., temperature extremes, physical activity, limited food) and without known antigenic challenge, can produce changes in parameters associated with nonspecific host defense.

In evaluating the effects of sleep deprivation on host defense, it is important to realize that the experimental conditions under which sleep deprivation is carried out often minimize or exclude other influences, including exposure to pathogens. In many circumstances, it is the immune status of the host that determines the clinical manifestations of illnesses (e.g., tuberculosis). It therefore must be determined whether immunocompetency in the sleep-deprived host is altered in the face of disease before it can be known whether sleep deprivation modifies resistance to infection. Further, many pathogens reside within the body itself. Whether the control of these pathogens is affected by short-term sleep deprivation is unknown, but there is evidence that their control is affected adversely by long-term sleep deprivation in the rat, as discussed subsequently.

Bacterial Products and Immunomodulators as Sleep Promoting Agents

In 1967, Pappenheimer, Miller, and Goodrich reported that when the cerebrospinal fluid of goats that had been sleep-deprived for 72 hours was injected into the cerebral ventricles of normal rats and cats, the animals slept much more, as indicated by a suppression of behavioral activity by 67% over a 6-hour period. The unknown sleep-promoting (i.e., somnogenic) factor was termed *Factor S*. The composition of Factor S isolated from the sleep-deprived goat cerebrospinal fluid, and subsequently from human urine and rabbit brain, was identified as a muramyl peptide (reviewed in Krueger & Majde, 1990). Muramyl peptides are peptidoglycans, part of the bacterial cell wall. Although they are not synthesized by the host, they have been shown to be present in normal mammalian tissues, and macrophages possess binding sites for them. Muramyl peptides administered to rabbits increase the amount of slow wave sleep during daylight hours from 40% to 60–70% over the course of 6 or more hours (Krueger, Pappenheimer, & Karnovsky, 1982). The state of the animal is consistent with true sleep rather than sedation. Muramyl peptides that are somnogenic also appear to be immunoactive, and under certain circumstances, they are pyrogenic. One muramyl peptide, muramyl dipeptide, is known to have several effects on macrophages in vitro, among them, increased bactericidal and tumoricidal activities and release of interleukin-1. Part of the pathway between muramyl peptides and sleep is believed to involve interleukin-1 (reviewed in Krueger & Karnovsky, 1987).

In laboratory animals, administration of interleukin-1 affects sleep in a similar manner to that of muramyl peptides, except that the onset of excessive slow wave sleep is earlier (reviewed in Krueger & Karnovsky, 1987). In humans peaks in interleukin-1 activity in the blood have been found during normal nighttime sleep (Gudewill et al., 1992; Moldofsky et al., 1989). Interleukin-1 stimulates interleukin-2 activity, and peaks in interleukin-2 activity have been found during the early part of sleep (Moldofsky et al., 1986, 1989), when slow wave sleep is most prevalent. Interleukin-1 and muramyl peptides induce the synthesis of other cytokines, such as tumor necrosis factor, which has also been found to be sleep promoting with a different time course than that of muramyl peptides and interleukin-1 (reviewed in Krueger & Majde, 1990). Muramyl peptides, interleukin-1, and viral ribonucleic acid (RNA) are effective stimuli for interferon-α2 (leukocytic), which enhances slow wave sleep in rabbits without greatly altering rapid eye movement (REM) sleep (reviewed in Krueger & Karnovsky, 1987).

The effects of immunogenic substances on the sleep of humans has been less thoroughly investigated, but they seem to be much the same as in animals. For example, Pollmächer and colleagues (1993) administered a low dose of endotoxin through intravenous cannulas in normal, healthy humans and allowed the participants to rest for 4 hours. The lights were then turned off at a normal bedtime hour, and the participants were permitted to sleep. The nighttime was associated with a significant increase in the amount of time spent in non-REM (NREM) sleep, whereas a decrease was found in the amount of both wakefulness and REM sleep. The increase in NREM sleep was accompanied by a mild elevation of core temperature (<1 °C above normal), and both were positively correlated with plasma concentrations of tumor necrosis factor–α, interleukin-6, cortisol, and adrenocorticotropic hormone (ACTH). The increase in NREM sleep was mostly attributable to an increase in Stage 2 rather than slow wave sleep (Stages 3 and 4). By comparison, intravenous administration of high doses of endotoxin to laboratory rabbits resulted in a period of enhanced slow wave sleep (a subcategory of NREM sleep) during the first 3 hours postinfusion, which was accompanied by a fever and suppression of REM sleep (Krueger, Kubillus, Shoham, & Davenne, 1986). Thus, although the sleep responses induced by endotoxin in humans and laboratory animals vary somewhat, the results are comparable to the extent that they suggest that common physiological mechanisms underlie the enhancement of NREM sleep in response to microbial products.

The immunogenic and somnogenic substances are also known pyrogens (i.e., endotoxin, muramyl peptides, interleukin-1, interferon, tumor necrosis factor, and prostaglandins). Yet the manifestations of fever and those of sleep can be separated. For example, administration of muramyl peptides in low doses to rats induces increases in both NREM and REM sleep but not fever, whereas administration in high doses enhances NREM sleep, decreases REM sleep, and produces a fever (reviewed in Krueger & Majde, 1994). Other evidence indicating that sleep and fever may be mediated by somewhat different pathways includes the following: (a) Fever can be induced by the administration of some forms of muramyl peptides that do not alter sleep; (b) febrile responses after administration of muramyl peptides and interleukin-1 can be blocked with antipyretics that do not block the sleep responses; and (c) prostaglandin D_2 administration is somnogenic in rats, yet it is also hypothermic (reviewed in Krueger & Karnovsky, 1987). Finally, manifestations of fever are dependent on the time of day, the dose, and the species observed. For example, administration of muramyl dipeptide during the day to rabbits increases the amount of sleep and induces fever, whereas at night it increases the amount of sleep without inducing fever (reviewed in Krueger & Majde, 1994).

Given the complex and intricate interactions among immunoregulatory factors and the expected cascade of cellular responses to stimulation, it is not surprising that many individual factors have the capacity to evoke sleep responses. The immunomodulators and the immunogenic substances are diffuse enough and their effects are multifarious enough to help explain how sleep, as a whole brain–body phenomenon, might be partially modulated when no anatomic center has been established and no one regulatory system has been identified as a sole controller of sleep. In addition to modulating the amount of sleep, immune-related factors induce the type of subtle physiological and biochemical processes that might underlie such everyday events as sleepiness, fatigue, and feelings of tiredness.

Antitumor and Antibody Responses During Short-Term Sleep Deprivation in Laboratory Animals

Bergmann, Kovar, Rechtschaffen, and Quintans (1994) tested the ability of sleep-deprived rats to reject cancer tumors. Rats were injected subdermally with carcinoma cells, which normally cause a tumor that is dissolved by the host in subsequent days. After 4 days of tumor growth, half of the rats were sleep-deprived for 8 hours. (Rats normally sleep 12 hours per day.) During the next 3 days, tumor growth was suppressed by 40–50% in sleep-deprived rats compared with undeprived rats. A repressed slope of tumor size in sleep-deprived rats continued through subsequent days. In this case, sleep deprivation appeared to have an adaptive advantage in combating subdermal foreign agents.

In a similar manner to sleep deprivation in humans, sleep deprivation in laboratory rats results in a progressive rise in the number of circulating WBCs, mostly neutrophils and monocytes, whereas the number of lymphocytes is eventually decreased (Everson, 1987). (However, the same was not reported in older studies of rabbits [Crile, 1921] or in adult dogs or puppies despite lethality [cited in Kleitman, 1963].) If sleep-deprived rats behave in a manner similar to humans, as suggested by the changes in leukocyte numbers, the tumor suppression possibly can be explained by increased concentrations of natural killer cells and cytokines that are known to have antitumor effects. At present, however, the concentrations of immunomodulators in sleep-deprived rats are not known.

Maladaptive aspects of short-term sleep deprivation were found by Brown, Pang, Husband, and King (1989), who investigated immunity in the respiratory tract of mice. Mice were twice inoculated with influenza virus through a feeding needle into the gastrointestinal tract and were allowed 7 days to develop antibody titers after each immunization. The mice were then challenged with live virus nasally. Half were subsequently sleep-deprived for 7 hours. Three days after the challenge, virus clearance from lung homogenates was complete for mice that had been allowed to sleep normally. In contrast, virus clearance from the lungs of mice that had been sleep-deprived was hardly better than that of mice that had never been immunized. Sleep deprivation did not appear to exacerbate virus replication, because the number of assayed plaque-forming units was similar to that found in nonimmunized mice, whether sleep-deprived or not. Rather, antibody titers were suppressed in immunized mice that were sleep-deprived compared with immunized mice that were allowed to sleep.

Brown, Price, King, and Husband (1989) also studied the effects of short-term sleep deprivation of 8 hours on the secondary antibody response in rats. Fourteen days in advance of study, rats were injected subcutaneously with sheep red blood cells (SRBCs). On the day of study, rats were once again injected with SRBCs and then deprived of sleep or allowed to sleep normally. At the beginning of the experimental period, one-third of each of these groups received a dose of one of the following: saline (placebo), interleukin-1, or muramyl dipeptide. The combined effects of sleep deprivation and placebo resulted in a reduction in antibody production compared with the normal sleep and placebo condition. If the sleep deprivation was combined with treatments of either interleukin-1 or muramyl dipeptide, however, there was no reduction in antibody production. These data suggest that stimulation of the immune system by exogenous interleukin-one and muramyl dipeptide overcame the suppressant effects of sleep deprivation on antibody production.

Benca et al. (1989) studied rats that were sleep-deprived until a moribund state developed; they found no group differences in lymphocyte proliferation or production of antibodies in vitro compared with rats that were either yoked to the experimental arousal structures and partially sleep-deprived (yoked control) or housed separately and allowed to sleep normally (surgery-control). Splenic lymphocytes were challenged with the T-independent B-cell antigen, lipopolysaccharide (i.e., endotoxin), and the T-cell mitogen, Con A. B-cell antibody responses were determined by stimulation in vitro with SRBCs or heat-killed rough pneumococcus. On the whole, the plaque-forming cell responses were highly variable among subjects within each group. The investigators then tested the ability of one sleep-deprived rat to mount an antibody response in vivo. After this rat had progressed through 9 days of sleep deprivation, two standard antigens were injected, and the splenic lymphocytes were harvested after another 5 days of sleep deprivation (i.e., midway through the course of sleep deprivation). The plaque forming cell responses in the sleep-deprived rat were marked: B-cell proliferation responses were more than 2- and 20-fold greater than those of the comparison yoked- and surgery-control rats, respectively. The T-dependent lymphocyte proliferation responses in the sleep-deprived rat were nearly 2-fold greater than those of the yoked control and nearly 10-fold greater than those of the surgery control. Thus, the results did not reveal an impairment in lymphocyte function, and although they are preliminary, the in vivo findings provide a clue that the immune system might be markedly activated at a time that is not otherwise associated with distinct abnormalities of other physiological parameters.

Host Defense During Long-Term Sleep Deprivation in Laboratory Rats

Sleep deprivation in laboratory rats has been prolonged to allow its pathophysiological consequences to unfold and to determine their mediation and clinical significance. The course of prolonged sleep deprivation has a syndromic nature: Rats develop consistent signs, only at varying rates, and the consequences are eventually sufficient to cause death (reviewed in Rechtschaffen, Bergmann, Everson, Kushida, & Gilliland, 1989). Identification of the first system to fail (i.e., a pathophysiological change of obvious clinical significance) might indicate which regulatory system is particularly vulnerable to sleep deprivation. The identity of this system remained a mystery for many years. Recently, it was established that the high lethality of sleep deprivation is due to a breakdown in host defense that allows pathogens that the body normally controls to infect the bloodstream (i.e., blood poisoning), presumably resulting in a deadly cascade of toxic reactions (Everson, 1993). Because this type of disease process does not spontaneously occur in normal animals with competent immune systems, it is important to place this finding within the context of other known effects of sustained sleep deprivation.

The average duration of sleep deprivation required for rats to reach a state of severe morbidity is about 3 weeks (Everson, Bergmann, & Rechtschaffen, 1989). A progressive increase in peripheral energy expenditure, manifested by increased food intake and loss of body weight, is consistently found. Several causes of the hypercatabolism have been ruled out, including diabetes, malabsorption of calories, changes in gross locomotor behavior, and changes in total body water (Bergmann et al., 1989; Everson, Bergmann, & Rechtschaffen, 1989). Other symptoms include the early development of skin dermatoses (Kushida et al., 1989) and development of anemia (normocytic) and hypoalbuminemia (Everson, Bergmann, & Rechtschaffen, 1988). Attempts to alleviate the negative energy balance by feeding sleep-deprived rats a diet augmented with fat and calories delay or attenuate development of several symptoms (e.g., weight loss) and prolong survival by an average of 7 days (40%; Everson & Wehr, 1993). These findings indicate that several symptoms are, in part, secondary to the energy debt that is induced by sleep deprivation. Core temperature increases mildly to 0.4–0.5 °C above baseline levels during the first half of the experimental period and declines to normal and below-normal levels during the second half of the experimental period (Bergmann et al., 1989). In spite of the high energy expenditure, sleep-deprived rats exhibit heat-seeking behavior (Prete, Bergmann, Holtzman, Obermeyer, & Rechtschaffen, 1991), suggesting that the eventual decline in body temperature is due to a disruption of autonomic processes responsible for heat retention.

Changes include a progressive increase in plasma hormone concentrations of both norepinephrine and epinephrine (Bergmann et al., 1989; Pilcher, Bergmann, Fang, Refetoff, & Rechtschaffen, 1990), indicating sympathetic activation in response to the increased energy requirements. Plasma thyroid hormones, however, decline to pathologically low concentrations (Everson & Reed, 1995). Mild increases in plasma corticosteroids are sometimes found during the second half of the experimental period (Bergmann et al., 1989), but the levels often remain normal (Everson & Reed, 1995). When increases are present, they appear to be reciprocal to the declines in body temperature and body weight and therefore suggest compensatory adjustments to thermoregulatory demands and increased energy requirements.

In the later stages of sleep deprivation, some rats permitted to sleep do not have rebound sleep; rather, their health continues to deteriorate and they die. In survivors, recovery sleep is marked by quick reversal of changes in neuroendocrine parameters and energy expenditure and a regaining of health (Everson, Gilliland, et al., 1989).

The blood of sleep-deprived rats was cultured to look for pathogenic organisms, because the sleep-deprived state has a strong resemblance to states of toxicity, as suggested by several observations. First, important structural changes had not been found in morphological and histopathological examinations of tissues, including the brain (Everson, 1993; Everson, Bergmann, & Rechtschaffen, 1989; Gilliland, Wold, Wollmann, Eschenbach, & Rechtschaffen, 1984). Second, changes in clinical chemistry and hematological parameters either were within normal limits or showed no disturbance of much diagnostic value (Everson & Wehr, 1993). In addition, the quick reversal of pathologies with subsequent sleep suggested that the lethal factor or factors were not likely to be cell death, neuronal degeneration, or other physiological changes that cause permanent damage or from which it would take a long time to recover. The sleep-deprived rat eventually resembles a cancer patient, with hypercatabolism and the appearance of bodily wasting, yet no tumors have been found. In patients with cancer, cytokine activation in response to the tumor is believed to underlie the excessive energy requirements. In the absence of a tumor, microbes are likely inducers of this clinical profile.

Blood samples were obtained for cultures when the sleep-deprived rats developed a life-threatening state marked by an emaciated, weak appearance and a drop in core temperature over 24 hours to 1 °C below baseline. In sleep-deprived rats, a drop in core temperature of this magnitude precedes moribund processes, whereas it is not considered severe if induced in animals by other means. The rats were ambulatory, however, and they had consumed food within the previous 24 hours. At this point, a systemic infection by important species of bacteria has the attribute of pathogenicity because it is antecedent to, rather than a consequence of, eventual incapacitation. Bacteria were cultured from the heart blood of 5 of 6 sleep-deprived rats and none of 10 yoked- and surgery-control rats (Everson, 1993). The significance of the lack of a positive blood culture in the sixth sleep-deprived rat is unclear because of the limitations inherent in blood cultures and the possibility of infection by a nonbacterial pathogen, such as a virus or a fungus, which can evoke similar metabolic derangements. The pathogens that were identified were all opportunistic and facultative anaerobes that are indigenous to the host and the environment and included both gram-negative rods and gram-positive cocci known to be highly lethal once they infect the bloodstream.

Several events would be expected to occur over days or weeks to culminate in a state whereby virulent, opportunistic microbes are allowed into the bloodstream. The systemic infection itself would not be expected to be other than a late development because it represents, in effect, the failure of the host defense system. Viewed in retrospect, many of the features of prolonged sleep deprivation are suggestive of a septic challenge that is chronic in nature. First of all, a state of immunosuppression is suggested by the fact that the systemic infection was not accompanied by fever and the tissue responses were poor compared with those typically found in most infectious disease states. The development of skin dermatosis, which begins early during deprivation, also suggests immunosuppression. The dermatoses progress to lesions that are large and necrotic but not inflamed. Skin dermatoses are often the first external manifestation of an immunocompromised host (reviewed in Weinberg & Swartz, 1987). Additionally, most sleep deprivation symptoms can be found in chronic septic states, for example, sympathetic activation, suppressed plasma thyroid hormone concentrations, increased plasma alkaline phosphatase, and hypercatabolism (reviewed in Everson, 1993). Challenges to host defense as important as those that culminate in systemic infection would be expected to induce the release of cytokines, known for their highly catabolic effects (Tracey, Lowry, & Cerami, 1988; reviewed in Zentella, Manogue, & Cerami, 1991). A role for cytokines as mediators of the hypercatabolism of sleep deprivation therefore becomes a distinct possibility. When they are overactivated (even in the absence of an identifiable pathogen), cytokines can cause a cascade of deleterious consequences. Finally, processes that accompany bacteremia provide a likely explanation for the development of hypothermia. Hypothermia associated with bacteremia is characterized by a high cardiac index and low vascular resistance, indicating that heat loss is due to impaired vasoconstriction (Morris, Chambers, Morris, & Sande, 1985). Thus, a breakdown in host defense provides an explanation for several sleep-deprivation-induced effects, such as hypothermia and mortality without apparent structural damage, and provides a starting place from which to determine mediation of other effects, such as skin dermatoses and hypercatabolism.

Still, there are many potential causes of decreased resistance to infection, and alterations in the immune complex might be evoked only secondarily in response to other pathophysiology. For instance, the hypercatabolic state might be caused by physiological changes that are not directly associated with the immune system and that might rob energy from vital processes. Indeed, several sleep deprivation symptoms are secondary to the high energy expenditure (Everson & Wehr, 1993) and resemble symptoms of malnutrition (e.g., weight loss, hypoalbuminemia), in which infection is always a high risk. Also, the progressive decline in plasma thyroid hormone concentrations would be expected to affect metabolism, tissue repair (e.g., of the skin), and body temperature. The hypothyroxinemia and hypothermia, together, could decrease resistance to infection, particularly if impaired thermoregulatory mechanisms preclude fever, which has been shown to be associated with increased survival rate during infection in animals (Kluger & Vaughn, 1978). These peripheral signs are further reflected by the ability of sleep deprivation to lower the functional activity of several cerebral structures that are known to be foci for thermoregulation, endocrine regulation, and host defense (Everson & Reed, 1995; Everson, Smith, & Sokoloff, 1994). Future studies are therefore required to determine whether an impairment in the immune system per se is the utmost predisposing factor in the breakdown of host defense. In the meantime, the findings provide a critical end-point marker by which to gauge earlier physiological changes.

The prediction of which sleep-deprived rats will live and which will die when permitted to sleep once again, as well as the time course of subsequent recovery or deterioration, may depend on the type of infecting pathogen. As Toth, Krueger, and colleagues have shown (discussed in the next section), physiological responses to microbial challenge vary depending on the type of pathogen that is introduced.

Sleep Responses to Infection

To examine the relationship between infection and changes in sleep, Toth and Krueger injected rabbits with various pathogens and recorded the resulting changes in sleep. They then evaluated whether the changes in amount of sleep reflected either recovery from the infection or clinical deterioration. Rabbits were inoculated intravenously with one of four pathogens: *Staphylococcus aureus* (gram-positive), *Streptococcus pyogenes* (gram-positive), *Escherichia coli* (gram-negative), and *Candida albicans* (fungal) (Toth & Krueger, 1988, 1989; Toth, Tolley, & Krueger, 1993). The resulting changes in sleep parameters varied in response to the different types of microbes, as do other physiological responses, such as fever and hematological parameters. Inoculation with *S. aureus, S. pyogenes,* and *C. albicans* resulted in a period of enhanced slow wave sleep, which occurred after a delay of a few hours, followed by a period of suppressed slow wave sleep. Inoculation with *E. coli* resulted in the same biphasic pattern of slow-wave-sleep enhancement followed by suppression, but the time course was different in that the enhancement was larger and earlier and the subsequent suppression was longer.

Changes in sleep parameters after inoculation with microbes depends on not only the type of microbe but also whether it is alive or dead and how it gets into the body. In the case of *E. coli*, the heat-killed form was as effective as the live form in producing the sleep changes. In contrast, the same doses of *S. pyogenes* and *C. albicans* in heat-killed forms failed to alter normal sleep, whereas high doses of heat-killed *S. aureus* resulted in the same sleep effect as the live form. With regard to the route of administration, intravenous inoculation of either *Pasteurella multocida* or *E. coli* (both gram-negative) results in similar time-dependent changes in sleep responses. However, when *P. multocida* is administered intranasally, the resulting changes in sleep responses resemble those observed after intravenous inoculation with the gram-positive bacteria, in which the period of sleep enhancement occurs after several hours (Toth & Krueger, 1988, 1989, 1990; Toth et al., 1993).

To explain these findings, the investigators hypothesized that the buildup of products of various bacteria and fungi, such as muramyl peptides, endotoxin, and polysaccharides, stimulates immune responses that result in the release of immunomodulators, which in turn modulate the changes in sleep. This would explain the latency period of 2–4 hours after inoculation and before slow wave-sleep enhancement, which is due to a time-dependent series of physiological reactions within the mounting of an immune response; these reactions would not occur as instantaneously as the presence of the microbes themselves. The subsequent period of slow-wave-sleep suppression below basal levels could be due to sleep-suppressing physiological reactions downstream from the initial reactions, possibly the production and release of corticotropin-releasing factor, α-melanocyte-stimulating hormone, and glucocorticoids (Toth et al., 1993). Whether the heat-killed forms were effective in producing an effect on amount of sleep is likely to be dependent on (a) the composition of the cell wall of the microbe (e.g., amount and molecular arrangement of muramyl peptides and presence or absence of endotoxin); (b) whether proliferation by the microbe is necessary to provide a sufficient challenge to the host to evoke the stimuli that induce sleep; and (c) whether antibodies directed to the microbe are present before the experimental challenge (Toth & Krueger, 1988).

After administration of microbes, a robust enhancement of slow-wave-sleep intensity and duration and a reduction in subsequent sleep suppression were associated with less severe clinical signs and a more favorable prognosis (Toth et al., 1993). In general, the higher the infective dose of microbes, the less the slow-wave-sleep enhancement. Yet among animals matched for infective dosages of microbes, there was still a positive relationship between slow-wave-sleep enhancement and clinical outcome. On the one hand, animals that are less ill after an injection of microbes may be comparatively better able to sleep. On the other hand, sleep and processes related to it might directly convey recovery advantage and affect the clinical outcome.

In humans, sleep abnormalities are found during infectious disease. For example, in a study of asymptomatic patients infected with human immunodeficiency virus (HIV), Norman, Chediak, Kiel, and Cohn (1990) reported decreased sleep efficiency and increased nocturnal awakenings but also a large increase in slow wave sleep in 6 of 8 patients during the second half of the night, a period during which slow wave sleep usually declines. Wiegand et al. (1991) also studied asymptomatic HIV-infected persons and found sleep disturbances but not an augmentation of amount of slow wave sleep. Differences between studies in the amount of slow wave sleep found in HIV-positive patients may be due to several factors, such as the age of the patients and the underlying progression of the illness, along with the fact that HIV infects the central nervous system, which might result in differential effects on sleep mechanisms in the brain. As yet, there are too few studies of infectious disease states to permit effective separation of sleep disturbances that may be unique from those that occur with many clinical and psychiatric conditions. On the other hand, many other clinical conditions are associated at some level with inflammatory processes and immune-related factors.

In conclusion, sleep deprivation is generally considered to create circumstances that predispose to illness. A convergence of scientific evidence indicates that short-term sleep deprivation in humans induces the first line of host defense without the presence of a known antigen and that long-term sleep deprivation in the laboratory rat results in a breakdown of host defense. Other evidence indicates that sleep deprivation alters in important ways the immune system's response to antigen and specific challenges, such as the presence of carcinoma cells. Links between sleep and the immune system have also been established by studies that suggest multiple ways in which immune-related variables may modify sleep and, conversely, are modified by sleep. Researchers are just beginning to understand the ways in which sleep deprivation affects the immune system and how immune-related variables may mediate pathophysiological changes. The rich nature of the interactions between the immune complex and sleep promises to hold answers to untold questions about health and disease processes.

REFERENCES

Åkerstedt, T., Palmblad, J., de la Torre, B., Marana, R., & Gillberg, M. (1980). Adrenocortical and gonadal steroids during sleep deprivation. *Sleep, 3,* 23–30.

Benca, R. M., Kushida, C. A., Everson, C. A., Kalski, R., Bergmann, B. M., & Rechtschaffen, A. (1989). Sleep deprivation in the rat: VII. Immune function. *Sleep, 12,* 47–52.

Bergmann, B. M., Everson, C. A., Kushida, C. A., Fang, V. S., Leitch, C. A., Schoeller, D. A., Refetoff, S., & Rechtschaffen, A. (1989). Sleep deprivation in the rat: V. Energy use and mediation. *Sleep, 12,* 31–41.

Bergmann, B., Kovar, S., Rechtschaffen, A., & Quintans, J. (1994). Effect of brief sleep deprivation on tumor growth in the rat. *Sleep Research, 23,* 403.

Brown, R., Pang, G., Husband, A. J., & King, M. G. (1989). Suppression of immunity to influenza virus infection in the respiratory tract following sleep disturbance. *Regional Immunology, 2,* 321–325.

Brown, R., Price, R. J., King, M. G., & Husband, A. J. (1989). Interleukin-1 β and muramyl dipeptide can prevent decreased antibody response associated with sleep deprivation. *Brain, Behavior, and Immunity, 3,* 320–330.

Crile, G. W. (1921). Studies in exhaustion: An experimental research. *Archives of Surgery, 2,* 196–220.

Dinges, D. F., Douglas, S. D., Zaugg, L., Campbell, D. E., McMann, J. M., Whitehouse, W. G., Orne, E. C., Kapoor, S. C., Icaza, E., & Orne, M. T. (1994). Leukocytosis and natural killer cell function parallel neurobehavioral fatigue induced by 64 hours of sleep deprivation. *Journal of Clinical Investigation, 93,* 1930–1939.

Everson, C. A. (1987). *Total sleep deprivation in the rat: Biochemical and physiological changes* (pp. 79–81). Unpublished doctoral dissertation, University of Chicago.

Everson, C. A. (1993). Sustained sleep deprivation impairs host defense. *American Journal of Physiology, 265,* R1148–R1154.

Everson, C. A., Bergmann, B. M., & Rechtschaffen, A. (1988). Hypoalbuminemia and anemia in totally sleep deprived rats. *Sleep Research, 17,* 314.

Everson, C. A., Bergmann, B. M., & Rechtschaffen, A. (1989). Sleep deprivation in the rat: III. Total sleep deprivation. *Sleep, 12,* 13–21.

Everson, C. A., Gilliland, M. A., Kushida, C. A., Pilcher, J. J., Fang, V. S., Refetoff, S., Bergmann, B. M., & Rechtschaffen, A. (1989). Sleep deprivation in the rat: IX. Recovery. *Sleep, 12,* 60–67.

Everson, C. A., & Reed, H. L. (1995). Pituitary and peripheral thyroid hormone responses to thyrotropin-releasing hormone during sustained sleep deprivation in freely moving rats. *Endocrinology, 136,* 1426–1434.

Everson, C. A., Smith, C. B., & Sokoloff, L. (1994). Effects of sustained sleep deprivation on local rates of cerebral energy metabolism in freely moving rats. *Journal of Neuroscience, 14,* 6769–6778.

Everson, C. A., & Wehr, T. A. (1993). Nutritional and metabolic adaptations to prolonged sleep deprivation in the rat. *American Journal of Physiology, 264,* R376–R387.

Gilliland, M., Wold, L., Wollmann, R., Eschenbach, K., & Rechtschaffen, A. (1984). Pathology in sleep deprived rats is not reflected in histologic abnormalities. *Sleep Research, 13,* 190.

Gudewill, S., Pollmächer, T., Vedder, H., Schreiber, W., Fassbender, K., & Holsboer, F. (1992). Nocturnal plasma levels of cytokines in healthy men. *European Archives of Psychiatry and Clinical Neuroscience, 242,* 53–56.

Horne, J. (1988). *Why we sleep: The functions of sleep in humans and other mammals* (pp. 13–103). New York: Oxford University Press.

Kleitman, N. (1963). *Sleep and wakefulness* (pp. 215–229). Chicago: University of Chicago Press.

Kluger, M. J., & Vaughn, L. K. (1978). Fever and survival in rabbits infected with *Pasteurella mutocida. Journal of Physiology (Cambridge), 282,* 243–251.

Krueger, J. M., & Karnovsky, M. L. (1987). Sleep and the immune response. *Annals of the New York Academy of Sciences, 496,* 510–516.

Krueger, J. M., Kubillus, S., Shoham, S., & Davenne, D. (1986). Enhancement of slow-wave sleep by endotoxin and lipid A. *American Journal of Physiology, 251,* R591–R597.

Krueger, J. M., & Majde, J. A. (1990). Sleep as a host defense: Its regulation by microbial products and cytokines. *Clinical Immunology and Immunopathology, 57,* 188–199.

Krueger, J. M., & Majde, J. A. (1994). Microbial products and cytokines in sleep and fever regulation. *Critical Reviews in Immunology, 14,* 355–379.

Krueger, J. M., Pappenheimer, J. R., & Karnovsky, M. L. (1982). The composition of sleep-promoting factor isolated from human urine. *Journal of Biological Chemistry, 257,* 1664–1669.

Krueger, J. M., Walter, J., Dinarello, C. A., Wolff, S. M., & Chedid, L. (1984). Sleep-promoting effects of endogenous pyrogen (interleukin-1). *American Journal of Physiology, 246,* R994–R999.

Kuhn, E., Brodan, V., Brodanová, M., & Ryšánek, K. (1969). Metabolic reflections of sleep deprivation. *Activitas Nervosa Superior, 11,* 165–174.

Kushida, C. A., Everson, C. A., Suthipinittharm, P., Sloan, J., Soltani, K., Bartnicke, B., Bergmann, B. M., & Rechtschaffen, A. (1989). Sleep deprivation in the rat: VI. Skin changes. *Sleep, 12,* 42–46.

Moldofsky, H., Lue, F. A., Davidson, J. R., & Gorczynski, R. (1989). Effects of sleep deprivation on human immune functions. *FASEB Journal, 3,* 1972–1977.

Moldofsky, H., Lue, F. A., Eisen, J., Keystone, E., & Gorczynski, R. M. (1986). The relationship of interleukin-1 and immune functions to sleep in humans. *Psychosomatic Medicine, 48,* 309–318.

Morris, D. L., Chambers, H. F., Morris, M. G., & Sande, M. A. (1985). Hemodynamic characteristics of patients with hypothermia due to occult infection and other causes. *Annals of Internal Medicine, 102,* 153–157.

Norman, S. E., Chediak, A. D., Kiel, M., & Cohn, M. A. (1990). Sleep disturbances in HIV-infected homosexual men. *AIDS, 4,* 775–781.

Palmblad, J., Cantell, K., Strander, H., Fröberg, J., Karlsson, C.-G., Levi, L., Granström, M., & Unger, P. (1976). Stressor exposure and immunological response in man: Interferon-producing capacity and phagocytosis. *Journal of Psychosomatic Research, 20,* 193–199.

Palmblad, J., Petrini, B., Wasserman, J., & Åkerstedt, T. (1979). Lymphocyte and granulocyte reactions during sleep deprivation. *Psychosomatic Medicine, 41,* 273–278.

Pappenheimer, J. R., Miller, T. B., & Goodrich, C. A. (1967). Sleep-promoting effects of cerebrospinal fluid from sleep-deprived goats. *Proceedings of the National Academy of Sciences of the United States of America, 58,* 513–517.

Pilcher, J. J., Bergmann, B. M., Fang, V. S., Refetoff, S., & Rechtschaffen, A. (1990). Sleep deprivation in the rat: XI. The effect of guanethidine-induced sympathetic blockade on the sleep deprivation syndrome. *Sleep, 13,* 218–231.

Pollmächer, T., Schreiber, W., Gudewill, S., Vedder, H., Fassbender, K., Wiedemann, K., Trachsel, L., Galanos, C., & Hosboer, F. (1993). Influence of endotoxin on nocturnal sleep in humans. *American Journal of Physiology, 264,* R1077–R1083.

Prete, F. R., Bergmann, B. M., Holtzman, P., Obermeyer, W., & Rechtschaffen, A. (1991). Sleep deprivation in the rat: XII. Effect on ambient temperature choice. *Sleep, 14,* 109–115.

Rechtschaffen, A., Bergmann, B. M., Everson, C. A., Kushida, C. A., & Gilliland, M. A. (1989). Sleep deprivation in the rat: X. Integration and discussion of the findings. *Sleep, 12,* 68–87.

Toth, L. A., & Krueger, J. M. (1988). Alteration of sleep in rabbits by *Staphylococcus aureus* infection. *Infection and Immunity, 56,* 1785–1791.

Toth, L. A., & Krueger, J. M. (1989). Effects of microbial challenge on sleep in rabbits. *FASEB Journal, 3,* 2062–2066.

Toth, L. A., & Krueger, J. M. (1990). Somnogenic, pyrogenic, and hematologic effects of experimental pasteurellosis in rabbits. *American Journal of Physiology, 258,* R536–R542.

Toth, L. A., Tolley, E. A., & Krueger, J. M. (1993). Sleep as a prognostic indicator during infectious disease in rabbits. *Proceedings of the Society for Experimental Biology and Medicine, 203,* 179–192.

Tracey, K. J., Lowry, S. F., & Cerami, A. (1988). Cachectin: A hormone that triggers acute shock and chronic cachexia. *Journal of Infectious Diseases, 157,* 413–420.

Weinberg, A. N., & Swartz, M. N. (1987). Gram-negative coccal and bacillary infections. In T. B. Fitzpatrick, A. Z. Eisen, K. Wolff, I. M. Freedberg, & K. F. Austen (Eds.), *Dermatology in general medicine: Textbook and atlas* (pp. 2121–2136). New York: McGraw-Hill.

Wiegand, M., Möller, A. A., Schreiber, W., Krieg, J. C., Fuchs, D., Wachter, H., & Holsboer, F. (1991). Nocturnal sleep EEG in patients with HIV infection. *European Archives of Psychiatry and Clinical Neuroscience, 240,* 153–158.

Zentella, A., Manogue, K., & Cerami, A. (1991). The role of cachectin/TNF and other cytokines in sepsis. In A. Sturk, S. J. H. van Deventer, J. W. ten Cate, H. R. Büller, L. G. Thijs, & J. Levin (Eds.), *Bacterial endotoxins: Cytokine mediators and new therapies for sepsis* (pp. 9–24). New York: Wiley-Liss.

Immunology Source Bibliography

Benjamini, E., & Leskowitz, S. (1991). *Immunology: A short course.* New York: Wiley-Liss.

Bona, C. A., & Bonilla, F. A. (1990). *Immunology for medical students.* New York: Harwood Academic.

Brostoff, J., Scadding, G. K., Male, D. K., & Roitt, I. M. (1991). *Clinical immunology.* Philadelphia: Lippincott.

Mudge-Grout, C. L. (1992). *Immunologic disorders*. St. Louis, MO: Mosby–Year Book.

Oppenheim, J. J., & Shevach, E. M. (Eds.). (1990). *Immunophysiology: The role of cells and cytokines in immunity and inflammation*. New York: Oxford University Press.

Sigal, L. H., & Ron, Y. (Eds.). (1994). *Immunology and inflammation: Basic mechanisms and clinical consequences*. New York: McGraw-Hill.

Stites, D. P., Stobo, J. D., & Wells, J. V. (Eds.). (1987). *Basic & clinical immunology* (6th ed.). Norwalk, CT: Appleton & Lange.

V

Sleep Disorders Across the Life Span

Children and Sleep

Jodi A. Mindell

I n discussing sleep and sleep disorders, it is important to look at age-related differences. This chapter discusses the ways in which sleep is different in children when compared with adults and provides a review of the most common sleep disorders experienced by children and adolescents.

Physiology and Development of Sleep

Children's sleep patterns are distinctly different from those of adults, and these sleep patterns change as children mature and develop. Sleep patterns begin to develop in the uterus, before birth. A fetus of 6 or 7 months' gestation experiences REM sleep, with non-REM (NREM) sleep beginning shortly afterward. By the end of the eighth month of gestation, sleep patterns are well established.

Instead of discussing REM and NREM sleep, as is done with adults, researchers studying sleep in infants classify the sleep as either active or quiet. During active-REM sleep, which is equivalent to REM sleep in adults, infants may move their arms or legs, cry, or whimper, and their eyes may be partly open. Their breathing is irregular and their eyes may dart back and forth under their eyelids. During quiet–NREM sleep, which corresponds to NREM sleep in adults, infants are behaviorally quiescent. Their breathing is regular, and they lie very still. However, they may have an occasional startle response or make sucking movements with their mouth.

Another difference between sleep of infants and adults is in how their sleep patterns are organized. Infants have polyphasic sleep periods; that is, they have many sleep periods throughout the day. Adults typically have only one sleep period, lasting about 8 hours (although there are many adults who continue to nap). A newborn infant typically sleeps for 3–4 hours and awakens only to be fed. This results in about seven sleeping and waking periods per day. Also, sleep is equally spaced throughout the day, with no clear differentiation between daylight and nighttime hours. This phenomenon is often cause for dismay in parents.

As infants get older, their sleep begins to consolidate and they begin to sleep less. For example, typical newborns sleep 17–18 hours a day, but by 1 month of age, infants sleep 16–17 hours, and by 3 or 4 months, they sleep about 15 hours a day. At this age, their sleep is consolidated into about four or five sleep periods. Two-thirds of babies' sleep now happens at night; babies at this age are already beginning to have a diurnal pattern of daytime wakefulness and nighttime sleep. At 6 months, infants have fewer daytime sleep periods, and sleep gets progressively longer at night. Whereas newborn infants sleep almost three-quarters of the time, 6-month-olds sleep only one-half of the time, for about 13 hours per day. At this age, the longest sustained daily sleep period is about 7 hours. Many children of this age wake for brief periods but can put themselves back to sleep. Thus, many parents who assume their child is sleeping for periods of 10–12 hours continuously may be inaccurate in their assessment. Their child may be waking for brief periods of time without disrupting anyone. By 24 months of age, toddlers' sleep has been reduced to about 12 hours per day, with most children continuing to take naps during the day, and by 4 years of age, children sleep about 10–12 hours per day, consisting chiefly of nighttime sleep with one daytime nap. The amount of sleep gradually decreases throughout childhood and adolescence, until it reaches the average 8 hours of sleep per night experienced by adults.

Another important aspect of the sleep of infants and young children is the nap. As an infant ages, the amount of nap time decreases. At 4 months of age, most children are taking either two or three naps per day. By 6 months, most (nearly 90%) children are only taking two naps per day, and by 15 months, almost half of all children are taking just one nap per day. In addition, the time of day in which the nap occurs affects the type of sleep involved in the nap. Early naps, occurring midmorning, have more active–REM sleep, and afternoon naps have more quiet–NREM sleep. It has been found that naps are beneficial: Children who nap have longer attention spans and are less fussy than their nonnapping counterparts. Some parents, concerned about their child's nighttime sleeping habits, try to get their child to sleep more at night by depriving their child of a nap. This practice is not effective and may in fact be detrimental. Also, evidence shows that keeping children up during the day does not help them sleep more at night.

Not only is the organization of infants' and children's sleep different from that of adults, but also its type and structure differ. For example, about 50% of the sleep of newborns is active–REM sleep, whereas REM sleep constitutes only about 20–25% of adults' sleep. As in adults, active–REM sleep is cyclical, but in comparison to the 90-minute cycle of adults, infants' cycles are 60 minutes long. Also, infants may have an active–REM period immediately on falling asleep, which is unusual for adults to experience. Quiet–NREM sleep in infants is also different from NREM sleep of adults. First, infants do not have the characteristic Stages 1, 2, 3, and 4 experienced by adults. Also, quiet–NREM sleep accounts for a smaller proportion of total sleep time. Quiet–NREM sleep accounts for 50% of total sleep time in infants, but almost 75% of adult sleep is spent in NREM. These differences between infants' and adults' sleep patterns in the type and structure of sleep quickly dissipate. By 3 months of age, the sleep stages of infants begin to resemble those of adults. For example, by 3 or 4 months, there is mature Stage 2 spindle activity, which consists of short bursts of rapid brain activity. Also, the spontaneous K complex, characterized by large slow waves, develops at 6 months. Other changes include a decrease in REM sleep and an increase in NREM sleep; by 6 months of age, REM sleep accounts for 30% of the time sleeping and NREM for 70% of the time, more like adult sleep. REM sleep continues to decrease throughout childhood, and in adolescence there is a significant dropoff of deep slow wave sleep.

Assessment

There are several methods used to assess infants', children's, and adolescents' sleep, some unique to these age groups. Polysomnography may be performed in the laboratory, as it is with adults. The child stays overnight at a sleep laboratory, and numerous physiological measures are extensively recorded. This method has several disadvantages, including concerns about how much the infant's or child's sleep in a laboratory setting resembles sleep at home and the expenses associated. More sophisticated and less cumbersome methods to study sleep in infants and children have been developed. In early studies, sleep was behaviorally observed, and determinations were made about the infants' state of sleep or wakefulness. Other studies have incorporated the use of videorecordings into behavioral observation, otherwise known as *time-lapse video somnography*. The videotapes can be accurately scored for different sleep–wake states, such as quiet sleep, active sleep, and awake time. Another method entails the use of a pressure-sensitive crib pad, which records infants' respiration and body movements. From these measures, active–REM, quiet–NREM, and wakefulness can be determined. A recent innovation has been the use of actigraphy. An *actigraph* is an instrument that children wear on their wrist, much like a watch. The actigraph keeps track of the child's movements and can measure the duration, stages, and quality of sleep.

Common Childhood Sleep Disorders

Approximately 25% of children experience some type of sleep disturbance (e.g., Lozoff, Wolf, & Davis, 1975; Richman, 1981; Richman, Stevenson, & Graham, 1975). The most common of these sleep problems are difficulties falling asleep, frequent night wakings, nighttime fears, nightmares, night terrors, enuresis, bruxism, and headbanging (e.g., Dollinger, 1982; Salzarulo & Chevalier, 1983). Furthermore, most sleep disturbances tend to persist, especially from infancy to later childhood. That is, children do not typically "outgrow" these problems. Of all the behavioral problems experienced by children, sleep disturbances are the most persistent.

Sleep disorders in children fall within three major categories. The first category includes problems of "insomnia," or the child who does not sleep. The second includes sleep disorders involving excessive daytime sleepiness. The final category consists of the parasomnias, such as night terrors, sleepwalking, and headbanging.

Insomnia

Insomnia in children usually presents itself as a child who does not sleep sufficiently. This sleeplessness may be the consequence of difficulties going to bed, trouble falling asleep at night, or nighttime awakenings.

Insomnia as found in adults does not usually occur in children; instead, it is often the result of factors such as negative sleep associations, adjustment problems, or other physiological sleep disturbances (e.g., sleep apnea or delayed sleep phase syndrome).

Bedtime problems. Many parents struggle with their child at bedtime. These bedtime struggles are often a source of considerable stress to both parents and children and can contribute to inadequate sleep for everybody in the family. Parents of children who have bedtime difficulties often report that they are depressed, anxious, and unhappy in their marriage. Bedtime problems are usually alleviated once limits are set by the parent and are highly amenable to behavioral treatments such as graduated extinction and the establishment of bedtime routines. Although sedative medications such as diphenhydramine (Benadryl) are commonly prescribed by pediatricians for these sleep problems, the drugs often result in a limited, short-term improvement (Richman, 1985).

Difficulties falling asleep at night can be related to children's nighttime fears. These nighttime fears, the most common fears experienced by children, are a normal, developmental occurrence in young children. Many of these fears are learned through simple conditioning. For example, the bedroom may be a source of anxiety for some children, especially if it is the place where the child is sent as punishment. Also, if the child has a nightmare or awakens distressed in the middle of the night, a parent typically comes into the room and turns on the light, causing the child to associate light with comfort and darkness with distress or nightmares. Although most children outgrow their nighttime fears, a variety of therapeutic techniques can be used, including guided imagery, relaxation training, and self-instruction.

Night wakings. Approximately 30% of young children have frequent nighttime awakenings. Although medical problems such as ear infections, allergies to cow's milk, or colic can contribute to nighttime awakenings, the majority of cases result from behavioral and learned factors. The primary cause of most night wakings is negative sleep associations. Behaviors or events that occur while falling asleep at bedtime, such as being rocked, sucking on a pacifier, or drinking from a bottle, promote sleep. However, when these objects or behaviors are not present, sleep is disturbed, and the result can be sleep-onset difficulties, frequent night wakings, or both. To understand this problem, it is important to realize that waking during the night is normal but that most children are able to return to sleep easily; these children are called "self-soothers." Other children, called "signalers," are unable to return to sleep until the conditions for sleep are reestablished. Behavioral interventions have been successful in treating these sleep-onset association disorders. One method that appears to involve little stress for parents is to intervene only at bedtime by establishing a positive bedtime routine and using graduated extinction. Parents use a simple checking method, waiting progressively longer periods of time before checking on their child. The goal of this method is to have the child fall asleep on his or her own at bedtime. Once the child is able to fall asleep on his or her own at bedtime, generalization occurs to reduce frequent night wakings.

Adjustment sleep disorder. Some difficulties sleeping are the result of a stressful event, problems in school, or an environmental change, sometimes called an *adjustment sleep disorder*. It is often seen in children following a move, after the death of a relative, or before the first day of school. The duration of the sleep problem is usually several days, although in some cases, often associated with ongoing stressors, it may last as long as several months.

In general, treatment for an adjustment sleep disorder is not necessary, because the problem resolves naturally over time. If treatment is sought for longer term sleep problems, psychological therapies usually focus on the disrupting events. With resolution of the precipitating event, the sleep problems typically dissipate and sleep returns to normal.

Excessive Daytime Sleepiness

Excessive daytime sleepiness in children is usually the result of inadequate sleep, a schedule disorder, or a physiological disturbance such as sleep apnea or narcolepsy.

Inadequate sleep. The most common cause of sleepiness in children and adolescents is an inadequate amount of sleep. Often adequate amounts of sleep are forsaken for children's active school and social schedules. Sports, after-school activities, and part-time jobs (especially early-morning newspaper routes) are given precedence over an early bedtime and adequate sleep. Adults in children's lives are often models for these poor sleep habits. Many touted role models also exhibit inadequate sleep, such as Olympian gymnasts and ice-skaters, whose schedules include 4:30 a.m. practice times and homework started at 10:00 or 11:00 at night. Sleep deprivation frequently contributes to school absences and tardiness, falling asleep in school, fatigue, and irritability. Sleep deprivation can also be tragic, because it is related to the increasing numbers of fatalities that are the result of driving accidents caused by falling asleep at the wheel. These types of car accidents are especially common in the adolescent and young adult populations.

The primary role of the clinician for this type of sleep problem is to help the entire family understand and acknowledge the impact of inadequate sleep. Behavioral contracts can be beneficial in helping children and adolescents get enough sleep both during the week and on weekends. Family priorities may need to be shifted to ensure that all members are getting sufficient sleep on a nightly basis.

Delayed sleep phase syndrome. Adolescents and many younger children enjoy staying up late at night. This practice becomes problematic, however, when their sleep–wake schedule becomes greatly shifted. The end result is delayed sleep phase syndrome (DSPS), with symptoms of sleep-onset insomnia and extreme difficulty awakening at a desired time in the morning. Approximately 7% of adolescents are sleep-phase-delayed. DSPS often begins with staying up late at night, sleeping late, or taking late afternoon naps. This process often begins on weekends, holidays, or summer vacations. Many children and adolescents with this sleep disorder have difficulties in school, primarily because of chronic absenteeism, tardiness, or sleepiness at school.

The primary mode of treatment for this disorder is chronotherapy. The first step in this program is stabilizing sleep at the phase-delayed times, for example 3:00 a.m. to noon. For the next week the sleeping period is delayed by 3 hours every day until the desired sleeping times occur. For example, on Night 1 sleep is to occur from 6:00 a.m. to 3:00 p.m., and on Night 2, from 9:00 a.m. until 6:00 p.m. The imposed scheduling of sleep must be strictly followed for treatment to be effective. Once sleep is occurring at the appropriate times, the new schedule must be rigidly adhered to; it is easy for these individuals to return to a delayed sleep phase pattern. Some adolescents are resistant to treatment; in those cases, psychological issues need to be addressed.

Sleep apnea. As discussed in previous chapters, obstructive sleep apnea syndrome (OSAS) involves repetitive episodes of upper airway obstruction during sleep that often cause a reduction in blood oxygen saturation. The clinical appearance of OSAS in children is quite different from that found in adults. The typical adult is obese, snores, and is excessively sleepy during the day. In contrast, the primary cause of OSAS in children is enlarged tonsils and adenoids. Children with OSAS may or may not be obese, and they do not always snore. Parents of children with OSAS may simply report that their child is a restless sleeper who often sleeps in unusual positions (usually to try to keep the airway open). There may also be reports of noisy breathing and a history of problems with tonsils or ear infections. Also, little is known about the impact of even brief episodes of apnea that do not meet published criteria for obstructive sleep apnea. Unfortunately, there are few normative studies of children that include pulmonary functioning. However, frequent brief arousals over a long period of time can have a significant impact on the quality of sleep and daytime functioning.

For children, the mean age at time of diagnosis is 7 years, with an increased prevalence in boys. Certain categories of children are at high risk for sleep apnea, including those with maxillofacial abnormalities, micrognathia, cleft palate, or Down's syndrome. Children who are morbidly obese are also at increased risk for sleep apnea.

The most common treatment is surgery to remove the airway obstruction, that is, a tonsillectomy, adenoidectomy, or both. These procedures relieve symptoms in about 70% of children. Other recommended treatments include weight loss and the use of pharmacological agents. Furthermore, nasal continuous positive airway pressure (NCPAP) may be an appropriate treatment for some children with sleep apnea.

Narcolepsy. Narcolepsy is a chronic disorder characterized by excessive sleepiness, often presenting itself as repeated episodes of naps or lapses into sleep of short duration throughout the day. Other common symptoms of narcolepsy are muscle paralysis (cataplexy and sleep paralysis) and dream imagery (hypnagogic and hypnopompic hallucinations). Although traditionally the onset of narcolepsy was thought to be late adolescence or early adulthood, there is increasing evidence that symptoms may begin in childhood.

Diagnosis of narcolepsy in children is more difficult than in adults. Particularly in younger children, sleepiness may be the only initial symptom, with no history of the other traditional symptoms. Furthermore, mild symptoms of cataplexy can be difficult to identify in children and may be evident only in retrospect following the diagnosis. Likewise, hypnagogic hallucinations can be difficult to elicit from a child's history. Even findings of polysomnography may not be conclusive. With prepubertal children and adolescents, repeat studies may be necessary before a final diagnosis is reached.

Treatment of narcolepsy in children and adolescents is similar to treatment of adults. Education and counseling of the patient and family are important, as is education of teachers and others in the school system. The child or adolescent must adhere to a regular sleep schedule with good sleep habits, which may include scheduled naps. Medications may also be beneficial, with use of short-acting stimulant medication for treatment of daytime sleepiness and of REM-suppressant medications for cataplexy, if necessary. Unfortunately, most studies of pharmacological treatments for narcolepsy have involved adults; few studies have included children.

Parasomnias

Parasomnias are unusual behaviors that occur during sleep. These include sleepwalking, night terrors, confused partial arousal, nightmares, and enuresis. Headbanging and bruxism are also commonly observed parasomnias in children.

Partial arousals. Sleepwalking, sleep talking, and night terrors are all variations of partial arousals from deep (usually Stages 3 and 4) sleep. Partial arousals occur during the transition from slow wave sleep (usually occurring during the first 1–3 hr after sleep onset) to lighter sleep, REM sleep, or a brief arousal. These transition episodes can consist of sleep talking, sleepwalking, confused arousals, or night terrors. The episodes typically last from 2 to 10 minutes, but they can be longer. During these episodes, the child is essentially asleep, and he or she usually has no memory of the event in the morning. During the event, the child appears disoriented and confused and may even seem terrified. The child usually does not recognize his or her parents and often resists attempts to be soothed or held. Some children may even become combative when parents attempt to calm them. Attempting to wake the child is often unsuccessful and may prolong the event. Rather, these episodes usually resolve naturally, with a rapid return to deep sleep. These partial arousals are common in children, with resolution as the child gets older.

Studies indicate a genetic component to these sleep disturbances, because there is usually a family history. Although many times parents are concerned that their child is severely anxious or depressed and that these nighttime episodes are a manifestation of psychological difficulties, this is rarely the case. Studies indicate that there is little relationship between these events and childhood anxiety or depression. Partial arousals, however, can be exacerbated or induced by fever and some medications, such as lithium, fluphenazine (Prolixin), and desipramine. Chaotic sleep schedules, sleep deprivation, and stress are also frequent contributors to partial arousals.

The most important aspects of treatment for these sleep disturbances are reassurance to the family and institution of safety precautions. Education about the nature and significance of these episodes is vital for all members of the family. Safety measures, such as erecting gates and locking all windows and doors, are essential. Behavioral treatments, including reinforcement and hypnosis, can be successful. Furthermore, medications such as a bedtime dose of a benzodiazepine or tricyclic antidepressant can also be helpful in significantly decreasing deep sleep, which is when these partial arousals are most likely to occur. When the medication is discontinued, however, there is often a rebound effect. Medication may be recommended when partial arousals or night terrors are extremely frequent or highly disruptive to the family or when the behavior puts the child or others in danger. For example, one child seen at a sleep disorders center had night terrors repetitively, every night, and several times attacked other family members, including his younger siblings. In this instance, medication was recommended and was successful in decreasing the frequency and intensity of the events.

Nightmares. Nightmares are frightening dreams that result in an awakening. In contrast to night terrors and other partial arousal disturbances, they occur primarily during REM sleep, which is usually in the second half of the night. Nightmares are common in children between the ages of 3 and 6 years, and many children continue to have them on a sporadic basis. Although a small percentage of children continue to have nightmares throughout adolescence and sometimes into adulthood, most nightmares decrease over time. Once awake, the child is usually frightened but is consolable by a parent and can recall the dream in vivid detail. Children often have difficulty returning to sleep following a nightmare. Most nightmares are related to fears of the dark, falling, or death. An increase in nightmares often occurs following a stressful period or traumatic event, such as an automobile accident or the death of a relative or friend. In addition, medications may be associated with nightmares, including some beta-blockers and antidepressants.

Treatment for nightmares focuses on anxiety reduction techniques such as relaxation and imagery, often combined with other behavioral strategies such as systematic desensitization or response prevention. Dream reorganization has also been successfully used. This treatment technique involves systematic desensitization combined with coping self-statements and guided rehearsal of mastery endings to dream content. For most families, however, reassurance that nightmares are part of normal child development is beneficial and all that is necessary, which decreases the likelihood that the child will be treated as though psychologically disturbed.

Enuresis. Enuresis is diagnosed when persistent bed-wetting occurs after age 5. Bed-wetting occurs in approximately 30% of 4-year-olds, 10% of 6-year-olds, 5% of 10-year-olds, and 3% of 12-year-olds. Primary enuresis, which is a continuous enuretic condition, comprises 70–90% of all cases. Secondary enuresis, in which the child has had at least 3–6 months of dryness, constitutes the remaining 10–30% of all cases.

Enuresis is undoubtably the best studied sleep disorder of children. Several behavioral treatments are highly successful. The most popular and effective technique is the bell-and-pad system, which sounds a bell when bed-wetting occurs. This method was developed by Mowrer and Mowrer in 1938. Reported success rates for this technique have been as high as 75%. Other treatment approaches for enuresis include bladder training, response prevention and contingency management, hypnosis, and dietary control, such as a reduction in caffeine intake. Typically, a comprehensive treatment program is used, incorporating a number of components such as bladder-stretching exercises, visual sequencing (imagining the behaviors required to get out of bed and urinate in the bathroom), a nightly waking schedule, positive practice, and an alarm activated by wetness.

For some, tricyclic antidepressants may be prescribed. Imipramine can be successful in controlling enuresis in up to 70% of cases. However, on withdrawal from the medication, few children stay dry. Because of the potential cardiotoxic effects of this drug and the high relapse rate following its withdrawal, it is usually not recommended for use over long periods of time. Another drug that has been used with success is desmopressin (DDAVP), an analogue of antidiuretic hormone (vasopressin). Desmopressin successfully treats 70% of cases with minimal side effects but also almost always leads to relapse following discontinuation. Because desmopressin is much more expensive and has higher relapse rates than other treatments, it may be the treatment of choice only when used on a short-term or as-needed basis.

Other behaviors during sleep. Many children fall asleep while rocking their body, rolling back and forth, or banging their head. These behaviors are common in infants, with 60% of 9-month-olds exhibiting one of these behaviors. Approximately one-quarter of infants continue to engage in one of these behaviors, and approximately 5% of children continue after 2 years. The behavior usually disappears by 4 years of age, although it can persist through adolescence and into adulthood.

Most of these rhythmic movement disorders occur at sleep onset, beginning with drowsiness. A recurrence of the behavior may be observed during the night at sleep stage transitions. These behaviors, which are similar to those occurring in a sleep-onset association disorder, help the child to fall asleep and return to sleep after waking up during the night. They usually last 5–15 minutes but can last as long as 4 hours. The activity is rapid, with a reported range of 19–21 bangs or rocks per minute.

Injuries are uncommon, and treatment typically is not instituted because the behavior is usually benign and self-limiting. Measures may need to be taken to alleviate the disruption this behavior may be having on other family members' sleep. Behavior modification programs can be successful. Benzodiazepines and tricyclic antidepressant medications may also be helpful when the behavior is highly disruptive to others or for short durations, such as while on family vacations or overnight outings. A psychiatric and neurological evaluation may be indicated when these behaviors persist beyond 3 years of age.

Conclusion

It is important to be educated about sleep and to have a thorough understanding of sleep disorders, because these disorders are commonly experienced by children and adolescents. Many childhood sleep problems are highly amenable to treatment, but unfortunately they are usually underdiagnosed and undertreated.

REFERENCES

Dollinger, S. L. (1982). On the varieties of childhood sleep disturbance. *Journal of Clinical Child Psychology, 11,* 107–115.

Lozoff, B., Wolf, A. W., & Davis, N. S. (1985). Sleep problems seen in pediatric practice. *Pediatrics, 75,* 477–483.

Mowrer, O. H., & Mowrer, W. M. (1938). Enuresis: A method for its study and treatment. *American Journal of Orthopsychiatry, 8,* 436–459.

Richman, N. (1981). A community survey of characteristics of one to two year olds with sleep disruptions. *Journal of the American Academy of Child Psychiatry, 20,* 281–291.

Richman, N. (1985). A double-blind drug trial of treatment in young children with waking problems. *Journal of Child Psychology and Psychiatry, 4,* 591–598.

Richman, N., Stevenson, J. E., & Graham, P. J. (1975). Behavior problems in three-year-old children: An epidemiological study in a London borough. *Journal of Child Psychology and Psychiatry, 12,* 5–33.

Salzarulo, P., & Chevalier, A. (1983). Sleep problems in children and their relationships with early disturbances of the waking-sleeping rhythms. *Sleep, 6,* 47–51.

23

Sleep and Aging

Donald L. Bliwise

The discrimination between health and disease as it is relevant for sleep is nowhere highlighted better than in a discussion of aging. Epidemiologists make distinctions between diseases that are age-related (have a distinct window of opportunity for developing) versus diseases that are age-dependent (have an increased chance of developing as one ages). Many chronic diseases are age-related, for example, heart disease, stroke, certain forms of cancer, and arthritis. With the possible exception of narcolepsy (see chapters 3 and 6), which has its peak incidence in the teens and twenties, most sleep disorders are also age-related. That is, an individual is more likely to demonstrate conditions such as sleep apnea, periodic leg movements, and phase advance of the sleep–wake cycle as one becomes older. Similarly, medical and neurologic diseases such as Alzheimer's disease (AD) and Parkinson's disease (PD) that are highly prevalent in the elderly often have marked associated sleep disturbance. Frequently, these can be devastating for family and other caregivers, as well as extraordinarily refractory to behavioral and to pharmacological treatments.

When discussing aging, the issue of "normality" always arises. Normality can be discussed as a purely statistical phenomenon by reference to the midpoint of a distribution, the most common occurrence in a distribution, or the arithmetic mean. Normality may also refer to a Gaussian distribution per se. When discussing age-related changes in physiological function, however, normality typically refers to absence of disease, whereas the presence of disease is, by definition, associated with morbidity, mortality, or both. Although readers new to the field of sleep disorders may find that the thoroughness of this volume attests otherwise, the field of sleep is so new that data on normality in a statistical sense vastly outweigh knowledge of associated morbidities. This is particularly true for such sleep-specific diseases as sleep apnea. By way of example, probably close to 100 controlled behavioral intervention studies have been performed on individuals with insomnia (see chapter 16 in this volume). However, to date not a single controlled clinical trial has been performed for sleep apnea in individuals of any age, let alone the aged, where the prevalence of the condition may be extraordinarily high. The reasons for this are complex and involve cost, adequacy of and compliance with treatment, uncertainty regarding length of follow-up with which to assess outcomes, and the range of potential outcomes to assess. Insofar as sleep apnea is concerned, the field of sleep disorders has probably reached a stage similar to that of the field of cardiovascular disease 40 years ago. This appears a daunting prospect for behavioral scientists, but it also invites participation by individuals interested in this area. There is much to learn about both health and disease associated with the aging process, and sleep provides a wonderful opportunity to examine issues related to psychological and physical function as well as issues of mechanism.

The psychologist interested in gerontology who begins to inquire and probe regarding sleep disturbance in his or her older clients is likely to encounter a wide variety of common, yet often diverse, sleep complaints. Psychologists often equate "sleep disturbance" with "insomnia," but the psychologist entering this area should be aware that sleep-related complaints are often very complex, usually necessitate more detailed history-taking, and may involve not only nocturnal, but also daytime, symptoms. By way of example, sleep latency insomnia is very common in the younger population but less so in the elderly, among whom sleep maintenance insomnia predominates. Even in the case of the latter, however, distinctions must be made between complaints involving awakening repeatedly and returning to sleep relatively easily (suggestive of intermittent events disturbing sleep) versus awakenings followed by prolonged periods of wakefulness (suggestive of circadian rhythm abnormalities or affective disorder). Inquiry must always be made regarding whether the poor sleep is characterized by feelings of restlessness and agitation specifically confined to the lower limbs (restless legs syndrome). Sleep specialists also typically examine specific types of sleep–wake complaints with a particular concern for their physiological bases. For example, daytime sleepiness in the older adult may be a manifestation of age-related changes in circadian rhythms (see chapter 2 in this volume), but it may also be reflective of nocturnal sleep fragmentation. Sleep fragmentation itself may be related to periodic leg movement, sleep apnea, or upper airway resistance syndrome. Finally, the complexity of evaluating a particular sleep related symptom is underscored by the situation in which the patient's symptoms come to the clinician's attention because of individuals other than the patient himself or herself. Typical situations here include the adult child who witnesses breath holding and snoring during sleep (suggestive of sleep apnea) in an aged parent, or the elderly spouse who becomes aware that their partner thrashes and flails his or her limbs in a potentially injurious manner during sleep.

Some specific prevalence figures provide a glimpse of the magnitude of the widespread nature of sleep–wake disturbance in the elderly. Self-reported snoring has been estimated to occur in about 50% of men and 40% of women at age 60; both figures represent substantial increases over the prevalence reported at age 40 in men (30%) and women (20%). There is some suggestion that after age 80 snoring prevalence may decrease, possibly reflecting household living status or, conceivably, mortality. The fact that snoring is related to sleep apnea, apart from whether an individual lives alone (D. Bliwise, Nekich, & Dement, 1991), is consistent with the latter. By far the most common sleep-related symptom experienced by the geriatric population is difficulty maintaining sleep. Some data have indicated that as many as 65% of the over-60 population experiences at least mild trouble with this symptom, whereas 25% to 35% experience more of a problem falling asleep. In some reports, problems falling asleep have been more closely associated with the occurrence of periodic leg movements (D. Bliwise, Petta, Seidel, & Dement, 1985) and depression (D. Bliwise, King, Harris, & Haskell, 1992; Friedman, Brooks, D. Bliwise, & Yesavage, 1993). Gender differences exist for both of these symptoms, with women reporting more complaints than men. This is a somewhat paradoxical situation relative to findings in the sleep lab, where older men have consistently more disturbed nocturnal sleep as measured polysomnographically.

To summarize the preceding discussion, sleep-related symptoms are exceedingly common and will rank high on the list of conditions that the psychologist is likely to encounter in inpatient or outpatient settings. In this chapter, I summarize some of the changes known to occur in sleep with advancing years, including both normative alterations in sleep architecture as well as several sleep "pathologies" commonly encountered in the aged population. Throughout the chapter, I make reference to relevant results from our own "normal" population, the Bay Area Sleep Cohort (BASC), which is a group of 256 individuals (mean age at entry = 65.2 ± 9.2) who underwent nocturnal polysomnography and have been followed over time. In many respects, this sample represents an example of "customary" or "usual" aging inasmuch as only individuals with acute and serious medical conditions and dementia were excluded from participation at entry. Descriptive and demographic data on the sample are provided in Table 1, and a more thorough description of the sampling will be made at the end of this chapter.

Table 1

Description of Bay Area Sleep Cohort (BASC)

Variable	*M*	*SD*	Percentage
Demographics/Health			
Gender			
Male (*n* = 83)			32
Female (*n* = 173)			68
Age	65.2	9.2	
Height in centimeters	166.4	9.2	
Weight in kilograms	68.6	13.1	
Metric body mass index (BMI)	24.7	3.9	
Systolic blood pressure	138.6	19.4	
Diastolic blood pressure	80.4	10.9	
Self-reported health rating			
Excellent			34.8
Good			53.2
Fair			10.6
Poor			1.4
Education level			
Under 7 years			1.1
Junior high			2.1
Partial high school			5.3
High school			17.0
Partial college			27.1
Standard college degree			22.3
Completed graduate/			
Professional training			25.0
Marital status			
Single			6.7
Married			55.4

Variable	M	SD	Percentage
Separated			2.6
Divorced			13.5
Divorced & remarried			0.5
Widowed			18.1
Widowed & remarried			3.1
Using psychoactive medication			16.9
Using cardiovascular, lipid Reducing, Insulin, and/or Respiratory stimulating medication			25.0
Using aspirin and/or Anti-inflammatory medication			18.8
Women using estrogen			15.1

Polysomnographic Measures

Total sleep time (in minutes)	359.7	89.8	
Sleep efficiency (%)	73.7	15.4	
Stage 1	14.6	10.9	
Stage 2	59.7	13.5	
Stages 3 and 4	6.9	8.5	
REM %	17.7	6.9	
Respiratory Disturbance Index (RDI)	4.5	9.9	
Periodic Leg Movements Index (PLMSI)	14.2	25.5	
PLMS with arousal index	5.5	15.2	

Self-Report Sleep Measures (% Positive)

Disturbed nocturnal sleep			47.0
Daytime fatigue			43.6
Snoring			32.8
Loud snoring			15.8
Holding breath/Stop breathing			4.9
Experience pain or discomfort			30.6
Falling asleep during movies, TV, travel, and/or listening to stereo			78.2
Teeth grinding			15.0
Restless legs			21.9
Leg twitching			19.8

A final theme in this chapter will be the interplay between so-called "somatic" and psychological factors in the sleep changes seen in old age. In clinical practice, it becomes of considerable importance to guard against the otherwise strong temptation to "psychologize" or otherwise overinterpret the poor sleep of old age as an indicator of suboptimal mental health. In fact, in the elderly there is considerable evidence that the vast majority of sleep-related symptoms (even those involving insomnia) are *not* related to mental disorders, at least to the extent that a preexisting mental health condition leads to poor sleep. I will summarize some of the evidence suggesting that medical disease plays a major role in the sleep disturbance seen in late life. For more complete coverage of this topic, the reader is directed to several other recent reviews encompassing the spectrum of medical (D. Bliwise, 1993) and neurological (D. Bliwise, 1994a) disease. Following this, I will return to the psychological literature on sleep disturbance in the elderly.

Normative Age-Related Changes Intrinsic to Sleep

Many studies have described the age-related differences in polysomno-graphic sleep patterns. Most of these data are cross-sectional, and even in those few studies where longitudinal data have been reported (Hoch et al., 1994; Hoch, Reynolds, Kupfer, & Berman, 1988), results are limited by the features of the particular population under study. For example, there are no studies examining different cohorts (of the same age) sequentially over time to allow for sorting out the influence of histori-cal change from developmental change (Schaie, 1986). Although we do not yet fully understand all of the historical factors that might affect sleep in an elderly individual, it is not at all inconceivable that physio-logical variables (customary diet, exercise, cumulative medication usage) as well as psychosocial variables (earlier life trauma, financial strain) now may well affect older individuals differently from how they did in the past and how they will in the future. In all likelihood, sleep will not be inured to such changes. It is also important to point out that most age differences described in this section may represent "custom-ary" or "normal" aging, but they do not represent "successful" aging as proposed by Rowe and Kahn (1987). The latter is thought to represent optimization of the aging process without the contribution of chronic disease or its treatment. Although far less is known about sleep patterns in such optimal or "best possible case" aging, I will make reference to studies embracing this definition.

Age differences in sleep patterns have been reviewed elsewhere (D. Bliwise, 1993) but can be briefly summarized here. Changes in the architecture of sleep (see chapters 1 and 8) described in adults are well appreciated in the elderly. Stage 1 sleep typically occupies a higher proportion of total sleep time in the older person relative to even middle aged adults. Stage 1 is generally considered to be a transitional stage indicating sleep disturbance. In the BASC, our participants averaged 14.6% of their sleep in Stage 1 (see Table 1). Sleep efficiency, the proportion of the night in bed actually asleep, also decreases. Mean sleep efficiency in the BASC was 73.7%. Additionally, changes in the so-called microarchitecture have also been described, consisting of brief arousals in the electroencephalogram (EEG), typically bursts of alpha activity of 2 to 15 seconds in duration (Carskadon, Brown, & Dement, 1982) that are further evidence of the instability of the sleep–wake state in the aged human. In most other species that have been examined to date, including mice, rats, and cats, similar age differences in sleep consolidation have been noted (D. Bliwise, 1993).

An area of particular interest to psychologists, particularly because of its relationship to the experience of dreaming, may be age differences in REM sleep. As discussed in chapter 1, relationships between REM sleep and dreaming have been the subject of intensive investigation by psychologists and psychophysiologists who have been interested in examining physiological correlates of different aspects of the dream experience. Of relevance here is that many older people experience changes in the quality and quantity of dreaming in late life. Age differences in dreaming have been explored within the sleep laboratory using awakenings from REM sleep (Zepelin, 1981), and the results are consistent with data from the midlife developmental personality literature showing a predominance of passive, dependent themes in men. In women more aggressive, assertive themes may be apparent. Despite these results, findings on physiologically measured REM sleep changes with aging have been far less impressive. Many studies have reported no age differences whatsoever in REM percentage (REM%) as a function of total sleep time (D. Bliwise, 1993), although a few reports have suggested a very slight lowering of REM% in the elderly. In the BASC mean REM% was 17.7% (Table 1). More recently, additional longitudinal data from a study of "successful" aging did not show significant changes in REM%, density, or latency over time (Hoch et al., 1994). As a final note to REM sleep in this section, it is important to observe that REM sleep may undergo more dramatic changes in certain neurologic diseases of the senium, including Alzheimer's disease (AD) and Parkinson's disease (PD).

From the physiological perspective, perhaps one of the most interesting age-related changes in sleep involves Stages 3 and 4 sleep, typically termed *delta* or *slow wave sleep* (SWS). In our cohort, Stages 3 and 4 occupied only about 7% of total time asleep. As described in chapters 1 and 8, these stages are often considered to represent the deepest and soundest stages of sleep and have the highest auditory arousal threshold to certain types of stimuli relative to other sleep stages. Numerous physiological accompaniments to these stages have been described, including release of growth hormone and autonomic activation, as indexed by skin resistance, and increases subsequent to exercise. Most significant for this chapter is that SWS decreases with age. However, the age at which decline has been first noted is considerably younger (20s) than is typically ascribed to most other psychological or physiological changes in the nervous system associated with aging (D. Bliwise, 1993). Sophisticated EEG quantification techniques have suggested that the decline in these stages primarily reflects a decrease in the amplitude (voltage), rather than any change in wavelength, of the delta waves during sleep (Smith, Karacan, & Yang, 1977). Also of note is that at every age in adulthood, women have significantly more SWS relative to men. This finding appears particularly paradoxical in view of the evidence that women typically have more sleep complaints than men. The functional significance of delta activity during sleep remains obscure. Extracerebral factors, such as head size and skull thickness may play a role; however, at least some cross-sectional data suggest that those persons aging "optimally" may in fact be the individuals who retain maximal amounts of Stages 3 and 4 sleep into old age (Buysse et al., 1992; Hoch et al., 1994).

Sleep Pathologies Common in the Aged

One of the initially alarming discoveries made in the field of sleep disorders over the last 15 years was that many specific pathophysiologic conditions (e.g., sleep apnea, periodic leg movements) are highly prevalent in otherwise healthy older adults. First, it should be stressed that these conditions may occur in the presence of specific diseases. For example, disordered breathing in sleep is more likely to occur in chronic obstructive pulmonary disease, congestive heart failure, hypertension, and renal disease; however, it may also occur in a purely idiopathic form. The best prevalence data to date suggest that 24% of the independently living elderly population have at least mild sleep apnea (Ancoli-Israel et al., 1991a). Similarly, periodic leg movements in sleep (PLMS) are more likely to occur in PD, osteoarthritis of the hips or lower limbs, restless legs syndrome, and fibromyalgia, although they may also occur in the absence of such conditions. In the San Diego prevalence study (Ancoli-Israel et al., 1991b), the prevalence of PLMS was estimated at about 45%. The widespread prevalence of these conditions has engendered controversy as to whether these so-called "pathologies" have any meaning at all.

Particularly for the elderly, one outcome that has been the focus of considerable research insofar as sleep apnea is concerned is mortality. If sleep apnea is associated with adverse cardiovascular events and oxygen desaturation during the night, is it conceivable that so-called "natural" death during sleep might be reflecting such pathophysiological events. Some inferential evidence for a potential role of sleep apnea in mortality comes from the study of Mitler, Hajdukovic, Shafor, Hahn, and Kripke (1987), who reported that among over 4,500 consecutive deaths in New York City, deaths from cardiovascular causes in the over-65 population showed a temporal specificity with a marked peak at about 6:00 a.m. Deaths from cancer showed no such pattern that argued against "discovery artifact" (elderly individuals living alone being discovered the morning after they had died) playing a major role in producing these results. Because REM sleep is more likely to occur in the hours immediately prior to morning awakening and because sleep apnea tends to be more severe during REM sleep, these results could be interpreted as consistent with the hypothesis that sleep apnea leads to death during sleep.

Although no prospectively designed controlled clinical trials have conclusively demonstrated a role for sleep apnea in mortality, at least several other studies have provided evidence that elderly individuals with sleep apnea were more likely to die of cardiovascular causes during sleep. D. Bliwise, N. Bliwise, et al. (1988) reported that among the BASC, individuals with even mild levels of sleep disordered breathing tended to be more likely to die within a 5-year follow-up relative to individuals without sleep apnea, the resulting univariate odds ratio being approximately 2.7 (95% confidence interval .95 to 7.47).

Additionally, among the 20 nontraumatic deaths reported in this study, individuals dying from cardiovascular causes were more likely to die during the period of midnight to 8:00 a.m. than individuals who died from cancer and other causes. In a more infirm population, Ancoli-Israel, Klauber, Kripke, Parker, and Cobarrubias (1989) reported that among nursing home patients with sleep apnea (recorded with an ambulatory recording monitor; see chapter 7), those individuals with high levels of sleep apnea were likely to die sooner. These results, although far from conclusive, do raise the possibility that sleep apnea could be a (preventable) cause of death in old age.

Results suggesting a role of sleep apnea in cardiovascular outcomes need not be as dramatic as mortality. In the BASC, we found a trend between use of all types of cardiovascular medication and higher Respiratory Disturbance Index levels (see Table 2). In a 30- to 60-year-old population, Hla et al. (1994) reported that individuals with sleep apnea had higher 24-hour blood pressure values than individuals without sleep apnea. Despite these findings, results from a carefully screened, healthy cohort of older individuals have been unable to show relationships between either measured blood pressure or medication status and sleep apnea using either cross-sectional or longitudinal data (Berry et al., 1987; Phillips, Berry, Schmitt, Harbison, & Lipke-Molby, 1994).

Unlike sleep apnea, where clear cardiovascular morbidity and mortality may be associated with the condition, the situation with PLMS may be more tenuous. First, a number of studies in nonclinical, aged populations have had trouble showing that these events have any pattern of symptoms associated with them (Ancoli-Israel et al., 1991b; Dickel & Mosko, 1990), although in clinical populations, the relationship between these movements and restless legs symptoms (Hening et al., 1986) is strong. Part of the problem may be that far less is known about the mechanisms controlling the appearance of these movements during sleep than is known about the mechanistic basis for disordered breathing in sleep. Although some studies have noted reflex abnormalities in PLMS patients (Wechsler, Stakes, Shahani, & Busis, 1986), most studies examining neurologic dysfunction in these patients have been negative.

In the BASC, the mean number of PLMS per hour of sleep was 14.2 (± 25.5), and the mean number of PLMS with arousal per hour of sleep was 5.5 (± 15.2), indicating that an exceedingly large number of elderly individuals demonstrated these movements during sleep. The prevalence of cases exceeding a value of 5.0 was 44.5% of all such movements and 22.6% for movements with arousal. In our cohort,

Table 2

Relationships Between Chronic Medication Use and Polysomnographic Measures in Bay Area Sleep Cohort (BASC)

| | Class of Medication | | | |
Variable	CV	Psych	Anti-Inflammatory	Estrogen
Total Sleep Time		2.15**		
Sleep Efficiency				
Stage 1%	1.75*H	2.01**		
Stage 2%		2.89***H		
Stages 3 & 4%	1.67*	3.22***		
REM%				
Total RDI	1.86*H	2.19**		
PLMS Index	3.09***H	1.69*		2.80***
PLMS with Arousal Index				2.41**

Note. Values in table are for *t* tests with two-tailed probabilities of 0.10 or less comparing individuals receiving/not receiving a particular medication. CV = cardiovascular; Psych = psychoactive; RDI = Respiratory Disturbance Index; PLMS = periodic leg movements in sleep.
*p<.10 **p<.05 ***p<.01
HHigher value in group receiving medication.

associations with polysomnographically defined PLMS were noted for cardiovascular medication (positive) and use of estrogen, progesterone, or both in women (negative), the latter at least raising the possibility that such medications might be protective for this condition.

Sleep in Medical Conditions Common for the Geriatric Population

The large number of chronic diseases experienced by elderly individuals and the consequent use of medication lead to a host of factors that can directly or indirectly disturb sleep. Regarding the latter, at the most general level, the number of medications (nonpsychoactive) used by an elderly individual correlates well with the severity of his or her sleep disturbance (Morgan, Healey, & Healey, 1989). Medications such as beta blockers (Kostis & Rosen, 1987), theophylline (Merlotti et al., 1992), analgesics, and nonsteroidal anti-inflammatories (Murphy, Badia, Myers, Boecker, & Wright, 1994) have been associated with disturbed sleep. All of these medications are used by large segments of the elderly population. In the BASC, trends for higher Stage 1 and lower Stages 3 and 4 sleep associated with cardiovascular medication use were noted (Table 2).

Insofar as medical diseases are concerned, a wide variety of conditions may disrupt sleep, although the mechanisms involved may be complex. One interesting Swedish study noted that any identified individuals using the health care system for any disease (as determined by registry in an automated medical record-keeping system) were more likely to report insomnia (Hanson & Ostergren, 1987). This finding has also been documented using multivariate models by Gislason and Almqvist (1987), who reported that when somatic diseases were controlled statistically, some types of insomnia complaints showed no age-related increase and some even showed a decrease with age. Finally, a sleep lab study showed that among elderly individuals who had not sought health care, minimal levels of sleep disturbance were seen (Vitiello, Prinz, Avery, et al., 1990). Specific conditions relevant for the geriatric population shown to disrupt sleep include renal disease (Kimmel, Miller, & Mendelson, 1989), gastrointestinal illness (Gerard, Collins, Dore, & Exton-Smith, 1978), respiratory disease (Mant & Eyland, 1988), chronic pain and fibromyalgia (Leigh, Hindmarch, Bird, & Wright, 1988), and menopause (Ballinger, 1976; Brugge, Kripke, Ancoli-Israel, & Garfinkel, 1989; see chapter 25).

Relevant to all of these diseases is that the sleep of the older person is more likely to be disrupted by any factor external to sleep (e.g., noise) relative to the sleep of a younger person, even within Stage 2 (Zepelin, McDonald, & Zammit, 1984). Thus the sleep of the older person is intrinsically lighter than that of the younger sleeper, even when "correcting" for lack of delta sleep. This means that the net effect of such conditions that introduce additional causes of interruption (pain, chronic nocturnal cough, the unpleasant sensation of acid backing into esophagus, autonomic flushing) is probably additive.

One medical cause of sleep disturbance for the older population is frequent nocturnal urination (nocturia). An analysis of the possible mechanisms underlying this widespread symptom serve to illustrate at once how complex and interdependent sleep-related symptoms can be. Awakenings to urinate represent a common phenomenon in the sleep of the elderly. Prevalence data suggest that about 50% of the geriatric population awakens at least twice during the night to urinate (Brocklehurst, Fry, Griffiths, & Kalton, 1971), and among 10 self-reported causes of awakenings, nocturia was by far the most common (Gerard et al., 1978). In one study (Friedman, D. Bliwise, Tanke, Salom, & Yesavage, 1992) it was reported that in elderly women, awakenings to urinate were significant discriminators of individuals who reported too little sleep or those reporting frank "insomnia." Why these results occurred only in women was unclear, though the finding may be related to the higher prevalence of urge incontinence in women (Burgio et al., 1994). It is also of note that among elderly community dwelling women, sleep disturbance *and* incontinence were among the most significant predictors of perceived health functioning (Kutner, Schechtman, Ory, Baker, & FICSIT Group, 1994). Asplund and Åberg (1992) have reported that daytime fatigue in the elderly was related to the number of awakenings during the night for micturition.

The reasons why nocturia affects sleep are probably multiply determined. As mentioned earlier, because sleep is more likely to be disturbed by any stimuli (presumably external *or* internal) it may be that the sensation of a partially filled bladder has more impact on the sleep of the older person. In the Burgio et al. (1994) study, nocturnal incontinence was not only more common in women, but also in individuals with congestive heart failure, those suffering from nocturnal shortness of breath, and those individuals using sleep medication. The last suggests that normal arousal responses, at least insofar as bladder function is concerned, may be militated through use of these medications. A somewhat different but complimentary perspective was provided by a sleep-laboratory-based study that examined the occurrence of patient-initiated requests for use of the bathroom over the course of a night in the sleep laboratory (Pressman et al., 1993). In this report, the majority of such requests were associated with awakenings occurring after the termination of an episode of sleep apnea. Thus, it may well be that elderly individuals whose predominant symptoms involve frequent nocturnal urination may be at risk for having sleep apnea, with the former serving as an unrecognized proxy for the latter. On the other hand, it may well be that sleep apnea itself leads to greater urine output overnight. For example, such diuresis in sleep apnea could represent the effects of elevated levels of atrial natriuretic factor produced by the heart in response to pooling of fluid in the pulmonary circulation (Partinen et al., 1991). Finally, patients with sleep apnea who are treated with diuretics may have increased urinary production related to their medication even apart from the disease per se.

The issue of nocturia in the elderly is thus highly relevant for the psychologist who may be encountering older persons with the complaint of poor sleep. First, specific inquiry should always be made regarding this aspect of the patient's sleep, especially probing for whether sleep is likely to be disturbed by other phenomena (e.g., noise, variations in ambient temperature). Awakenings to void should not be confused with or attributed to awakenings due to psychological distress, even though an individual may have distressing ruminations associated with being unable to return to sleep following awakenings for micturition. Second, inquiry about diseases or medications that could lead to increased nocturia should be made. Finally, specific questions regarding sleep apnea should always be made in the case of an elderly man or woman with such a complaint.

Just as systemic medical diseases affecting the elderly can influence sleep via a variety of complex mechanisms, the presence of various neurologic diseases may also serve to disrupt sleep (D. Bliwise, 1994a). Two of the most prevalent neurodegenerative conditions in old age, AD and PD, may disturb sleep by interfering with normal mechanisms regulating sleep and circadian rhythms. Although studies are far from conclusive (and also extraordinarily difficult to perform technically because of the nocturnal exacerbation of agitation often seen in such patients; D. Bliwise, 1994b), some points of convergence seem to exist. First, there is now good evidence that in AD patients, the extent of their dementia is associated with the amount of wakefulness seen during the nocturnal recording and possibly with the amount of sleep seen during the daytime hours (Prinz, Vitaliano, et al., 1982; Vitiello, Prinz, Williams, Frommlet, & Ries, 1990). Stages 3 and 4 sleep may be absent and REM sleep parameters may also be decreased at more severe levels of illness (D. Bliwise, Tinklenberg, et al., 1989). Sleep apnea has been subject to several investigations in AD, largely with conflicting results (D. Bliwise, 1989; D. Bliwise, Yesavage, Tinklenberg, & Dement, 1989). The possibility of disturbance in circadian rhythmicity in AD, leading to so-called sundowning or day–night reversal, has received a modicum of support (Okawa et al., 1991) and may be partially alleviated by bright light exposure (Satlin, Volicer, Ross, Herz, & Campbell, 1992), but the syndrome is probably affected by many factors (D. Bliwise, 1994b). The sleep disturbance of PD patients may be more profound than in AD (D. Bliwise et al., 1995) and may be characterized by excessive motor activity (and PLMS) during sleep (Irbe, Rye, & D. Bliwise, 1994). The prevalence of sleep problems in PD patients has been reported to be over 90%. High-dosage L-dopa is often assumed to be involved in this sleep dysfunction, although more recent work has suggested that these effects may be seen regardless of patients' medication status (D. Bliwise et al., 1995; Comella, Tanner, & Ristanovic, 1993), thus leaving open the possibility that diminished inhibitory output from the basal ganglia throughout brainstem structures may be involved. For both AD and PD, sleep disturbance is exceedingly difficult to treat, and neuroleptic medication is often used as a last resort. Customary hypnotics are ineffective, and other treatment modalities, such as exposure to outdoor light (Satlin et al., 1992) or daytime sleep restriction, may also warrant systematic trials.

Psychological Factors in Sleep in the Elderly

Given the large number of physiological challenges to the integrity of uninterrupted nocturnal sleep and consequent sustained daytime wakefulness, it is easy to overlook psychological factors as being salient in sleep disturbance in late life. For the purposes of this chapter, in fact, I have to this point perhaps overstated the former to emphasize that sleep is a neurobehavioral state subjected to and indeed controlled by the central nervous system in concert with a variety of other organ systems in the body. The significance of these somatic factors notwithstanding, it is important to bear in mind that psychological influences on sleep disturbance in late life should not be overlooked, most certainly not by psychologists. In our BASC participants, usage of psychoactive medications was correlated with higher amounts of stage 1 sleep and lower stages 3 and 4 (Table 2), as well as with the presence of sleep latency or sleep maintenance problems (Table 3).

Although the *Diagnostic and Statistical Manual of Mental Disorders, 4th Edition (DSM-IV;* American Psychiatric Association, 1994) now includes the diagnosis of primary insomnia (see chapter 27), there has long been clear evidence that insomnia is often associated with psychiatric disorder. Early studies with the Minnesota Multiphasic Personality Inventory (MMPI) indicated that predominately middle-aged insomniacs were

Table 3

Relationships Between Chronic Medication Use and Self-Report Sleep Measures in Bay Area Sleep Cohort (BASC)

Variable	CV	Psych	Anti-Inflammatory	Estrogen
			Class of Medication	
Disturbed Nocturnal Sleep		6.06***[H]		
Daytime Fatigue		5.27**[H]		
Snoring				
Loud Snoring		4.19**		
Holding Breath/ Stop Breathing	4.05**[H]		3.35*	
Experience Pain or Discomfort		7.19***[H]		

Trouble Falling
  Asleep During
  Movies, and/or TV, Travel,
  Listening to Stereo
				2.87*[H]

Teeth Grinding				
Restless Legs				
Leg Twitching				

Note. Values in table are for chi-squares, with probabilities of 0.10 or less indicating differences in the distribution of individuals receiving/not receiving a particular medication. CV = cardiovascular; Psych = psychoactive.
*p<.10 **p<.05 ***p<.01
[H]Higher proportion in group receiving medication.

likely to have elevated profiles, particularly on the neurotic triad (Scales 1, 2, and 3; Kales, Caldwell, Preston, Healey, & Kales, 1976). A subsequent study using the MMPI-168 reported that such elevations did not occur in older insomniacs (Roehrs, Lineback, Zorick, & Roth, 1982), but the questionable validity of such short forms of the MMPI left open some doubt as to whether the association between psychopathology and insomnia was weaker in old age. N. Bliwise, D. Bliwise, and Dement (1985) reported, for example, that although a somewhat lower proportion of older, relative to younger, insomniacs exceeded a *T*-score of 70 on clinical scales of the MMPI, a substantial portion of such individuals still showed pathological elevations on a number of the clinical scales. Later work by N. Bliwise (1992) showed similar results using the Symptoms Checklist–90 (SCL-90) comparing older women who sleep well with those who sleep poorly. In a study of older poor sleepers, Friedman et al. (1993) reported that depressive mood (as measured with the BDI) and trait anxiety (as measured with the anxiety facet of the Neuroticism subscale of the NEO Personality Inventory) but not state anxiety (as measured with the Spielberger State-Trait Anxiety Inventory) were correlated with measures of poor sleep as defined on a sleep log. Of interest in this study was that actigraphic estimates of total sleep time (see chapter 7) showed positive correlations with these measures of anxiety and depression. In other words, elderly individuals with poor sleep may lie in bed motionless, and these characteristics are associated with feelings of tension and dysphoria.

On further consideration, there are a number of reasons to think that psychological factors may be extremely important in the sleep of the elderly. Major life transitions and life stresses such as retirement, financial strain, or relocation probably play a major role in the disruption of sleep. For some cohorts, particular historical trauma may play an important role in the development of such symptoms in late life. For example, one study emphasized the development of insomnia in Holocaust survivors (Rosen, Reynolds, Yeager, Houck, & Hurwitz, 1991). Particular attention in recent years has focused on the polysomnographic correlates of bereavement in late life as possible causes of disturbed sleep in the elderly. It is not an uncommon circumstance for the elderly person to, one by one, lose a spouse, a best friend, and a long-time golfing partner. Bereavement following death of a spouse is estimated to result in depression in as many as 10% to 20% of elderly individuals (Pasternak et al., 1992).

There is some evidence, although far from incontrovertible, that major depression may be associated with polysomnographic abnormalities in all age groups (see chapter 27 of Benca, Obermeyer, Thisted, & Gillin, 1992), including the elderly (Reynolds et al., 1992). Such changes may include shortened REM latency, elevated REM%, and early-morning awakening, with the REM markers often being considered "trait-like" biomarkers with genetic loading for development of depression. Recent polysomnographic studies have shown that when elderly, bereaved individuals develop an initial-onset major depression in late life, even in the absence of any prior depressive episodes, they manifest polysomnographic changes somewhat similar to those in non-bereaved depression (Reynolds et al., 1992). These findings were not seen in elderly individuals who experienced "subsyndromal" depression, although the latter individuals did show evidence of sleep fragmentation and elevated Stage 1 Sleep (Pasternak et al., 1992). In another study, however, this investigative team reported that selected aspects of REM sleep (computerized measurement of REM density) remained elevated for as long as 23 months after bereavement (Reynolds et al., 1993) in elderly individuals who did not meet Research Diagnostic Criteria/ Schedule for Affective Disorders criteria for major depression. Taken together, these data suggest that late-life bereavement may lead to changes in polysomnographic measures that are compatible with, and possibly precursors for, major depression in late life.

Sleep in an Aged Population: The Bay Area Sleep Cohort

BASC is a group of 256 individuals recruited between the years of 1974 and 1985 for research studies in the Sleep and Aging Program at Stanford University Medical Center directed by me in research supported by the National Institute on Aging. The sample was originally recruited as a convenience sample of individuals ages 40 or older at entry who resided in the San Francisco Bay area (generally the mid-peninsula region) who were interested in becoming research volunteers in a study of aging and sleep. At entry, few stipulations were made of these participants other than that they must have been willing to undergo at least one night of in-lab nocturnal polysomnography. Individuals with known neurodegenerative diseases at the time of entry, such as PD or AD, were excluded from the study. Additionally, individuals were required to have been free from current or past cancer, free from prior myocardial infarct or stroke, and stable medically (e.g., no renal or hepatic failure). No restrictions were made on current use of medication including cardiovascular (diuretics, beta blockers), thyroid replacement, or estrogen or progesterone preparations. Individuals using psychoactive medications were included, and in fact individuals with insomnia (many of whom used such medications) were actively recruited at various points over the course of the study (see Table 1). No restrictions were made on alcohol or tobacco use except that patients were required to avoid alcohol on the day and evening prior to their laboratory night. Other details regarding a description of the cohort on entry are shown in Table 1. Subsets of the BASC have been reported in a number of publications, including cross-sectional analyses of risk factors for sleep disordered breathing (D. Bliwise et al., 1987), symptoms of PLMS (D. Bliwise, Petta, et al., 1985), night-to-night variability in both sleep apnea and PLMS (D. Bliwise, Benkert, & Ingham, 1991; D. Bliwise, Carey, & Dement, 1983; Bliwise, Carskadon, & Dement, 1988), and daytime alertness with the MSLT (D. Bliwise, 1991). Preliminary longitudinal studies with BASC have demonstrated that increased sleep disordered breathing was associated with progressive neuropsychological impairment (D. Bliwise, Carskadon, Seidel, Nekich, & Dement, 1991), decreased forced vital capacity (D. Bliwise, 1994c), and 5-year mortality (D. Bliwise, N. Bliwise, et al., 1988). An advantage of this cohort is that none of the individuals have elected to undergo treatment for sleep apnea, and thus the group offers the unique opportunity to examine the natural history of this sleep pathology. In the future, we will continue to follow members of the BASC to determine whether incident sleep apnea is associated with other adverse outcomes over still longer periods of time.

Conclusion

This chapter has provided a brief overview of how sleep is influenced by aging and its associated diseases. The multifaceted nature of variables affecting sleep in old age cannot be overstated, as medical disease, psychological issues, specific sleep pathology, and intrinsic age-dependent changes in sleep physiology all interact. The health psychologist working with sleep disorders in a geriatric setting must be cognizant of these many issues influencing the nighttime and daytime wellbeing of the elderly person.

REFERENCES

American Psychiatric Association. (1994). *Diagnostic and statistical manual of mental disorders* (4th ed.). Washington, DC: Author.

Ancoli-Israel, S., Klauber, M. R., Kripke, D. F., Parker, L., & Cobarrubias, M. (1989). Sleep apnea in female nursing home patients: Increased risk of mortality. *Chest, 96,* 1054–1058.

Ancoli-Israel, S., Kripke, D. F., Klauber, M. R., Mason, W. J., Fell, R., & Kaplan, O. (1991a). Sleep disordered breathing in community dwelling elderly. *Sleep, 14*, 486–495.

Ancoli-Israel, S., Kripke, D. F., Klauber, M. R., Mason, W. J., Fell, R., & Kaplan, O. (1991b). Periodic limb movements in sleep in community dwelling elderly. *Sleep, 14*, 496–500.

Asplund, R., & Åberg, H. (1992). Health of the elderly with regard to sleep and nocturnal micturition. *Scandinavian Journal of Primary Health Care, 10*, 98–104.

Ballinger, C. B. (1976). Subjective sleep disturbance at the menopause. *Journal of Psychosomatic Research, 20*, 509–513.

Benca, R. M., Obermeyer, W. H., Thisted, R. A., & Gillin, J. C. (1992). Sleep and psychiatric disorders: A meta-analysis. *Archives of General Psychiatry, 49*, 651–668.

Berry, D. T. R., Phillips, B. A., Cook, Y. R., Schmitt, F. A., Gilmore, R. L., Patel, R., Keener, T. M., & Tyre, E. (1987). Sleep-disordered breathing in healthy aged persons: Possible daytime sequelae. *Journal of Gerontology, 42*, 620–626.

Bliwise, D. L. (1989). Neuropsychological function and sleep. *Geriatric Clinics of North America, 5*, 381–394.

Bliwise, D. L. (1991). Cognitive function and SDB in aging adults. In S. T. Kuna, P. M. Suratt, & J. E. Remmers (Eds.), *Sleep and respiration in aging adults* (pp. 237–243). New York: Elsevier.

Bliwise, D. L. (1993). Sleep in normal aging and dementia. *Sleep, 16*, 40–81.

Bliwise, D. L. (1994a). Sleep in dementing illness. In *Annual Review of Psychiatry*, (Vol. 13, pp. 757–777). Washington, DC: American Psychiatric Press.

Bliwise, D. L. (1994b). What is sundowning? *Journal of the American Geriatrics Society, 42*, 1009–1011.

Bliwise, D. L. (1994c). Development of sleep disordered breathing and changes in body weight over time in an elderly population. *Sleep Research, 23*, 234.

Bliwise, D. L., Benkert, R. E., & Ingham, R. H. (1991). Factors associated with nightly variability in sleep-disordered breathing in the elderly. *Chest, 100*, 973–976.

Bliwise, D. L., Bliwise, N. G., Partinen, M., Pursley, A. M., & Dement, W. C. (1988). Sleep apnea and mortality in an aged cohort. *American Journal of Public Health, 78*, 544–547.

Bliwise, D. L., Carey, E., & Dement, W. C. (1983). Nightly variation in sleep-related respiratory disturbance in older adults. *Experimental Aging Research, 9*, 77–81.

Bliwise, D. L., Carskadon, M. A., & Dement, W. C. (1988). Nightly variation of periodic leg movements in sleep in middle-aged and elderly individuals. *Archives of Gerontology and Geriatrics, 7*, 273–279.

Bliwise, D. L., Carskadon, M. A., Seidel, W. F., Nekich, J. C., & Dement, W. C. (1991). MSLT-defined sleepiness and neuropsychological test performance do not correlate in the elderly. *Neurobiology of Aging, 12*, 463–468.

Bliwise, D. L., Feldman, D. E., Bliwise, N. G., Carskadon, M. A., Kraemer, H., North, C. S., Petta, D. F., Seidel, W. F., & Dement, W. C. (1987). Risk factors for sleep disordered breathing in heterogeneous geriatric populations. *Journal of the American Geriatrics Society, 35,* 132–141.

Bliwise, D. L., King, A. C., Harris, R. B., & Haskell, W. L. (1992). Prevalence of self-reported poor sleep in a healthy population aged 50–64. *Social Science and Medicine, 34,* 49–55.

Bliwise, D. L., Nekich, J., & Dement, W. C. (1991). Relative validity of self-reported snoring as a symptom of sleep apnea in a sleep clinic population. *Chest, 99,* 600–608.

Bliwise, D., Petta, D., Seidel, W., & Dement, W. (1985). Periodic leg movements during sleep in the elderly. *Archives of Gerontology and Geriatrics, 4,* 273–281.

Bliwise, D. L., Tinklenberg, J., Yesavage, J. A., Davies, H., Pursley, A. M., Petta, D. E., Widrow, L., Guilleminault, C., Zarcone, V. P., & Dement, W. C. (1989). REM latency in Alzheimer's Disease. *Biological Psychiatry, 25,* 320–328.

Bliwise, D. L., Watts, R. L., Watts, N., Rye, D. B., Irbe, D., & Hughes, M. (1995). Nocturnal disruptive behavior in Parkinson's disease and Alzheimer's Disease. *Journal of Geriatric Psychiatry and Neurology, 8,* 107–110.

Bliwise, D. L., Yesavage, J. A., Tinklenberg, J., & Dement, W. C. (1989). Sleep apnea in Alzheimer's disease. *Neurobiology of Aging, 10,* 343–346.

Bliwise, N. G. (1992). Factors related to sleep quality in healthy elderly women. *Psychology and Aging, 7,* 83–88.

Bliwise, N. G., Bliwise, D. L., & Dement, W. C. (1985). Age and psychopathology in insomnia. *Clinical Gerontologist, 4,* 3–9.

Brocklehurst, J. C., Fry, J., Griffiths, L., & Kalton, G. (1971). Dysuria in old age. *Journal of the American Geriatrics Society, 19,* 582–592.

Brugge, K. L., Kripke, D. F., Ancoli-Israel, S., & Garfinkel, L. (1989). The association of menopausal status and age with sleep disorders. *Sleep Research, 18,* 208.

Burgio, K. L., Locher, J. L., Ives, D. G., Hardin, J. M., Newman, A. B., & Kuller, L. (1994). Nocturnal enuresis in older adults. *Gerontologist, 34,* 321.

Buysse, D. J., Browman, K. E., Monk, T. H., Reynolds, C. F., III, Fasiczka, A. L., & Kupfer, D. J. (1992). Napping and 24-hour sleep/wake patterns in healthy elderly and young adults. *Journal of the American Geriatrics Society, 40,* 779–786.

Carskadon, M. A., Brown, E. D., & Dement, W. C. (1982). Sleep fragmentation in the elderly: Relationship to daytime sleep tendency. *Neurobiology of Aging, 3,* 321–327.

Comella, C. L., Tanner, C. M., & Ristanovic, R. K. (1993). Polysomnographic sleep measures in Parkinson's disease patients with treatment-induced hallucination. *Annals of Neurology, 34,* 710–714.

Costa, P. A., Jr., & McCrae, R. R. (1985). *NEO personality inventory manual.* Odessa, FL: Psychological Assessment Resources.

Dickel, M. J., & Mosko, S. S. (1990). Morbidity cut-offs for sleep apnea and periodic leg movements in predicting subjective complaints in seniors. *Sleep, 13*(2), 155–166.

Derogatis, L. R., Lipman, R. S., Rickels, K., Uhlenhuth, E. H., & Cowi, L. (1974). The Hopkins Symptom Checklist (HSCL): a measure of primary symptom dimensions. In P. Pichot (Ed.), *Psychological measurements in Psychopharmacology: Vol. 7: Modern problems in pharmacopsychiatry (pp. 79–110)*. Basel: Karger.

Friedman, L. F., Bliwise, D. L., Tanke, E. D., Salom, S. R., & Yesavage, J. A. (1992). A survey of self-reported poor sleep and associated factors in older individuals. *Behavior, Health and Aging, 2*(1), 13–20.

Friedman, L., Brooks, J. O., III, Bliwise, D. L., & Yesavage, J. A. (1993). Insomnia in older adults: Relations to depression and anxiety. *The American Journal of Geriatric Psychiatry, 1*, 153–159.

Gerard, P., Collins, K. J., Dore, C., & Exton-Smith, A. N. (1978). Subjective characteristics of sleep in the elderly. *Age and Ageing, 7*(Suppl.), 55–63.

Gislason, T., & Almqvist, M. (1987). Somatic diseases and sleep complaints. *Acta Medica Scandinavica, 221*, 475–481.

Hanson, B. S., & Ostergren, P. O. (1987). Different social network and social support characteristics, nervous problems and insomnia: Theoretical and methodological aspects on some results from the population study men born in 1914 Malmo, Sweden. *Social Science Medicine, 25*, 849–859.

Hening, W. A., Walters, A., Kavey, N., Gidro-Frank, S., Cote, L., & Fahn, S. (1986). Dyskinesias while awake and periodic movements in sleep in restless legs syndrome: Treatment with opioids. *Neurology, 36*, 1363–1366.

Hla, K. M., Young, T. B., Bidwell, T., Palta, M., Skatrud, J. B., & Dempsey, J. (1994). Sleep apnea and hypertension: A population-based study. *Annals of Internal Medicine, 120*, 382–388.

Hoch, C. C., Dew, M. A., Reynolds, C. F., III, Monk, T. H., Buysse, D. J., Houck, P. R., Machen, M. A., & Kupfer, D. J. (1994). A longitudinal study of laboratory- and diary-based sleep measures in healthy "old old" and "young old" volunteers. *Sleep, 17*, 489–496.

Hoch, C. C., Reynolds, C. F., Kupfer, D. J., & Berman, S. R. (1988). Stability of EEG sleep and sleep quality in healthy seniors. *Sleep, 11*, 521–527.

Irbe, D., Rye, D. B., & Bliwise, D. L. (1994). Sinemet in advanced Parkinson's disease (PD): Effects on sleep-related movements and tremor. *Sleep Research, 23*, 368.

Kales, A., Caldwell, A. B., Preston, T. Z., Healey, S., & Kales, J. D. (1976). Personality patterns in insomnia. *Archives of General Psychiatry, 33*, 1128–1134.

Kimmel, P. L., Miller, G., & Mendelson, W. B. (1989). Sleep apnea syndrome in chronic renal disease. *The American Journal of Medicine, 86*, 308–314.

Kostis, J. B., & Rosen, R. C. (1987). Central nervous system effects of b-adrenergic-blocking drugs: The role of ancillary properties. *Circulation, 75*, 204–212.

Kutner, N. G., Schechtman, K. B., Ory, M. G., Baker, D. I., & the FICSIT Group (1994). Older adults' perceptions of their health and functioning in relation to sleep disturbance, falling, and urinary incontinence. *Journal of the American Geriatrics Society, 42*, 757–762.

Leigh, T. J., Hindmarch, I., Bird, H. A., & Wright, V. (1988). Comparison of sleep in osteoarthritic patients and age and sex matched healthy controls. *Annals of Rheumatic Diseases, 47*, 40–42.

Mant, A., & Eyland, E. A. (1988). Sleep patterns and problems in elderly general practice attenders: An Australian survey. *Community Health Studies, 12*(2), 192–199.

Merlotti, L., Halpin, D., Maglio, R., Roehrs, T. A., Rosenthal, L. D., Wittig, R. M., & Roth, T. (1992). Dose effects of theophylline on nocturnal sleep and daytime alertness. *Sleep Research, 21*, 63.

Mitler, M. M., Hajdukovic, R. M., Shafor, R., Hahn, P. M., & Kripke, D. F. (1987). When people die: Cause of death versus time of death. *American Journal of Medicine, 82*, 266–274.

Morgan, K., Healey, D. W., & Healey, P. J. (1989). Factors influencing persistent subjective insomnia in old age: A follow-up study of good and poor sleepers aged 65–74. *Age and Ageing, 18*, 117–122.

Murphy, P. J., Badia, P., Myers, B. L., Boecker, M. R., & Wright Jr., K. P. (1994). Nonsteroidal anti-inflammatory drugs affect normal sleep patterns in humans. *Physiology & Behavior, 55*, 1063–1066.

Okawa, M., Mishima, K., Hishikawa, Y., Hozumi, S., Hori, H., & Takahashi, K. (1991). Circadian rhythm disorders in sleep-waking and body temperature in elderly patients with dementia and their treatment. *Sleep, 14*, 478–485.

Partinen, M., Telakivi, T., Kaukiainen, A. Salmi, T., Färkkilä, M., Saijonmaa, O., & Fyhrquist, F. (1991). Atrial natriuretic peptide in habitual snorers. *Annals of Medicine, 23*, 147–151.

Pasternak, R. E., Reynolds, C. F., III, Hoch, C. C., Buysse, D. S., Schlernitzauer, M., Machen, M., & Kupfer, D. J. (1992). Sleep in spousally bereaved elders with subsyndromal depressive symptoms. *Psychiatry Research, 43*, 43–53.

Phillips, B. A., Berry, D. T. R., Schmitt, F. A., Harbison, L., & Lipke-Molby, T. (1994). Sleep-disordered breathing in healthy aged persons: Two- and three-year follow-up. *Sleep, 17*, 411–415.

Pressman, M. R., Figueroa, W. G., Kendrick-Mohamed, J., Smith, B. M., Jakubowski, G., Greenspon, L. W., & Peterson, D. D. (1993). Causes of night waking in adults: Pressure to urinate or sleep disorders? *Sleep Research, 22*, 252.

Prinz, P. N., Vitaliano, P. P., Vitiello, M. V., Bokan, J., Raskind, M., Peskind, E., & Gerber, C. (1982). Sleep, EEG and mental function changes in senile dementia of the Alzheimer type. *Neurobiology of Aging, 3*, 361–370.

Reynolds, C. F., III, Hoch, C. C., Buysse, D. J., Houck, P. R., Schlernitzauer, M., Frank, E., Mazumdar, S., & Kupfer, D. J. (1992). Electroencephalographic sleep in spousal bereavement and bereavement-related depression of late-life. *Biological Psychiatry, 31*, 69–82.

Reynolds, C. F., III, Hoch, C. C., Buysse, D. J., Houck, P. R., Schlernitzauer, M., Pasternak, R. E., Frank, E., Mazumdar, S., & Kupfer, D. J. (1993). Sleep after spousal bereavement: A study of recovery from stress. *Biological Psychiatry, 34*, 791–797.

Roehrs, T., Lineback, W., Zorick, F., & Roth, T. (1982). Relationship of psychopathology to insomnia in the elderly. *Journal of the American Geriatrics Society, 30*, 312–315.

Rosen, J., Reynolds, C. F., Yeager, A. L., Houck, P. R., & Hurwitz, L. F. (1991).

Sleep disturbances in survivors of the Nazi Holocaust. *American Journal of Psychiatry, 148*, 62–66.

Rowe, J. W., & Kahn, R. L. (1987). Human aging: Usual and successful. *Science, 237*, 143–149.

Satlin, A., Volicer, L., Ross, V., Herz, L., & Campbell, S. (1992). Bright light treatment of behavioral and sleep disturbances in patients with Alzheimer's disease. *American Journal of Psychiatry, 149*, 1028–1032.

Schaie, K. W. (1986). Beyond calendar definitions of age, period and cohort: The general developmental model revisited. *Developmental Review, 6*, 252–277.

Smith, J. R., Karacan, I., & Yang, M. (1977). Ontogeny of delta activity during human sleep. *Electroencephalography and Clinical Neurophysiology, 43*, 229–237.

Spitzer, R., Endicott, J., Robins, E. (1978). Research diagnostic criteria. *Archives of General Psychiatry, 35*, 776–782.

Vitiello, M. V., Prinz, P. N., Avery, D. H., Williams, D. E., Ries, R. K., Bokan, J. A., & Khan, A. (1990). Sleep is undisturbed in elderly, depressed individuals who have not sought health care. *Biological Psychiatry, 27*, 431–440.

Vitiello, M. V., Prinz, P. N., Williams, D. E., Frommlet, M. S., & Ries, R. K. (1990). Sleep disturbances in patients with mild-stage Alzheimer's Disease. *Journal of Gerontology: Medical Sciences, 45*, M131–M138.

Wechsler, L. R., Stakes, J. W., Shahani, B. T., & Busis, N. A. (1986). Periodic leg movements of sleep (nocturnal myoclonus): An electrophysiological study. *Annals of Neurology, 19*, 168–173.

Zepelin, H. (1981). Age differences in dreams. I: Men's dreams and thematic apperceptive fantasy. *International Journal of Aging and Human Development, 12*, 171–186.

Zepelin, H., McDonald, C. S., & Zammit, G. K. (1984). Effects of age on auditory awakening thresholds. *Journal of Gerontology, 39*, 294–300.

Sleep and Pregnancy

Gila Hertz

A lthough complaints about sleep disturbances during pregnancy are common, they are often overlooked by physicians. It is only recently that scientific research has focused on the incidence and causes of sleep complaints in pregnancy and on the consequences of disturbed sleep for the well-being of the mother and infant. A separate diagnostic entity, *pregnancy-associated sleep disorder*, has been proposed in the most recent edition of the *International Classification of Sleep Disorders* (Diagnostic Classification Steering Committee, 1990).

Studies investigating gender differences in sleep variables and sleep complaints have found that, in general, women report more disturbed sleep and increased sleep latency compared with men, use more sleeping pills, and are more sensitive to environmental factors affecting their sleep. Polysomnographic studies have confirmed a small but consistent finding of a longer sleep latency in women. Differences in sleep architecture between men and women have been found to be minimal and include longer rapid eye movement (REM) latency in women and lighter sleep in terms of increased Stages 1 and 2 in men. In general, men experience increased respiratory disturbance during sleep, although this gender gap narrows with increasing age. Some of the described gender differences in sleep have been explained by biological distinctions such as differences in genetic predisposition, sexual hormones, and reproductive systems; by psychosocial factors; and by acquired gender differences regarding lifestyle and health habits.

465

During pregnancy, sleep complaints are practically universal and probably reflect the drastic changes in all these aspects combined. In this chapter, sleep patterns during normal pregnancy are described, followed by a review of the existing literature concerning sleep and common complications of pregnancy.

Sleep in Normal Pregnancy

Subjective Complaints

There have been surprisingly few studies of the prevalence of sleep complaints in pregnancy and the implications for maternal and fetal health. One of the earliest studies investigating the prevalence of sleep complaints in pregnancy was prompted by the tragedy of the hypnotic thalidomide in Europe in the early 1960s. A subjective survey of sleep of 100 British women who were 38 or more weeks pregnant was carried out by Schweiger (1972). Sixty-eight of the women reported some change in their sleep during pregnancy. About 50% of the women surveyed reported decreased total sleep time and increased awakenings from sleep. Sleep problems increased fivefold from the first to the third trimester. In 12 women, severe sleeping problems required treatment with hypnotics. The most frequent complaints were general discomfort, including backache, urinary frequency, fetal movements, spontaneous arousals, heartburn, and leg cramps.

In a much later study, Hertz et al. (1992) similarly reported frequent awakenings, low back pain, leg cramps, and morning headaches as the most common causes of sleep disturbances in 12 women who were at 30–38 weeks of gestation. In this report, the most common reason for nocturnal awakenings was the need for bathroom trips. There were no reported difficulties falling asleep in this group.

Lee and De Joseph (1992) investigated self-reported sleep disturbances and levels of vitality in 25 pregnant and 29 postpartum employed women. The pregnant women complained of difficulty in both initiating and maintaining sleep, whereas the postpartum women reported problems maintaining sleep but not falling asleep. As in previous reports, the most common reason for midsleep awakening in the pregnant group was urinary frequency, followed by leg cramps and nightmares. Heartburn and backaches, commonly reported during late pregnancy, were not frequent in this group, which included only 8 women in their last trimester. In addition to sleep difficulties, about 50% of both groups in this study reported daytime fatigue and diminished vitality. The authors attributed these surprisingly high figures to the added stress of employment commitment and cautioned against generalization of these results to nonemployed childbearing women.

Polysomnographic Studies

Karacan, Agnew, Williams, Webb, and Ross (1968) were the first to investigate sleep electroencephalography (EEG) during pregnancy. They studied 7 women during late pregnancy and the early postpartum period and compared them with nonpregnant controls. The pregnant group had a longer sleep latency compared with the controls, although their reported mean sleep latency of 21 minutes is considered within normal limits. The pregnant group also demonstrated frequent awakenings, shorter sleep times, and a marked reduction in Stage 4 sleep. Immediately after delivery, there was a suppression of REM sleep, which returned to normal levels by the second week of the postpartum period. The authors discussed the possible relationship between the observed reduction in Stage 4 sleep and postpartum depression and suggested that the sleep changes should provide "a prognostic index in forthcoming emotional disturbances."

Hertz et al. (1992) recently studied 12 women in their third trimester with complete polysomnography for one night. Seven women returned for a postpartum study. Their study confirmed the presence of increased waking after sleep onset and decreased sleep efficiency compared with age-matched nonpregnant controls. There was also a reduction noted in REM sleep in the pregnant group. Unlike previous studies, however, in this study slow wave sleep (Stages 3 and 4 combined) did not decrease significantly in the pregnant group. In addition, sleep latency did not differ from that of controls, suggesting a pattern seen in individuals experiencing sleep-maintenance insomnia. In the postpartum study, waking after sleep onset decreased to a minimum and sleep efficiency returned to normal high levels, although slow wave sleep and REM sleep remained lower than the nonpregnant control values. However, subjective complaints of frequent awakenings persisted during the postpartum study, with the discomfort, aches, and pains associated with pregnancy now replaced by the newborn-handling activities. Thus, it appears that in the laboratory, with the mother away from her child, sleep efficiency rapidly improves, although the recovery of altered sleep architecture was slower to occur. Indeed, sleep studies performed at home with ambulatory recording devices confirmed the presence of increased wake time and reduced sleep efficiency in the postpartum phase (Lee, Zaffke, McEnany, & Hoehler, 1994).

Little is known about sleep patterns during early pregnancy. Fatigue and daytime sleepiness have been the primary complaints during early pregnancy and were thought to be related to increased circulating progesterone. (Lee et al., 1994) There have been two longitudinal studies of sleep throughout pregnancy. Driver and Shapiro (1992) recorded sleep patterns of 5 healthy women between 8 and 16 weeks' gestation as well as every 2 months until parturition and at 1 month postpartum. REM sleep time decreased during the last 2 months of pregnancy, and waking time after sleep onset increased. Sleep Stage 4 remained constant throughout the initial phases of pregnancy and increased toward the last few weeks. Finally, there was no change in sleep-onset latency. In contrast, Lee et al. (1994) found that when measured against a prepregnancy baseline, sleep onset was slightly reduced at 12 weeks' gestation, although it was not clear whether these differences were significant.

In summary, findings of sleep studies have been inconsistent, in part because of the small samples studied. Nevertheless, common features, at least in late stages of pregnancy, point to a pattern of sleep typically described by patients with sleep-maintenance insomnia: increased waking time after sleep onset, decreased sleep efficiency, reduced REM sleep, and often decreased slow wave sleep. Although some of the discomfort, aches, and pains associated with pregnancy have been determined to be causes of nocturnal awakenings, the direct effects of hormonal changes on sleep architecture during pregnancy have not yet been studied. Fatigue and daytime sleepiness are commonly reported in the first period of pregnancy. Further studies with objective measures such as the Multiple Sleep Latency Test (MSLT) are needed to confirm the presence of daytime sleepiness in pregnancy.

Sleeping Positions During Pregnancy

The relation of sleeping position to sleep patterns in pregnancy is of special interest because owing to the added weight and discomfort, women may be limited in their choice of position and in the number of postural shifts they can make during sleep. Furthermore, it has been shown that assuming a supine position, particularly during the last trimester, may pose risks for mother and fetus. In the supine position, the enlarged uterus compresses the inferior vena cava, resulting in reduced cardiac output. The combination of obstructed vena cava with supine position also has been postulated as the mechanism that produces nocturnal back pain in pregnancy, as discussed later in this chapter. Finally, sleep-disordered breathing has been found to worsen significantly in the supine sleeping position. Therefore, avoiding this position during sleep can be protective against such risks. Indeed, studies have shown that during late pregnancy, few women assume supine and prone positions during sleep. In a study of 52 pregnant women, all beyond the 30th week of gestation, only 1 woman adopted a supine position (Mills, 1994). Similarly, Hertz et al. (1992) reported significantly less time spent in both supine and prone sleeping positions during late pregnancy compared with the postpartum period. During the first weeks of pregnancy, however, the rate of sleeping in the supine position is higher and stands at 34%. The reported rate for sleep in the prone position is low even during the first weeks of gestation, but after 16 weeks when the abdomen is prominent, only a few women assume that position (Ogita et al., 1990).

Sleep Disorders in Pregnancy

Sleep-Disordered Breathing

A number of anatomic changes in the airways, thoracic cage, and respiratory muscles take place during pregnancy that can potentially affect breathing during sleep. The diaphragm is pushed upward by the enlarging uterus, resulting in decreased functional residual capacity, particularly in the supine position. These changes, along with increased nasal mucus, increase airway resistance, which can lead to hypoxemia. Fortunately these factors are typically counterbalanced by increased ventilatory rate, widening of the rib cage, and decreased abdominal tone, possibly related to increased circulating progesterone. Nevertheless, studies have shown that pregnant women have mild hypoxemia when in the supine position compared with a sitting position. During sleep, a recumbent position and a further decrease in muscle tone could worsen oxygen saturation.

There have been a few studies examining breathing patterns during sleep in pregnancy. Brownell, West, and Kryger (1986), studying 6 healthy women in their third trimester with polysomnography, found no evidence of significant sleep-disordered breathing and oxygen desaturation. In fact, when compared with postpartum studies, a decrease in the apnea–hypopnea index has been reported during pregnancy.

Hertz et al. (1992), in their study of 12 pregnant women, confirmed a lack of significant sleep apnea in late pregnancy, although periodic breathing was common during REM sleep and one woman demonstrated sleep apnea of moderate degree. In contrast, this group had a mild but significant decrease in oxygen saturation compared with the nonpregnant controls. The saturation values were significantly correlated with the time spent in a supine sleeping position. Feinsilver and Hertz (1992) proposed that some of the observed changes in sleep parameters during pregnancy might prove protective against sleep-disordered breathing. For example, the observed decrease in REM sleep and the reduced time spent in supine position during late pregnancy could provide protection against nocturnal desaturation.

In spite of the relatively low incidence of sleep-disordered breathing during pregnancy, there have been several reports of severe sleep apnea requiring intervention (Hastie, Prowse, Perks, Atkins, & Blunt, 1989; Kowall, Clark, Nino-Marcia, & Powell, 1989). Sleep-disordered breathing may be exacerbated or even precipitated by pregnancy (Kowall et al., 1989; Sherer, Caverly, & Abramowitz, 1991). In one case, excessive daytime sleepiness developed at about 35 weeks' gestation. Regular "uterine activity" on cardiotocography was identified as loud snoring and periods of apnea. Polysomnography after delivery confirmed the presence of severe obstructive sleep apnea (Sherer et al., 1991).

Obesity, sleep apnea, and even snoring during pregnancy have been identified as risk factors for fetal complications. Joel-Cohen and Schoenfeld (1978) reported on three pregnant women who were obese snorers and had clinical diagnoses of sleep apnea. Fetal monitoring showed significant acidosis and heart rate changes related to apneic episodes. Charbonneau, Falcone, and Cosio (1991) similarly described a 32-year-old woman in her last trimester of pregnancy who presented with severe apnea and oxygen desaturation as well as significant cardiac arrhythmias. External cardiotocography showed normal fetal heart rate that persisted through treatment with nasal continuous positive airway pressure (CPAP). Nevertheless, at Week 39 of pregnancy, the woman gave birth to a newborn with growth retardation. The impact of snoring alone on fetal outcome was studied in 67 women in late pregnancy. Snoring was reported by 31% of the patients. In this group, the fetal complication rate was 43%, whereas the nonsnorers had a 22% complication rate. In this study, however, reported snoring was not verified by objective measures, and the contribution of other potential risk factors such as obesity was not assessed (Schutte et al., 1994).

Restless Legs Syndrome and Periodic Leg Movements

Restless legs syndrome (RLS) and periodic leg movements (PLM) are idiopathic disorders that can cause profound sleep disruption. RLS, a waking disorder that usually occurs before sleep onset, is associated with discomfort in the calves causing restlessness in the legs, which is relieved by movement. PLM, occurring during sleep, involve isolated periodic movements of the lower limbs and are usually followed by arousal from sleep. In severe cases, frequent leg movements can cause significant sleep interruption, resulting in complaints of insomnia or excessive sleepiness. In his initial account of the condition, Ekbom (1960) noted a relatively high prevalence of RLS during pregnancy. However, no polysomnographic studies have documented increased nocturnal leg movements in pregnancy. Hertz et al. (1992) observed no significant RLS or PLM in any of the 12 pregnant women studied. However, 2 women who returned for a postpartum study exhibited PLM of moderate severity at that time but not on the prepartum recording. The authors suggested that night-to-night variability might account for the lack of PLM on the prepartum study. Many different conditions have been associated with RLS, including diabetes, iron deficiency anemia, uremia, and malnutrition. All these conditions when present during pregnancy can precipitate or exacerbate existing RLS. Polysomnographic investigation of abnormal limb movements in complicated pregnancy could shed more light on the pathophysiology underlying such movements. Leg cramps, which have been reported in about 20% of pregnant women and are discussed later, should be distinguished from PLM and RLS.

Narcolepsy

Narcolepsy is a lifelong neurological disorder that involves an uncontrollable urge to fall asleep. A detailed description of narcolepsy can be found elsewhere in this volume. Although in most cases there are no definitive precipitants to narcolepsy, a number of precipitating factors, including pregnancy, have been suggested. Pregnancy and childbirth have been identified in 4 cases of a series of 100 patients with narcolepsy. Other factors identified include head injury, infectious disease, and emotional shock (Parkes et al., 1974).

Little research has been done on sleep patterns of patients with narcolepsy during pregnancy. Sleep disturbances can be expected to occur in such patients during pregnancy because fragmented and disturbed nighttime sleep has been frequently observed in patients with narcolepsy. In addition, other sleep disorders such as sleep apnea and periodic leg movements are not uncommon in narcolepsy. Because most patients with narcolepsy rely on stimulant and antidepressant medication to maintain daytime alertness and to control cataplexy, the cessation of medication during pregnancy can cause excessive sleepiness or cataplexy, which may result in injury. In addition, withdrawal from medication may also affect sleep patterns; some psychotropic medications have suppressive effects on REM sleep. Two case reports have described no adverse fetal outcome in women with narcolepsy who continued to take amphetamine throughout pregnancy and during nursing. Despite these findings, caution must be used in the administration of medication during pregnancy because the long-term effects of these medications are unknown.

Sleepwalking and Night Terrors

Both sleepwalking and night terrors are parasomnias, also known as disorders of arousal, which occur mainly during slow wave sleep. The prevalence of sleepwalking in adults is about 1%. In most individuals with sleepwalking, a greater amount of slow wave sleep (Stages 3 and 4) is seen on the polysomnogram. Sleepwalking and night terrors have rarely been reported in pregnancy. This fact has been related to findings from polysomnographic studies in pregnancy describing a decrease or no change in slow wave sleep compared with that of normal controls.

However, there have been two reports of sleepwalking and night terrors during pregnancy that suggest that pregnancy plays a role in the course of these parasomnias. Snyder (1986) reported a case of a 23-year-old woman with a history of sleep terrors who experienced increased intensity of the episodes during the initial part of her pregnancy. After the third week of gestation, the episodes were virtually eliminated. Snyder hypothesized that the sudden cessation in night terror episodes might have resulted from a reduction in Stage 4 sleep. However, in another report, Berlin (1988) suggested that pregnancy can precipitate sleepwalking episodes. He described a 32-year-old woman with a history of childhood sleepwalking that stopped when she was 11 years old. The woman reported frequent sleepwalking episodes during her two pregnancies, but she was asymptomatic when not pregnant. The episodes in both pregnancies did not appear until the 10th week of gestation. Individual variability in sleep habits and lifestyle during pregnancy can account, at least in part, for these conflicting reports. Therefore, it seems likely that for individuals with a genetic predisposition, sleepwalking and night terrors may be triggered by the sleep deprivation and stress associated with pregnancy.

Pregnancy Complications Associated With Sleep Disturbances

Sleep in Preeclampsia

Preeclampsia complications occur in about 10% of all pregnancies. In this condition, hypertension, edema, and kidney disorders develop during the second half of the pregnancy. The added stress resulting from the risks associated with the condition combined with the absence of a regular sleep–wake schedule in women who are confined to bed can predispose women with preeclampsia to significant sleep disorders. The condition is more common in women with diabetes or existing kidney disease, and both conditions have been associated with an increased incidence of periodic leg movements. Nevertheless, little is known about sleep in this condition. Ekholm, Polo, Rauhala, and Ekblad (1992) studied the sleep of 9 women with preeclampsia and 9 women with normal term pregnancy. Subjective sleep complaints were similar in both groups and included multiple awakenings and reduced sleep quality. In the preeclampsia group, 2 women complained of teeth grinding and two women developed snoring. Objective measurements of sleep quality were performed by recording body movement activity with a static-charge-sensitive bed. Women in the preeclampsia group had a significantly higher number of body movements per night and left the bed more frequently than those in the control group. Two women in both groups had periodic leg movements. The authors concluded that sleep quality was poorer in the preeclampsia group, determined by the higher number of body movements.

Nocturnal Backache and Sleep-Related Leg Cramps

In his survey of sleep disturbances in 100 women during late pregnancy, Schweiger (1972) reported that 18% of the women complained that backache was responsible for their sleep alterations. Fast, Weiss, Sheilesh, and Hertz (1989) surveyed another 100 women who were at least 20 weeks pregnant at the time regarding their nocturnal backache complaints and sleeping habits. In this report, 67 women experienced backache during the night, and 36% reported waking up because of backache. Of interest was the lack of significant correlations between nocturnal backache and maternal weight and sleeping positions. The authors hypothesized that changes in venous collateral circulation during pregnancy can lead to compromised neural microcirculation within the vertebral bodies, hypoxemia, and irritation of spinal nerves, which result in night backache. Some support for this theory has been provided by the observation of a small but significant decrease in oxygen saturation during pregnancy (Hertz et al., 1992). The data from this study were further analyzed to determine the relationship between reported back pain during pregnancy and nocturnal desaturation. The group of 13 pregnant women was divided into two subgroups on the basis of reported nocturnal back pain (Fast & Hertz, 1992). In this analysis, the subgroup with pain exhibited a significant decrease in basal oxygen saturation and spent a longer time in a supine sleeping position compared with the group without pain. The authors suggested that the combination of inadequate collateral circulation with decreased basal oxygen saturation in the supine position during pregnancy compromised circulation to neural structures in the spine, which resulted in pain. In addition to decreased oxygen saturation, the subgroup with pain had a decreased amount of REM sleep and increased Stage 2 sleep. Sleep disturbances and increased waking may lead to musculoskeletal disturbances (Moldofsky, 1986). Whether disturbed sleep architecture plays a role in the production of nocturnal pain in pregnancy remains to be established.

The prevalence of reported leg cramps during sleep can be as high as 75% during the last trimester (Gupta, Schork, & Gay, 1992; Hertz et al., 1992). The occurrence of leg cramps at various times of the night was studied in 56 pregnant women. In the first trimester, a higher frequency of leg cramps was associated with sleep onset and time spent trying to fall asleep. However, during the third trimester, an increased frequency of leg cramps was reported during early morning and on awakening (Gupta, Schork, & Gay, 1992).

Emotional Changes

Emotional disturbances during childbearing and the early postpartum period are common. An association between sleep disturbances during pregnancy and postnatal blues has been proposed by a number of researchers, but there have been no polysomnographic studies to confirm such a correlation. About 9% of pregnant women and 12% of women in the postpartum period experience minor or major depression. The complaint of disturbed sleep is common in both depression and pregnancy. Sleep abnormalities in depression include increased wakefulness during sleep, early-morning awakening, and decreased slow wave sleep. Later studies have focused on specific REM changes that have been identified in patients with depression: decreased REM sleep latency and increased REM density (Kupfer, Ehler, & Frank, 1991).

Karacan (1969) suggested that the reduction of Stage 4 sleep observed during late pregnancy may be an indication of subclinical depression, which continues into the first few weeks of the postpartum period, when a recovery of Stage 4 occurs. It seems likely that hormonal changes have a direct effect on sleep architecture during pregnancy. Studies of sleep during the menstrual cycle have shown that a reduction in Stage 4 sleep occurs premenstrually when the levels of progesterone and estrogen are high (Ho, 1972). However, recent polysomnographic studies have not confirmed the findings of decreased Stage 4 sleep during late pregnancy (Driver & Shapiro, 1992; Hertz et al., 1992).

A possible link between REM sleep changes and depression has been proposed by Frank, Kupfer, Jacob, Blumenthal, and Jarrett (1987). These researchers studied 52 women with recurrent depression to determine the differences in sleep patterns between women with and without pregnancy-related affective episodes. In this study, the women who reported pregnancy- or postpartum-related depression had increased REM sleep and REM activity. These changes were accounted for almost entirely by the women with postpartum episodes. The authors concluded that the postpartum period may be more sensitive to sleep pattern changes associated with depressive episodes.

Postnatal psychosis, a form of bipolar mood disorder, occurs in approximately 1 in 500 births. Total sleeplessness on the first few postnatal days has been described as the first warning symptom of postnatal psychosis. This occurrence may assist in recognizing the problem, particularly because women who develop postnatal psychosis often have had no previous psychiatric illness (Jilbert & Sved Williams, 1994).

Pregnancy and Dreaming

Dreams about pregnancy or the unborn baby are reported by 67% of pregnant women, and the frequency of dreams increases with advancing gestational age. About 25% of women recall having had frightening dreams during pregnancy, and many report having had the same dream more than once. Some women reported having been upset by frightening dreams (Blake & Reiman, 1993). The content of the frightening dreams experienced by women during pregnancy frequently involved harm or threat to the baby or to the pregnant woman, or conflict with the baby's father. Compared with women without pregnancy-related dreams, women with dreams were further along in their pregnancy, were more likely to report receiving less emotional support than they wanted from the baby's father, and were having trouble sleeping (Blake & Reiman, 1992). This last finding might be related to a reported increase in the occurrence of REM sleep arousals in late pregnancy. Whether increased REM arousals produce more dream recall or the intense nature of pregnancy-related dreams causes REM arousals remains to be established.

Conclusion

Relatively little is known about the health significance of sleep disturbance in pregnancy. Pregnancy can pose a risk for developing sleep-disordered breathing, back pain, and leg cramps. It can trigger episodes of sleepwalking and periodic leg movements. Sleep disturbance during pregnancy also can be associated with frightening dreams, postpartum blues, and sometimes major depression and postnatal psychosis. Currently, polysomnographic data concerning sleep in pregnancy are sparse, and there are limited data available regarding the outcome of pregnancies of women who experience pregnancy-associated sleep disorders.

Data from a study of female residents who experienced significant sleep deprivation have suggested that sleep deprivation may be associated with increased risk for premature labor (Osborn, Harris, Reading, & Prather, 1990). Further investigation is warranted into the relationship between sleep qualities and health and general well-being during pregnancy. Future studies need to focus on early identification and management of sleep disorders during pregnancy as well as on identifying sleep deficit and promoting sleep hygiene during this vulnerable period in a woman's life.

REFERENCES

Berlin, R. M. (1988). Sleepwalking disorder during pregnancy: A case report. *Sleep, 11*, 298–300.

Blake, R. L., & Reiman, J. (1993). The pregnancy-related dreams of pregnant women. *Journal of the American Board of Family Practice, 6*, 117–122.

Brownell, L. G., West, P., & Kryger, M. H. (1986). Breathing during sleep in normal pregnant women. *American Review of Respiratory Disease, 133*, 38–40.

Charbonneau, M., Falcone, T., & Cosio, M. G. (1991). Obstructive sleep apnea during pregnancy. *American Review of Respiratory Disease, 144*, 461–463.

Diagnostic Classification Steering Committee. (1990). *International classification of sleep disorders: Diagnostic and coding manual.* Rochester, MN: American Sleep Disorders Association.

Driver, H. S., & Shapiro, C. M. (1992). A longitudinal study of sleep stages in young women during pregnancy and postpartum. *Sleep, 15*, 449–453.

Ekbom, K. (1960). Restless legs syndrome. *Neurology, 10*, 868–873.

Ekholm, E. M., Polo, O., Rauhala, E. R., & Ekblad, U. U. (1992). Sleep quality in preeclampsia. *American Journal of Obstetrics and Gynecology, 167*, 1262–1266.

Fast, A., & Hertz, G. (1992). Nocturnal low back pain in pregnancy: Polysomnographic correlates. *American Journal of Reproductive Immunology, 28*, 251–253.

Fast, A., Weiss, L., Sheilesh, P., & Hertz, G. (1989). Night backache in pregnancy. *American Journal of Physical Medicine and Rehabilitation, 68*, 227–229.

Feinsilver, S. H., & Hertz, G. (1992). Respiration during sleep in pregnancy. *Clinics in Chest Medicine, 13*, 637–644.

Frank, E., Kupfer, D. J., Jacob, M., Blumenthal, S. J., & Jarrett, D. B. (1987). Pregnancy-related affective episodes among women with recurrent depression. *American Journal of Psychiatry, 144*, 288–293.

Gupta, M. A., Schork, N. J., & Gay, C. (1992). Nocturnal leg cramps in pregnancy: A prospective study of clinical features. *Sleep Research, 21,* 294.

Hastie, S. J., Prowse, K., Perks, W. H., Atkins, J., & Blunt, V. A. (1989). Obstructive sleep apnea during pregnancy requiring tracheostomy. *Australia New Zealand Journal of Obstetrics and Gynecology, 29,* 365–367.

Hertz, G., Fast, A., Feinsilver, S. H., Albertario, C. A., Schulman, H., & Fein, A. M. (1992). Sleep in normal late pregnancy. *Sleep, 15,* 246–251.

Ho, A. (1972). Sex hormones and sleep of women. *Sleep Research, 1,* 184.

Jilbert, A. R., & Sved Williams, A. E. (1994). Postnatal psychosis: A patient's experience with comment by consulting psychiatrist. *Australian College of Midwives Incorporated, 7,* 26–30.

Joel-Cohen, S. H., & Schoenfeld, A. (1978). Fetal response to periodic sleep apnea: A new syndrome in obstetrics. *European Journal of Obstetrics, Gynecology and Reproductive Biology, 8,* 77–81.

Karacan, I., Agnew, H. W., Williams, R. L., Webb, W. B., & Ross, J. J. (1968). Characteristics of sleep patterns during late pregnancy and the postpartum periods. *American Journal of Obstetrics and Gynecology, 101,* 579–586.

Kowall, J., Clark, G., Nino-Marcia, G., & Powell, N. (1989). Precipitation of obstructive sleep apnea during pregnancy. *Obstetrics and Gynecology, 74,* 453–455.

Kupfer, D. J., Ehlers, C. L., & Frank, E. (1991). EEG sleep profiles and recurrent depression. *Biological Psychiatry, 30,* 645–655.

Lee, K. A., & De Joseph, J. F. (1992). Sleep disturbances, vitality, and fatigue among a select group of employed childbearing women. *Birth, 19,* 208–213.

Lee, K. A., Zaffke, M. E., McEnany, G., & Hoehler, K. (1994). Sleep and fatigue: Before, during, and after pregnancy. *Sleep Research, 23,* 126.

Madhulika, A., Gupta, M. A., Schork, N. J., & Gay, C. (1992). Nocturnal leg cramps of pregnancy: A prospective study of clinical features. *Sleep Research, 21,* 294.

Mills, G. H. (1994). Sleeping positions adopted by pregnant women of more than 30 weeks gestation. *Anesthesia, 49,* 249–250.

Moldofsky, H. (1986). Sleep and musculoskeletal pain. *American Journal of Medicine, 81,* 85–89.

Moorcroft, W. H. (1989). *Sleep, dreaming, and sleep disorders: An introduction.* Lanham, MD: University Press of America.

Ogita, S., Imanaka, M., Takebayashi, T., Nakai, Y., Fukumasu, H., Matsuo, S., Matsumoto, M., Tanaka, B., & Iwanaga, K. (1990). Significance of exercise and bedrest in pregnancy: Study on the lying postures of gravidas during sleep. *Annals of Physiological Anthropology, 9,* 93–98.

Osborn, L. M., Harris, D. L., Reading, J. C., & Prather, M. B. (1990). Outcome of pregnancies experienced during residency. *Journal of Family Practice, 31,* 618–622.

Parkes, J. D., Fenton, G., Struthers, G., Curzon, G., Kantameneni, B. D., Buton, B. H., & Record, C. (1974). Narcolepsy and cataplexy: Clinical features, treatment and cerebrospinal fluid findings. *Quarterly Journal of Medicine, 43,* 525–536.

Schutte, S., Del Conte, A., Doghramji, K., Gallagher, K., Oliver, R., Rose, C., Breuninger, W., De Los Santos, L., & Youakim, J. (1994). Snoring during pregnancy and its impact on fetal outcome. *Sleep Research, 23,* 325.

Schweiger, M. S. (1972). Sleep disturbances in pregnancy. *American Journal of Obstetrics and Gynecology, 114,* 879–882.

Sherer, D. M., Caverly, C. B., & Abramowitz, J. S. (1991). Severe obstructive sleep apnea and associated snoring documented during external tocography. *American Journal of Obstetrics and Gynecology, 165,* 1300–1301.

Snyder, S. (1986). Unusual case of sleep terror in a pregnant patient. *American Journal of Psychiatry, 143,* 391.

VI

Psychological Disorders
and Sleep

Sleep in Depression and Anxiety

J. Catesby Ware and Charles M. Morin

Common wisdom has not changed much in the last 200 years. Buchan wrote in 1799:

> Nothing more certainly disturbs our repose than anxiety. When the mind is not at ease, one seldom enjoys sound sleep. That greatest of human blessings flies the wretched, and visits the happy, the cheerful, and the gay. This is a sufficient reason why every man should endeavour to be as easy in his mind as possible when he goes to rest. Many, by indulging grief and anxious thought, have banished sound sleep so long, that they could never afterwards enjoy it. (p. 76)

Studies confirm Dr. Buchan's clinical observations that patients with psychopathology experience sleep difficulties at least during the acute phase of their illness. The usual belief is that anxiety produces difficulty falling asleep and depression results in early-morning awakenings. In clinical practice, complaints of difficulties falling and staying asleep are common among patients with anxiety, depression, or mixed anxiety–depressive disorders. Although no single sleep variable has absolute specificity for a particular psychiatric disorder, the pattern of sleep disturbances associated with affective disorders differs more reliably from normal sleep than from the sleep of other disorders (Benca, Obermeyer, Thisted, & Gillin, 1992).

Practical and Theoretical Problems

A number of practical and theoretical challenges make the study of psychopathology and sleep a difficult task. These issues are raised here so that they will be in mind when specific studies are discussed. First, depression and anxiety are a constellation of symptoms. Therefore, specific symptoms, including sleep complaints, vary considerably from patient to patient. Second, this symptom haze blurs the boundaries between anxious and depressed patients. Third, sleep disturbance is often part of the definition of depression and anxiety (e.g., see Exhibit 1 and the *Diagnostic and Statistical Manual of Mental Disorders*, 4th ed., *DSM-IV*, American Psychiatric Association, 1994). Fourth, patients' reports of disturbed sleep can vary widely from objective measures of their sleep. Depression affects both sleep and the ability to accurately estimate sleep. Depressed patients (and insomniacs) usually underestimate the length of their sleep (Bliwise, Friedman, & Yesavage, 1993; Carskadon et al., 1976). Finally, there is the need to consider the bidirectional nature of the relationship between sleep and mood disturbances, that is, to consider to what extent the sleep disturbance contributes to the psychopathology.

Cross-Sectional and Longitudinal Data

Sleep in Depressed and Anxious Patients

Many studies have described subjective and electroencephalographic (EEG) sleep features of patients with anxiety and depression. Although discrepancies among studies are more often the rule than the exception, consistent findings across investigations are summarized in Table 1. For comparative purposes, information about the sleep patterns in primary insomniacs and normal controls is also presented.

Kupfer and Foster (1972) first proposed that a reduced rapid eye movement (REM) latency was a biological marker for depression. Also, longer first REM sleep periods, less deep sleep, and more awakenings may occur in a depressed patient group. However, there is still controversy regarding the diagnostic specificity, sensitivity, and clinical utility of REM latency and other sleep markers for depression. Reduced REM sleep latency and increased percentages have occurred in studies of other psychopathologies. Likewise, not all depressed patients show

Exhibit 1

Summary of DSM-IV Diagnostic Criteria for Major Depression and Generalized Anxiety Disorder

Major Depression

(1) Depressed mood
(2) Markedly diminished interest or pleasure
(3) Significant weight loss or weight gain
(4) Insomnia or hypersomnia
(5) Psychomotor agitation
(6) Fatigue or loss of energy
(7) Feelings of worthlessness or excessive inappropriate guilt
(8) Diminished ability to think or concentrate, or indecisiveness
(9) Recurrent thoughts of death, suicidal ideation, or suicide attempt

Generalized Anxiety Disorder

(1) Excessive anxiety and worry (apprehensive expectation)
(2) Difficulty controlling the worry
(3) Anxiety/worry associated with three of more of the following symptoms:
   (a) restlessness or feeling keyed up or on edge;
   (b) being easily fatigued;
   (c) difficulty concentrating;
   (d) irritability;
   (e) muscle tension;
   (f) sleep disturbance (difficulty falling or staying asleep, or restless unsatisfying sleep)

a reduced REM latency or increased percentage of REM sleep. Several factors affect REM sleep, including age, the severity of the depressive illness, and the subtype of depression. For instance, REM latency decreases slightly with aging. Therefore, a shortened REM latency may be less of a specific marker of depression in late-life. Changes in REM sleep are generally more reliable in well-defined clinical samples of inpatients with more severe forms of endogenous depression (Reynolds & Kupfer, 1987).

Two studies demonstrate the difficulty of trying to separate the sleep patterns of generalized anxiety disorder (GAD) patients from those of

Table 1

EEG Sleep Abnormalities in Anxiety and Depression Relative to Insomnia Patients and Normal Controls

Sleep Parameters	Normal	Anxiety	Insomnia Complaint	Depression
Sleep-onset latency	5–15 min	↑	↑	↑
Wake after sleep onset	0–15 min	↑	↑	↑
Total sleep time	6.5–8 hrs	↓	↓	↓
Sleep efficiency	90% +	↓	↓	↓
REM latency	70–90 min	↔	↔	↓
% Stage 1	5%–10%	↑	↑	↔
% Stage 2	50%–60%	↑	↑	↔
% Stage 3–4	10%–15%	↓	↓	↓
% Stage REM	20%–25%	↔	↔	↑

Note. Normative values for a 35-year-old female without sleep or psychiatric disorders (Williams, Karacan, & Hursch, 1974). These values are only approximate and differ across gender and age groups. EEG = electroen-cephalographic

depressed patients. Reynolds et al. (1983) studied patients during a clinical episode of anxiety. The GAD patients averaged long sleep latencies (40 minutes), low sleep efficiencies (77%), low percentages of deep sleep (<4%), and increased intermittent wakefulness when compared with normal values. On most variables the anxiety patients were similar to patients with primary depression. The anxious group did have a longer REM sleep latency (the time from sleep onset to REM sleep onset) and a lower REM percentage than a depressed patient group. However, these patients may have been atypical because they were referred primarily by psychiatrists to other psychiatrists with recognized expertise in sleep disorders.

Rosa, Bonnet, and Kramer (1983) recruited study participants through newspaper ads and screened them for anxiety using clinical interviews and questionnaires. They obtained both subjective estimates and objective measurements of sleep. The GAD group had less sleep, less deep sleep, less REM sleep, a *shorter* REM latency, and a greater percentage of light sleep (Stage 1) than normal participants. Subjectively, the anxious group reported more awakenings and fewer hours of sleep. These changes are similar to findings from other GAD studies except for the shorter REM latency. The authors suggested that anxiety and depression was part of the same continuum.

Induction of Mood Disturbances

Although it is impossible to experimentally induce a GAD or major depressive episode, it is possible to induce stress (which may result in some degree of anxiety or other mood disturbances) and measure resulting changes in sleep patterns. A common sleep-altering event is the "first night effect." Sleep, a very personal time, is penetrated by unknown technicians and a variety of gadgets in unfamiliar surroundings that presumably induce stress and at least temporarily some symptoms of anxiety. On the first sleep-laboratory night, it takes the participant longer to fall asleep, REM sleep latency is longer, there is less deep sleep, and participant awaken more frequently. Assuming the first-night effect results from anxiety, then GAD patients may have less of a change in their sleep from the first to the second night because high levels of anxiety should occur on both nights (a ceiling effect; Reynolds, Shaw, Newton, Coble, & Kupfer, 1983).

Goodenough, Witkin, Koulack, and Cohen (1975) showed male participants a film depicting a series of operations on the penis during an aboriginal tribesman's initiation rite. Following the stress film, an adjective checklist demonstrated increased anxiety, depression, distrust, and hostility. Sleep latencies and dream anxiety content increased after the stress film. Dream anxiety content increased particularly in the participant with the greatest presleep anxiety increase. The duration of sleep, the number of REM periods, and the number of dreams did not differ from the travelogue control film group. In a daytime nap study of good sleepers (Gross & Borkovec, 1982), participants in one group were told they would have to give a short speech upon awakening, whereas control group members were not given such instruction. Those expecting to give a speech took significantly longer to fall asleep.

Examination of Insomnia Patients

If patients with depression and anxiety sleep poorly, then at least some of the patients complaining of insomnia should demonstrate depression or anxiety. Studies of insomnia patients reliably find significant levels of depression and anxiety. The 1979 National Survey of Psychotherapeutic Drug Use, as reported in Mellinger, Balter, and Uhlenhuth (1985), indicated that 35% of the respondents had had problems sleeping within the last year and that 17% of those surveyed were "bothered a lot" by the problem. Of this severe insomnia group, 42% had high anxiety levels and 25% had mixed anxiety and depression symptoms. Only 8% of those who had "never had" insomnia had high anxiety. When respondents with severe insomnia were classified according to *DSM-III* criteria (American Psychiatric Association, 1980), 13% had GAD (versus 3% for controls who had never had insomnia) and 21% had a major depression disorder (versus <1% for controls who had never had insomnia).

Descriptive studies of the psychological profile of insomniacs have found elevated measures of anxiety, dysphoria, worry, somatized tension, or neuroticism (Edinger, Stout, & Hoelscher, 1988; Hauri & Fisher, 1986; Kales, Caldwell, Soldatos, Bixler, & Kales, 1983). Two MMPI profiles (2-7-3; 1-2-3) have been reported with some consistency across investigations. These profiles also suggest depressed and anxious moods, a cognitive style characterized by excessive worrying and obsessive ruminations, internalization of psychological conflicts, and preoccupation with one's health.

Although the rate of psychopathology is reliably higher among insomniacs than it is in good sleepers, estimates vary depending upon the diagnostic criteria and the particular samples selected. For example, some studies (Kales et al., 1983) have relied on a single MMPI scale elevation (i.e., *T* score above 70) as evidence of psychopathology, whereas others (Jacobs, Reynolds, Kupfer, Lovin, & Ehrenpreis, 1988) have used the more stringent Research Diagnostic Criteria. Some estimates are also high because they are based on samples of psychiatric patients. Finally, there may be a tendency among health professionals to automatically link insomnia to depression and to overdiagnose psychiatric disorders.

Insomnia may not be as strongly associated with psychopathology in older adults as it is with younger people (Roehrs, Lineback, Zorick, & Roth, 1982). Although elderly poor sleepers report higher levels of depression and anxiety symptomatology than elderly good sleepers, the severity of these symptoms does not necessarily fall within a pathological range (Morin & Gramling, 1989). This suggests that insomnia alone may not be a good indicator of psychopathology in elderly persons, even though there is more psychopathology among individuals with sleep complaints than among good sleepers.

Temporal Relationship Between Sleep Disturbances and Psychopathology

In one study, 264 older adult study participants were questioned about four sleep problems: difficulties falling asleep, frequent awakenings in the night, early morning awakening, and feelings of not being rested in the morning. They completed several health and psychosocial measures, including the Depressive Adjective Check Lists, on eight separate occasions over a 3-year period (Rodin, McAvay, & Timko, 1988). In the final sample of 196 participants, depressed affect correlated with sleep disturbances even after controlling for age, gender, and health status. The probability of reporting moderate to severe sleep difficulties increased with the number of interviews at which a participant was depressed. Early-morning awakening was the problem most consistently related to depressed mood. A decrease in depressive symptomatology corresponded to a decrease in early-morning awakening.

In a longitudinal study of late-life depression, 1,577 community-resident elderly completed several psychosocial and health measures twice at a 2-year interval (Kennedy, Kelman, & Thomas, 1991). Participants whose depressive symptoms persisted over the 2-year period ($n = 97$) were compared with those whose symptoms remitted over the same interval ($n = 114$). The results showed that respondents with persistent depressive symptoms tended to be older, to experience declining health, and to report more sleep disturbances.

Because depression and anxiety strongly correlate with insomnia complaints, it is easy to accept that anxiety is the etiological factor in the insomnia, although one could argue that insomnia leads to depression and anxiety. Ford and Kamerow (1989), using the Diagnostic Interview Schedule, questioned 7,954 community respondents about sleep complaints and psychiatric symptoms as part of the National Institute of Health (NIMH) Epidemiologic Catchment Area Study. Forty percent of those with insomnia and 47% of those with hypersomnia had a psychiatric disorder compared with 16% of those without sleep complaints. The most common disorders in respondents with insomnia complaints were anxiety disorders (24%), major depression (14%), dysthymia (9%), and alcohol (7%) and drug abuse (4%).

A follow-up interview 1 year later found that the risk of developing a new major depression (and to a smaller extent new anxiety disorders) was greater among those who reported persistent insomnia from baseline to the second interview, compared with those whose insomnia had resolved during that time. A similar pattern occurred in those with continuing hypersomnia, but the number of new cases was substantially smaller. A number of hypotheses might explain the relationship, particularly between insomnia and depression. First, because insomnia is one of the diagnostic criteria, this positive relationship may represent an artifact of the measurement process. Second, sleep disturbance might be an epiphenomenon of the underlying psychiatric disorder, and its alteration would not change the course and eventual full manifestation of the depressive or anxiety disorder. Third, and perhaps the most parsimonious hypothesis, insomnia represents an early precursor in the clinical course of the disorder. Whether early treatment of insomnia might prevent the development of a full major depression remains to be determined.

Effects of Treatment

Treatment of Anxiety

If disturbed sleep is a common clinical feature of anxiety, then treatment of the underlying psychopathology should normalize sleep continuity and architecture. Unfortunately, there has been little effort at monitoring sleep improvement in outcome studies of anxiety disorders. On the other hand, if arousal accompanying anxiety is the etiological factor of the complaint of insomnia, treatment with relaxation or other techniques focused on reducing the arousal should improve sleep. These behavioral techniques are effective in some insomnia patients with a high degree of somatized anxiety and tension (Borkovec & Weerts, 1976). Because not all insomnia patients demonstrate high levels of physiological arousal, the treatment should be matched to the specific problem. For example, Hauri (1981) reported that biofeedback of frontalis electromyographic (EMG) activity produced greater reductions of sleep latency in subjects who were tense during baseline assessment, whereas feedback of sensorimotor rhythm activity produced better outcome in those who were already relaxed at baseline. A more recent attempt at tailoring interventions had little success in showing differential reductions of insomnia symptoms (Sanavio, 1988).

Treatment of Depression

Acute administration of most tricyclic antidepressants (TCA) or of monoamine oxidase inhibitors (MAOI) dramatically decreases the percentage of REM sleep, and prolongs the latency to the first REM sleep episode. The newer selective serotonin reuptake inhibiting (SSRI) antidepressant drugs such as fluoxetine (i.e., Prozac) and sertraline (i.e., Zoloft) also reduce REM sleep, although not to the extent of the MAOI and most of the TCA. Even behavioral reduction of REM sleep by awakening subjects when they enter REM sleep, effectively treats depression (Vogel, Vogel, McAbee, & Thrummed, 1980). Is the shortened REM sleep latency in depressed patients the mediating factor? The cause–effect relationship is not clear because not all antidepressants reduce REM sleep. Also, the ability of TCA to normalize sleep in depressed and anxious patients varies tremendously among drugs, without apparent differences in their antidepressant efficacy (Ware et al., 1989). Finally, with regular usage, REM sleep may recover but without an increase in depression.

Although numerous investigations have focused on the biological correlates of depression and its pharmacological treatment, a more recent line of innovative research has examined changes in REM sleep associated with psychological treatments of depression. Preliminary data suggest that cognitive-behavioral therapy for depression also may produce changes in REM sleep (Thase, Simons, Cahalane, & McGeary, 1991; Thase et al., 1994) and that such changes covary with a decrease in affect intensity during the day (Nofzinger et al., 1994).

Posttreatment Sleep

Does sleep normalize following adequate treatment of the underlying affective disorder? Although this often occurs, just as frequently sleep remains disrupted after the depression has lifted. For instance, patients previously hospitalized for unipolar depression still showed residual sleep disturbances relative to normal controls even 6 months after remission (Hauri, Chernik, Hawkins, & Mendels, 1974). Difficulties falling and staying asleep, as well as increased Stage 1 and decreased Stages 3 and 4 sleep, persisted in successfully treated depressed patients. Rush and his colleagues (1986) evaluated the sleep patterns of depressed patients during the depressive episode and 6 months after clinical remission. None of the REM sleep variables significantly changed from the depressive to the remission phases. There was a slight improvement in sleep efficiency and continuity, although these variables were not impaired initially. Collectively, these findings suggest that EEG-defined sleep impairments (particularly those of REM sleep) in depressed patients represent a "trait-like feature."

Treatment of Insomnia

There is some evidence that mood improvements covary with sleep improvements in controlled treatment studies of primary insomnia. Cognitive-behavioral interventions have produced reduction of depression and anxiety symptoms as well as decreased mood disturbances (Jacobs, Benson, & Friedman, 1993; Morin, Kowatch, Barry, & Walton, 1993). Because patients with significant depression or anxiety are usually excluded from these studies, mood improvement is usually modest but clinically meaningful. Similar mood changes have been reported in studies using pharmacological interventions.

Insomnia patients with concomitant psychopathology are typically excluded from treatment outcome studies of insomnia because it is presumed that they would not respond to a sleep-focused intervention. Although the primary treatment should focus on the underlying psychiatric disorders, recent evidence suggests that patients with insomnia secondary to psychopathology may still benefit from a sleep-focused intervention (Morin, Stone, McDonald, & Jones, 1994; Tan et al., 1987). For example, in a clinical replication series of 100 patients presenting to a sleep clinic for insomnia treatment (Morin et al., 1994), cognitive-behavioral therapy produced comparable increases in sleep efficiency from baseline to posttreatment across patients with primary insomnia (70% to 84%) and those whose insomnia was secondary to psychopathology (61% to 75%). Patients whose insomnia was associated with psychopathology (mostly affective and anxiety disorders) reported more severe sleep disturbances, both at baseline and at posttreatment, than psychophysiological insomniacs. Although there was little difference in the absolute levels of changes obtained on the various outcome measures, individuals with psychiatric disorders did not achieve the same sleep patterns at posttreatment as those in the other two subgroups. Whether long-term outcome correlates more with absolute change scores or to endpoint functioning is unclear.

Specific Sleep Events

More than just five stages compose a night of sleep. A large number of events occur that are not reflected in standard sleep staging. Depression and anxiety also affect some of these micro events. An as yet little-explored possibility is that these micro events may contribute to subjective reports of poor sleep independently of that reflected in sleep staging.

REM Density

A minute of REM sleep may have 2 or 20 eye movements. Measurements of the frequency of eye movements per unit of time (REM density) vary with mood. REM density is higher in dreams with stronger emotional content (Goodenough et al., 1975), greater following psychological stress (Zarcone & Benson, 1983), and greater in depressed patients (Kupfer, Coble, McPartland, & Ulrich, 1978). Increased REM density does not occur in anxious patients, at least to the degree that it does in depressed patients. Additionally, REM density increases when total sleep time is greater than one's normal range, a situation that is unlikely to occur in anxious patients (Aserinsky, 1973). As depression in nonmedicated patients resolves, REM density approaches normal, that is, eye movements become less frequent (Thase et al., 1994).

Sleep-Related Penile Erections (SRE)

Penile erections accompany REM sleep. In patients complaining of impotence, reduced SRE duration and rigidity indicate organic pathology (Ware, 1987). Anxiety and depression also may accompany an altered SRE pattern. There is greater variability in penile circumference during dreams with greater anxiety, and SRE in depressed patients may be abnormal. Even after treatment of depression, these abnormalities can remain, suggesting that SRE, like other REM sleep characteristics, may be trait markers for depression (Nofzinger et al., 1993).

Although there is little analogous work with women, sleep-related orgasm in women appears positively correlated with anxiety (Henton, 1976). Because sexual arousal may be more of a parasympathetic phenomenon and orgasm more of a sympathetic nervous system response, these reports are not incompatible with the idea that increased physiological arousal (sexual or otherwise) accompanies anxiety.

Bruxism

Numerous reports suggest that bruxism during sleep reflects psychological factors. Bruxism increases after days with stressful events and in subjects anticipating stressful events (Funch & Gale, 1980; Rugh & Solberg, 1975). Correlational studies examining psychological traits in bruxism patients report anxiety and depression as well as other emotional traits (Thaller, Rosen, & Saltzman, 1967; Vernallis, 1955).

Sleep bruxism occurs primarily in non-REM (NREM) sleep. However, patients with severe dental and facial pain, problems secondary to bruxism, have an increased rate of bruxism in REM sleep (Ware & Rugh, 1988). These REM-sleep bruxism patients are more likely to present with features of depression. Patients without dental and facial pain have the majority of their bruxism in NREM sleep, are likely to be anxious, and present with a sleep disturbance complaint.

Rocking

Sleep rocking is primarily an NREM sleep phenomenon that has received little scientific attention, although patients may rock vigorously for hours. The rocking may result in patients hitting their head against the mattress or the head of the bed. Nevertheless, the act of rocking may be comforting and perhaps prevents or competes with anxious thoughts and feelings (Ferber, 1985; Oswald, 1964).

Night Terrors and Sleepwalking

Although the etiology of these dramatic Stage 4 sleep behaviors remains elusive, several authors have suggested that night terrors are a violent release of uncontrolled anxiety (e.g., Fisher, Kahn, Edwards, Davis, & Fine, 1974). The MMPI profiles of night terror patients indicate high levels of anxiety as well as depression, aggression, obsessive-compulsive tendencies, and phobia (Kales, Kales, et al., 1980). In addition to genetic and developmental factors, psychological factors apparently play an important role, particularly in their maintenance beyond childhood. Kales, Soldatos, et al. (1980) found that more than a third of their night terror patients had "major life events" that preceded and possibly were factors in the occurrence of night terrors. Night terrors may respond to psychotherapy, hypnotherapy, dopaminergic agents, and diazepam (e.g., Valium). One explanation for the efficacy of diazepam is that it suppresses deep sleep, from which night terrors occur. Diazepam, an anxiolytic medication, may reduce the anxiety that triggers the arousal.

Dreams and Nightmares (Dream Anxiety Attacks)

Unlike night terrors, dreams and nightmares occur primarily from REM sleep. Dreams, if anything, are affect laden even in nonhumans. Admittedly, it is not easy to tell the content of an animal's dream. However, brain stem lesions in cats can abolish the paralysis that normally accompanies REM sleep. These cats, although judged to be asleep because of lack of response to environmental stimuli, myotic pupils, and relaxed nictitating membranes, frequently assume attack and defense postures suggesting fear and rage (Henley & Morrison, 1974). In human dream reports, the most common affect is anxiety, followed by anger and surprise (McCarley, 1983). In children, anxiety, and then aggression, are among the first dream affects to occur (DeMartino, 1955). Hartmann (1984), in his book *The Nightmare*, concludes, "One point on which there is agreement among many of the authors mentioned is that the nightmare involves some of the earliest, most profound anxieties" (p. 47).

Does psychopathology result in an increase in anxious dreams or nightmares? Anxieties can be incorporated into, and perhaps precipitate, nightmares. This certainly is the case of posttraumatic nightmares. On a less dramatic level, Orr, Dozier, Green, and Cromwell (1968) instructed study participants to awaken themselves at certain times during the night. All the participants who were successful at this task reported dreams with anticipation and apprehension, apparently as a result of their concern over performing the task successfully. In addition, Goodenough et al. (1975) found that presleep anxiety contributed to increased anxiety in dreams.

Sleep Talking

Somniloquy is not as clearly stage related as some other phenomena; and, it may initially seem far from the topic of depression and anxiety. However, there may be a relationship. In the experiment by Orr et al. (1968), three of the seven students instructed to awaken at specific times during the night had episodes of sleep talking apparently related to concern over the task of awakening. If transient stressors might result in sleep talking, the more powerful state of anxiety may increase sleep talking. Arkin (1981) concluded that sleep talking is not a sign of any specific psychopathological state, although he did report several cases in which emotional stress apparently precipitated sleep talking.

Effects of Disturbed Sleep

Sleep Deprivation Studies: The Production of Symptoms

What role does disturbed sleep play in the symptom complex associated with depression and anxiety? Numerous sleep deprivation studies have been carried out, but the circus-like atmosphere that often develops from the heroic efforts required to keep subjects awake may distort the effects. Nevertheless, some reliable effects occur. Several of these effects do fall within the symptom complex of anxiety listed in Exhibit 1.

Irritability. Irritability increases after sleep deprivation. Irritability is not only a common consequence in humans, it may occur in animals as well (see Kleitman, 1963). One of the most common symptoms besides sleepiness reported by the spouses of sleep apnea patients, who for years have had a fragmentation of their sleep as a result of the apnea periods, is irritability. This irritability improves following successful treatment of the apnea that results in a normalization of sleep.

Pain. Sleep deprivation may result in an increase in pain sensitivity (Cooperman, Mullin, & Kleitman, 1934) that may be relevant to the increased level of aches and pains that clinically anxious and depressed patients report. Even joint aches and pains may result from a specific deep sleep disturbance. Moldofsky and Scarisbrick (1976) were able to induce a muscculoskeletal pain syndrome by selectively depriving participants of deep sleep, a sleep state that is reduced in depressed patients.

Memory. Besides the obvious concentration problems occurring following sleep deprivation, sleep deprivation also results in an impairment in memory as reflected in diminished immediate recall and long term memory (Polzella, 1975). It is not entirely clear whether this is a problem with storage or retrieval. Research does indicate that REM sleep is important for certain types of learning (Karni, Tanne, Rubenstein, Askenasy, & Sagi, 1994). Therefore, the disturbance in REM sleep that often occurs with depression may have specific effects, particularly in patients treated with REM-sleep-altering antidepressant medications.

Autonomic activity. Although altered autonomic activity may occur in depression and anxiety, it is difficult to document any consistent changes in autonomic activity that are associated with sleep deprivation. Sleep deprivation increases heart rate in rats (Karadzic & Dement, 1967). Animals increase their food intake, become more aggressive, and become hypersexual (Morden, Conner, Mitchell, Dement, & Levine, 1968). Also, there is an increased excitability of the brain as indicated by a decrease in convulsion threshold. Following human sleep deprivation, reports indicate increase, decrease, and no change in the level of arousal as measured by autonomic activity. One may hypothesize an increased autonomic liability during sleep loss. However, even this has not been a reliable finding. After two or three days of sleep deprivation, extreme stimulation and constant muscle activity are required to keep subjects awake. This potentially interferes with the detection of subtle changes.

Sleep Deprivation and Mood Change

Treatment potential. Nondepressed individuals may develop mild depressive symptoms (dysphoria) following sleep deprivation. Conversely, sleep deprivation produces an antidepressant effect in some depressed patients. Approximately 60% of drug-free patients have an antidepressant response to a single night of sleep deprivation. However, 83% of unmedicated patients and 59% of medicated patients relapsed after a night of recovery sleep (Wu & Bunney, 1990). Thus, the effect of sleep deprivation on mood is relatively short-lived. Depressive symptoms are quick to return, even after a brief nap, especially if it contains REM sleep.

The effect on the mood of depressed patients is relatively the same with total, partial, or selective REM-sleep deprivation (see Gillin, 1983). Late partial sleep deprivation, for example, a patient is awakened at 2:00 a.m., produces superior results to early partial sleep deprivation in which the patient is *kept* awake until 2:00 a.m. and allowed to sleep the rest of the night. This finding is consistent with the hypothesis that the mood-altering effect of sleep deprivation is mediated by the suppression of REM sleep, which is more predominant in early morning hours.

The main advantages to using sleep deprivation as an antidepressant agent is that the intervention is inexpensive, noninvasive, and produces quick results. It can also be self-implemented, although the lack of motivation to stay awake through the night is a problem with severely depressed patients. Patients may need supervision; some mood-disorders centers in Europe run weekly sleep deprivation clinics where nurses, technicians, and other patients keep patients awake (Leibenluft & Wehr, 1992).

Diagnostic utility. Besides its potential applications in the treatment of mood disorders, sleep deprivation can serve a useful diagnostic function. For example, Reynolds et al. (1987) used sleep deprivation to distinguish elderly patients with depression and dementia from healthy normal controls. Whereas the pattern of slow wave sleep rebound is comparable across the three groups following sleep deprivation, REM rebound is more delayed among the depressed subgroup. A related study suggested that a positive response to sleep deprivation distinguished patients with depressive pseudodementia from those with primary degenerative dementia (Buysse et al., 1988). Given the high incidence of coexisting depressive symptoms and cognitive impairments in elderly people, sleep deprivation could have a useful diagnostic function.

Conclusion

Complementing Buchan's clinical observations, the empirical evidence indicates a high rate of comorbidity between sleep and psychiatric disorders, and particularly between insomnia, anxiety, and depression. What is less clear, however, is the cause–effect relationship. The natural course of insomnia often begins with anxiety resulting from stressful life events that results in insomnia and finally depression.

The data indicate that (a) anxiety increases sleep latency; the act of being anxious while in bed will forestall sleep as would engaging in any arousing activity or activity incompatible with sleep onset; (b) depression and anxiety increase the perception of a sleep disturbance more so than the standard polysomnographic variables reflect; (c) once an anxious patient is asleep, the basic sleep cycle as it is generally measured is completed in normal fashion, with the exception that if one awakens during the night, anxiety may prolong the awakening because of the occurrence of incompatible sleep behaviors; and (d) depression is more likely to alter the architecture of sleep, particularly REM-sleep parameters. In only a small number of patients is sleep not affected at all. Approximately 90% of depressed inpatients show some form of objective sleep disturbance, whereas 10% to 15% sleep efficiently (Reynolds & Kupfer, 1987). The latter feature is often more characteristic of the depressive phase in bipolar patients.

Depression and anxiety also appear to affect a number of specific sleep events. They can be associated with REM sleep (e.g., anxious dreams and eye movements), NREM sleep (e.g., night terrors, sleepwalking, and rocking), and both REM and NREM sleep (e.g., bruxism).

These effects are important because they indicate that sleep is not isolated from daytime concerns and worries. From the standpoint of understanding psychopathology, these changes also suggest that these states must have a fundamental physiological component to persevere not only through wakefulness but through NREM and REM sleep.

Finally, there is a great deal of interest in viewing EEG sleep as an important window into mood disorders. Particularly patients with the so-called "masked depression" may exclusively emphasize sleep disruptions, along with other neurovegetative symptoms, while denying affective symptomatology. In theory, a sleep study should provide a picture rich with useful clinical information that is otherwise not easily accessible to clinicians. Possibly, treatment advances may come from evaluating the patient's sleep and matching the treatment to the specific sleep disturbance.

REFERENCES

American Psychiatric Association, (1980). *Diagnostic and statistical manual of mental disorders* (3rd ed.). Washington, DC: Author.

American Psychiatric Association. (1994). *Diagnostic and statistical manual of mental disorders* (4th ed.). Washington, DC: Author.

Arkin, A. M. (1981). *Sleep talking: Psychology and psychophysiology.* Hillsdale, NJ: Erlbaum.

Aserinsky, E. (1973). Relationship of rapid eye movement density to the prior accumulation of sleep and wakefulness. *Psychophysiology, 10,* 545–558.

Benca, R. M., Obermeyer, W. H., Thisted, R. A., & Gillin, J. C. (1992). Sleep and psychiatric disorders: A meta-analysis. *Archives of General Psychiatry, 49,* 651–668.

Bliwise, D. L., Friedman, L., & Yesavage, J. A. (1993). Depression as a confounding variable in the estimation of habitual sleep time. *Journal of Clinical Psychology, 49,* 471–477.

Borkovec, T. D., & Weerts, T. D. (1976). Effects of progressive relaxation on sleep disturbance: An electroencephalographic evaluation. *Psychosomatic Medicine, 38,* 173–180.

Buchan, W. (1799). *Domestic medicine: Or, a treatise on the prevention and cure of diseases.* Philadelphia: Folwell.

Buysse, D. J., Reynolds, C. F., Kupfer, D. J., Houck, P. R., Hoch, C. C., Stack, J. A., & Berman, S. R. (1988). Electroencephalographic sleep in depressive pseudodementia. *Archives of General Psychiatry, 45,* 568–575.

Carskadon, M. A., Dement, W. C., Mitler, M., Guilleminault, C., Zarcone, V. P., & Spiegel, R. (1976). Self-reports versus sleep laboratory findings in 122 drug-free subjects with complaints of chronic insomnia. *American Journal of Psychiatry, 133*, 1382–1387.

Cooperman, N. R., Mullin, F. J., & Kleitman, N. (1934). Studies on the physiology of sleep, XI: Further observations on the effects of prolonged sleeplessness. *American Journal of Physiology, 107*, 589–593.

DeMartino, M. F. (1955). A review of literature on children's dreams. *Psychiatric Quarterly Supplement, 29*, 90–101.

Edinger, J. D., Stout, A. L., & Hoelscher, T. J., (1988). Cluster analysis of insomniacs' MMPI profiles: Relation of subtypes to sleep history and treatment outcome. *Psychosomatic Medicine, 50*, 77–87.

Ferber, R. (1985). *Solve your child's sleep problems.* New York: Simon & Schuster.

Fisher, C., Kahn, E., Edwards, S. A., Davis, D. M., & Fine, J. (1974). A psychophysiological study of nightmares and night terrors. III: Mental content and recall of Stage 4 night terrors. *Journal of Nervous and Mental Disease, 158*, 174–188.

Ford, D. E., & Kamerow, D. B. (1989). Epidemiologic study of sleep disturbances and psychiatric disorders: An opportunity for prevention? *Journal of the American Medical Association, 262*, 1479–1484.

Funch, D. P., & Gale, E. N. (1980). Factors associated with nocturnal bruxism and its treatment. *Journal of Behavioral Medicine, 3*, 385–397.

Gillin J. C. (1983). The sleep therapies of depression. *Progress in Neuropsychopharmacology and Biological Psychiatry, 7*, 351–364.

Goodenough, D. R., Witkin, H. A., Koulack, D., & Cohen, H. (1975). The effects of stress films on dream affect and on respiration and eye-movement activity during rapid-eye-movement sleep. *Psychophysiology, 12*, 313–320.

Gross, R. T., & Borkovec, T. D. (1982). Effects of cognitive intrusion manipulation on sleep-onset latency of good sleepers. *Behavior Therapy, 13*, 112–116.

Hartman, E. (1984). *The nightmare.* New York: Basic Books.

Hauri, P. J. (1981). Treating psychophysiologic insomnia with biofeedback. *Archives of General Psychiatry, 38*, 752–758.

Hauri, P. J., Chernik, D., Hawkins, D., & Mendels, J. (1974). Sleep of depressed patients in remission. *Archives of General Psychiatry, 31*, 386–391.

Hauri, P. J., & Fisher, J. (1986). Persistent psychophysiologic (learned) insomnia. *Sleep, 9*, 38–53.

Henley, K., & Morrison, A. R. (1974). A re-evaluation of the effects of lesions of the pontine tegmentum and locus coeruleus on phenomena of paradoxical sleep in the cat. *Acta Neurobiolgiae Experimentalis, 34*, 215–232.

Henton, C. L. (1976). Nocturnal orgasm in college women: Its relation to dreams and anxiety associated with sexual factors. *The Journal of Genetic Psychology, 129*, 245–251.

Jacobs, E. A., Reynolds, C. F., Kupfer, D. J., Lovin, P. A., & Ehrenpreis, A. B. (1988). The role of polysomnography in the differential diagnosis of chronic insomnia. *American Journal of Psychiatry, 145*, 346–349.

Jacobs, G. D., Benson, H., & Friedman, R. (1993). Home-based central nervous system assessment of a multifactor behavioral intervention for chronic sleep-onset insomnia. *Behavior Therapy, 24,* 159–174.

Kales, A., Caldwell, A. B., Soldatos, C. R., Bixler, E. O., & Kales, J. D. (1983). Biopsychobehavioral correlates of insomnia. II. Pattern specificity and consistency with the Minnesota Multiphasic Personality Inventory. *Psychosomatic Medicine, 45,* 341–356.

Kales, J. D., Kales, A., Soldatos, C. R., Caldwell, A. B., Charney, D. S., & Martin E. D. (1980). Night terrors: Clinical characteristics and personality patterns. *Archives of General Psychiatry, 37,* 1413–1417.

Kales, A., Soldatos, C. R., Caldwell, A. B., Kales, J. D., Humphrey, F. J., Charney, D. S., & Schweitzer, P. K. (1980). Somnambulism: Clinical characteristics and personality patterns. *Archives of General Psychiatry, 37,* 1406–1410.

Karadzic, V., & Dement, W. (1967). Heart rate changes following selective deprivation of rapid eye movement (REM) sleep. *Brain Research, 6,* 786–788.

Karni, A., Tanne, D., Rubenstein, B. S., Askenasy, J. J., & Sagi, D. (1994). Dependence on REM sleep of overnight improvement of a perceptual skill. *Science, 265,* 679–682.

Kennedy, G. J., Kelman, H. R., & Thomas, C. (1991). Persistence and remission of depressive symptoms in late life. *American Journal of Psychiatry, 148,* 174–178.

Kleitman, N. (1963). *Sleep and wakefulness.* Chicago: University of Chicago Press.

Kupfer, D. J., Coble, P., McPartland, R. J., & Ulrich, R. F. (1978). The application of EEG sleep for the differential diagnosis of affective disorders. *American Journal of Psychiatry, 135,* 69–74.

Kupfer, D. J., & Foster, F. G., (1972). Interval between onset of sleep and rapid-eye-movement sleep as an indicator of depression. *Lancet, 2,* 684–686.

Leibenluft, E., & Wehr, T. A. (1992). Is sleep deprivation useful in the treatment of depression? *American Journal of Psychiatry, 149,* 159–168.

McCarley, R. (1983). REM dreams, REM sleep, and their isomorphisms. In M. H. Chase & E. D. Weitzman (Eds.), *Sleep disorders: Basic and clinical research* (pp. 363–392). New York: Spectrum.

Mellinger, G. D., Balter, M. B., & Uhlenhuth, E. H. (1985). Insomnia and its treatment. *Archives of General Psychiatry, 42,* 225–232.

Moldofsky, H., & Scarisbrick, P. (1976). Induction of neurasthenic muscoskeletal pain syndrome by selective sleep stage deprivation. *Psychosomatic Medicine, 38,* 35–44.

Morden, B., Conner, R., Mitchell, G., Dement, W., & Levine, S. (1968). Effects of rapid eye movement (REM) sleep deprivation on shock-induced fighting. *Physiological Behavior, 3,* 425–432.

Morin, C. M., & Gramling, S. E. (1989). Sleep patterns and aging: Comparison of older adults with and without insomnia complaints. *Psychology of Aging, 4,* 290–294.

Morin, C. M., Kowatch, R. A., Barry, T., & Walton, E. (1993). Cognitive-behavior therapy for late-life insomnia. *Journal of Consulting and Clinical Psychology, 61,* 137–146.

Morin, C. M., Stone, J., McDonald, K., & Jones, S. (1994). Psychological management of insomnia: A clinical replication series with 100 insomnia patients. *Behavior Therapy, 25,* 291–309.

Nofzinger, E. A., Schwartz, R. M., Reynolds, C. F., Thase, M. E., Jennings, J. R., Frank, E., Fasiczka, A. L., Garamoni, G. L., & Kupfer D. J. (1994). Affect intensity and phasic REM sleep in depressed men before and after treatment with cognitive-behavioral therapy. *Journal of Consulting and Clinical Psychology, 62,* 83–91.

Nofzinger, E. A., Thase, M. E., Reynolds, C. F., Frank, E., Jennings, J. R., Garamoni, G. L., Fasiczka, A. L., & Kupfer, D. J. (1993). Sexual function in depressed men: Assessment by self-report, behavioral, and nocturnal penile tumescence measures before and after treatment with cognitive behavior therapy. *Archives of General Psychiatry, 50,* 24–30.

Orr, W. F., Dozier, J. E., Green, L., & Cromwell, R. I. (1968). Self-induced waking: Changes in dreams and sleep patterns. *Comprehensive Psychiatry, 9,* 499–506.

Oswald, I. (1964). Rocking at night. *Electroencephalography and Clinical Neurophysiology, 16,* 312–313.

Polzella, D. J. (1975). Effects of sleep deprivation on short-term recognition memory. *Journal of Experimental Psychology, 104,* 194–200.

Reynolds, C. F., & Kupfer, D. J. (1987). Sleep research in affective illness: State of the art circa 1987. *Sleep, 10,* 199–215.

Reynolds, C. F., Kupfer, D. J., Hoch, C. C., Houck, P. R., Stack, J. A., Berman, S. R., Campbell, P. I., & Zimmer, B. (1987). Sleep deprivation as a probe in the elderly. *Archives of General Psychiatry, 44,* 982–990.

Reynolds, C. F., Shaw, D. H., Newton, T. F., Coble, P. A., & Kupfer, D. J. (1983). EEG sleep in outpatients with generalized anxiety: A preliminary comparison with depressed outpatients. *Psychiatry Research, 8,* 81–89.

Rodin, J., McAvay, G., & Timko, C. (1988). A longitudinal study of depressed mood and sleep disturbances in elderly adults. *Journal of Gerontology, 43,* 45–53.

Roehrs, T., Lineback, W., Zorick, F., & Roth, T. (1982). Relationship of psychopathology to insomnia in the elderly. *Journal of American Geriatric Society, 30,* 312–315.

Rosa, R. R., Bonnet, M. H., & Kramer, M. (1983). The relationship of sleep and anxiety in anxious subjects. *Biological Psychology, 16,* 119–126.

Rugh, J. D., & Solberg, W. K. (1975). Electromyographic studies of bruxist behaviour before and during treatment. *Journal of California Dental Association, 3,* 56–59.

Rush, A. J., Erman, M. K., Giles, D. E., Schlesser, M. A., Carpenter, G., Vasavada, N., & Roffwarg, H. P. (1986). Polysomnographic findings in recently drug-free and clinically remitted depressed patients. *Archives of General Psychiatry, 43,* 878–884.

Sanavio, E. (1988). Pre-sleep cognitive intrusions and treatment of onset-insomnia. *Behaviour Research and Therapy, 26,* 451–459.

Tan, T. L., Kales, J. D., Kales, A., Martin, E. D., Mann, L. D., & Soldatos, C. R. (1987). Inpatient multidimensional management of treatment-resistant insomnia. *Psychosomatics, 28,* 266–272.

Thaller, J. L., Rosen, G., & Saltzman, S. (1967). Study of the relationship of frustration and anxiety to bruxism. *Journal of Periodontology, 38,* 193–197.

Thase, M. E., Reynolds, C. F., III, Frank, E., Jennings, J. R., Nofzinger, E., Fasiczka, A. L., Garamoni, G. L., & Kupfer, D. J. (1994). Polysomnographic studies of unmedicated depressed men before and after cognitive behavioral therapy. *American Journal of Psychiatry, 151,* 1615–1622.

Thase, M. E., Simons, A. D., Cahalane, J. F., & McGeary, J. (1991). Cognitive behavior therapy of endogenous depression: Part 1: An outpatient clinical replication series. *Behavior Therapy, 22,* 457–467.

Vernallis, F. F. (1955). Teeth-grinding: Some relationships to anxiety, hostility, and hyperactivity. *Journal of Clinical Psychology, 11,* 389–391.

Vogel, G. W., Vogel, F., McAbee, R. S., & Thrummed, A. J. (1980). Improvement of depression by REM sleep deprivation. *Archives of General Psychiatry, 37,* 247–253.

Ware, J. C., (1987). The evaluation of impotence: Monitoring periodic erections during sleep. In M. Erman (Ed.), *Psychiatric clinics of North America: Sleep disorders* (pp. 675–686). Philadelphia: Saunders.

Ware, J. C., Brown, F. W., Moorad, P. J., Pittard, J. T., & Cobert, B. (1989). Effects on sleep: A double-blind study comparing trimipramine to imipramine in depressed insomniac patients. *Sleep, 12,* 537–549.

Ware, J. C., & Rugh, J. D. (1988). Destructive bruxism: Sleep stage relationship. *Sleep, 11,* 172–181.

Williams, R. L., Karacan, I., & Hursch C. J. (1974). *Electroencephalography (EEG) of human sleep: Clinical applications.* New York: Wiley.

Wu, J. C., & Bunney, W. E. (1990). The biological basis of an antidepressant response to sleep deprivation and relapse: Review and hypothesis. *American Journal of Psychiatry, 147,* 14–21.

Zarcone, V. P., & Benson, K. L. (1983). Increased REM eye movement density in self-rated depression. *Psychiatry Research, 8,* 65–71.

Appendix A

The International Classification of Sleep Disorders

Classification Outline

1. Dyssomnias
   A. Intrinsic sleep disorders
   B. Extrinsic sleep disorders
   C. Circadian rhythm disorders
2. Parasomnias
   A. Arousal disorders
   B. Sleep–wake transition disorders
   C. Parasomnias usually associated with rapid eye movement (REM) sleep
   D. Other parasomnias
3. Medical–psychiatric sleep disorders
   A. Associated with mental disorders
   B. Associated with neurological disorders
   C. Associated with other medical disorders
4. Proposed sleep disorders

1. Dyssomias
   A. Intrinsic sleep disorders
      1. Psychophysiological insomnia
      2. Sleep-state misperception
      3. Idiopathic insomnia
      4. Narcolepsy
      5. Recurrent hypersomnia
      6. Idiopathic hypersomnia
      7. Posttraumatic hypersomnia
      8. Obstructive sleep apnea

    9. Central sleep apnea
   10. Central alveolar hypoventilation syndrome
   11. Periodic limb movement disorder
   12. Restless legs syndrome
   13. Intrinsic sleep disorder not otherwise specified
B. Extrinsic sleep disorders
    1. Inadequate sleep hygiene
    2. Environmental sleep disorder
    3. Altitude insomnia
    4. Adjustment sleep disorder
    5. Insufficient sleep syndrome
    6. Limit-setting sleep disorder
    7. Sleep-onset association disorder
    8. Food allergy insomnia
    9. Nocturnal eating (drinking) syndrome
   10. Hypnotic-dependent sleep disorder
   11. Stimulant-dependent sleep disorder
   12. Alcohol-dependent sleep disorder
   13. Toxin-induced sleep disorder
   14. Extrinsic sleep disorder not otherwise specified
C. Circadian rhythm sleep disorders
    1. Time zone change (jet lag) syndrome
    2. Shift work sleep disorder
    3. Irregular sleep–wake pattern
    4. Delayed sleep phase syndrome
    5. Advanced sleep phase syndrome
    6. Non-24-hour sleep–wake disorder
    7. Circadian rhythm sleep disorder not otherwise specified

2. Parasomnias
  A. Arousal disorders
    1. Confusional arousals
    2. Sleepwalking
    3. Sleep terrors
  B. Sleep–wake transition disorders
    1. Rhythmic movement disorder
    2. Sleep starts
    3. Sleep talking
    4. Nocturnal leg cramps

C. Parasomnias usually associated with REM sleep
1. Nightmares
2. Sleep paralysis
3. Impaired sleep-related penile erections
4. Sleep-related painful erections
5. REM sleep-related sinus arrest
6. REM sleep behavior disorder
D. Other parasomnias
1. Sleep bruxism
2. Sleep enuresis
3. Sleep-related abnormal swallowing syndrome
4. Nocturnal paroxysmal dystonia
5. Sudden unexplained nocturnal death syndrome
6. Primary snoring
7. Infant sleep apnea
8. Congenital central hypoventilation syndrome
9. Sudden infant death syndrome
10. Benign neonatal sleep myoclonus
11. Other parasomnia not otherwise specified

3. Medical–Psychiatric Disorders
A. Associated with mental disorders
1. Psychoses
2. Mood disorders
3. Anxiety disorders
4. Panic disorders
5. Alcoholism
B. Associated with neurological disorders
1. Cerebral degenerative disorders
2. Dementia
3. Parkinsonism
4. Fatal familial insomnia
5. Sleep-related epilepsy
6. Electrical status epilepticus of sleep
7. Sleep-related headaches
C. Associated with other medical disorders
1. Sleep sickness
2. Nocturnal cardiac ischemia
3. Chronic obstructive pulmonary disease

   4. Sleep-related asthma
   5. Sleep-related gastroesophageal reflux
   6. Peptic ulcer disease
   7. Fibrositis syndrome

4. Proposed Sleep Disorders
   1. Short sleeper
   2. Long sleeper
   3. Subwakefulness syndrome
   4. Fragmentary myoclonus
   5. Sleep hyperhidrosis
   6. Menstrual-associated sleep disorder
   7. Pregnancy-associated sleep disorder
   8. Terrifying hypnagogic hallucinations
   9. Sleep-related neurogenic tachypnea
   10. Sleep choking syndrome

Appendix B

Diagnostic and Statistical Manual (DSM-IV) Sleep Disorders Codes

Primary Sleep Disorders

Codes	Description
Dyssomnias	
307.42	Primary insomnia
307.44	Primary hypersomnia
347	Narcolepsy
780.59	Breathing-related sleep disorder
307.45	Circadian rhythm sleep disorder
	Delayed sleep phase type
	Jet lag type
	Shift work type
	Unspecified type
307.47	Dyssomnia not otherwise specified
Parasomnias	
307.47	Nightmare disorder
307.46	Sleep terror disorder
307.46	Sleepwalking disorder

Sleep Disorders Related to Another Mental Disorder

307.42	Insomnia related to another mental disorder
307.44	Hypersomnia related to another mental disorder

From *Diagnostic and Statistical Manual of Mental Disorders* (4th ed.), American Psychiatric Association, 1994.

Other Sleep Disorders

Sleep Disorder Due to General Medical Condition 780.xx

780.52	Insomnia type
780.54	Hypersomnia type
780.59	Parasomnia type
780.59	Mixed type

Substance Induced Sleep Disorder

291.8	Alcohol induced sleep disorder
292.89	Cocaine induced sleep disorder
292.89	Amphetamine induced sleep disorder
292.89	Caffeine induced sleep disorder
292.89	Sedative, hypnotic, and anxiolytic

Subtypes

Insomnia type
Hypersomnia type
Parasomnia type
Mixed type

Specify

With onset during intoxication
With onset during withdrawal

Appendix C

ICD-9-CM Sleep Disorders Codes

Code	Description
347	**Narcolepsy**
307.4	**Specific Disorders of Sleep of Nonorganic Origin**
307.40	Nonorganic sleep disorder, unspecified
307.41	Transient disorder of initiating or maintaining sleep
307.42	Persistent disorder of initiating or maintaining sleep
307.43	Transient disorder of initiating or maintaining wakefulness
307.44	Persistent disorder of initiating or maintaining wakefulness
307.45	Phase-shift disruption of 24-hour sleep–wake cycle
307.46	Somnambulism or night terrors
307.47	Other dysfunctions of sleep stages or arousal from sleep
307.48	Repetitive intrusion of sleep
307.49	Other
780.5	**Sleep Disturbances**
780.5	Sleep disturbances, unspecified
780.51	Insomnia with sleep apnea
780.52	Other insomnia
780.53	Hypersomnia with sleep apnea
780.54	Other hypersomnia
780.55	Disruptions of the 24 hour sleep–wake cycle
780.56	Dysfunctions associated with sleep stages or arousal from sleep
780.59	Other

From *The International Classification of Diseases, 9th Revision, Clinical Modification* (DHHS Publication No. DHS 89–1260). U.S. Government Printing Office, 1989.

Appendix D

CPT (Procedure) Codes
for Sleep Laboratory Studies

Sleep Testing

Sleep studies and polysomnography refer to the continuous and simultaneous monitoring and recording of various physiological and pathophysiological parameters of sleep for 6 or more hours with physician review, interpretation, and report. The studies are performed to diagnose a variety of sleep disorders and evaluate a patient's response to therapies such as nasal continuous positive airway pressure (NCPAP). Polysomnography is distinguished from sleep studies by the inclusion of sleep staging, which is defined to include a 1–4 lead electroencephalogram (EEG), electrooculogram (EOG), and submental electromyogram (EMG). Additional parameters of sleep include: 1) ECG; 2) airflow; 3) ventilation and respiratory effort; 5) extremity muscle activity motor activity–movement; 6) extended EEG monitoring; 7) penile tumescence; 8) gastroesophageal reflux; 9) continuous blood pressure monitoring; 10) snoring; 11) body positions, etc.

For a study to be reported as polysomnography, sleep must be recorded and staged.

95805   Multiple Sleep Latency Testing (MSLT): recording, analysis, and interpretation of physiological measurements of sleep during multiple nap opportunities
95807   Sleep study; 3 or more parameters of sleep other than sleep staging, attended by technologist

From *Physicians Current Procedural Terminology* (4th ed. rev.). American Medical Association, 1996.

95808 Polysomnography; sleep staging with 1–3 additional parameters of sleep attended by technologist

95810 Polysomnography; sleep staging with 4 or more additional parameters of sleep, attended by a technologist

Appendix E

Requirements, Eligibility, and Examination Process for Certification as a Clinical Sleep Specialist by the American Board of Sleep Medicine

Health professionals with a PhD have been eligible to sit for the American Board of Sleep Medicine Board Exams since its inception in 1978. Of the 800 doctoral-level health professionals certified by the ABSM, 100 are PhDs. Below is information for PhD applicants. This information is taken from the 1996–1997 pamphlet. Requirements and required fees may change with time, and potential applicants in 1998 and later should request current information for PhD applicants from the American Board of Sleep Medicine. The information below is reprinted with permission of the American Board of Sleep Medicine.

HISTORY OF THE AMERICAN BOARD OF SLEEP MEDICINE

In 1978, the Association of Sleep Disorders Centers formed a committee to produce an examination for the purpose of establishing and maintaining standards of individual proficiency in clinical polysomnography. This committee, which became the Examination Committee of the American Sleep Disorders Association, directed by Helmut S. Schmidt, MD, had certified 432 physicians and PhDs as Accredited Clinical Polysomnographers (ACPs) by the end of 1990.

Culminating many years of planning, the American Board of Sleep Medicine was incorporated by William C. Dement, MD, PhD, as an independent, nonprofit, self-designated Board on January 28, 1991. The 11 directors of the Board are nominated by the American Sleep Disorders Association and other professional associations that have a

515

significant role in sleep medicine. The Board directs all aspects of the certifying process. Committees of the Board review applications' credentials and produce and evaluate the 2-part examination.

As sleep medicine is a broad medical field, the Board has discontinued the term "ACP" and instead refers to its diplomates—individuals certified both before and after its establishment as an independent Board—as Board-certified sleep specialists.

THE AMERICAN BOARD OF SLEEP MEDICINE
Examination Process

The examination is administered in two parts:

PART I is a multiple-choice written examination administered in October of each year at several U.S. locations. Part I tests the general body of knowledge in sleep medicine and clinical polysomnography. It covers sleep-related subjects in physiology, neuroanatomy, biochemistry, pharmacology, endocrinology, psychophysiology, and psychopathology, as well as sleep–wake disorders (including etiology, epidemiology, symptomatology, diagnostic procedures, and treatment); sleep in other medical, psychiatric, and neurological disorders; patient safety issues; legal–medical issues; and the basic skills of monitoring, record reading, and interpretation.

Part I is divided into three multiple-choice sections. Booklet I emphasizes the basic science of sleep, and Booklet II emphasizes clinical disorders of sleep. Booklet III uses fragments of polysomnograms and other displays to examine pattern recognition, sleep stage scoring, artifact recognition, interpretation, and diagnosis and treatment.

A candidate who fails Part I may retake it within 2 years. After 2 years or two consecutive failures of Part I, a candidate must submit a complete, new application, including all documentation. The candidate must meet the eligibility requirements in effect at the time of the reapplication before being accepted to retake Part I.

Successful completion of Part I confers eligibility to take Part II, which is given at a single location in April of each year.

PART II consists of questions based on clinical and polygraphic data from a sleep center that emphasizes interpretation of sleep studies, diagnosis of sleep disorders, and patient management skills. Short-answer and essay questions are included that focus on record reading, interpretation, and the ability to make diagnostic clinical assessment and patient management decisions. Successful completion of Part II leads to certification in the specialty of sleep medicine.

A candidate who fails Part II may retake it within 2 years. After 2 years or two successive failures of Part II, the candidate must submit a new application, including all documentation, and must retake and pass Part I before being allowed to take Part II again. All references to diagnostic classification refer to the terminology established by the *International Classification of Sleep Disorders*, published by the American Sleep Disorders Association, 1990.

Examination composition: Examination items are prepared by members of the Part I and Part II Examination Committees and other individuals certified by the American Board of Sleep Medicine. All items undergo extensive review before inclusion in the examination.

Scoring: All scoring is done without knowledge of the candidate's identity, and all decisions concerning examination scoring are made prior to the matching of names and code numbers. Once the code is broken, no decisions or individual scores are changed.

Examination results: The results of the examination, including overall test score and scores for each individual section, are mailed to candidates 2–3 months after the examination data. Results are not available by telephone. Candidates may request verification of their scores for a $100 fee.

Application Procedure

Applications for the examination may be obtained from the American Board of Sleep Medicine. Please call or write to:

Judith Morton, Examination Coordinator
American Board of Sleep Medicine
1610 14th Street, Suite 302
Rochester, MN 55901

Phone: (507) 287-9819
Fax: (507) 287-6008
E-mail: jmorton@millcomm.com

The deadline for receipt of a complete application by the Board at the preceding address is March 1. A complete application is defined as a fully completed application form, all supporting documentation requested on the application form (excluding letters of reference), and the examination fee of $450 for Part I. Checks should be made payable to the American Board of Sleep Medicine. The applicant will receive acknowledgment of receipt of the application. If such notification has not been received, please notify the Board immediately at the address given.

All licensing requirements must be satisfied and training completed by June 30 of the year of the Part I examination.

Late applications: A nonrefundable fee of $200 is assessed for late applications. No applicants will be accepted after April 1.

Application review and appeal procedure: All applications are reviewed by the Credentialing Committee of the Board, which determines whether the applicant is accepted or rejected. A rejected applicant who believes he or she meets the eligibility requirements can appeal the Committee's decision by submitting a written request detailing the reasons for the appeal and enclosing a review fee of $100. The applicant's credentials will then be reviewed by the Board of Directors, whose decisions will be final. Requests for appeal must be received at the office of the American Board of Sleep Medicine, 1610 14th Street NW, Suite 302, Rochester, MN 55901, within 2 weeks following notification of the decision.

Refunds and withdrawals: If the applicant is rejected by the Board, $300 will be refunded to the applicant. If an accepted candidate withdraws from the examination (either Part I or Part II) at least 4 weeks prior to the examination date, $200 will be refunded.

A candidate who withdraws within 4 weeks of the examination is not entitled to a refund, except when the withdrawal is the result of a documented emergency. The candidate may apply for the $200 emergency late withdrawal refund by submitting proper documentation of the emergency.

A candidate who withdraws from either Part I or Part II must take that part at its next scheduled administration to maintain eligibility.

Eligibility Requirements

Please read these requirements carefully and use them to evaluate your qualifications. The Credentialing Committee will examine each application for evidence that all requirements have been fully met.

1. Ph.D. degree (or an equivalent degree) with doctoral specialization in a health-related field.
2. Two years of full-time supervised clinical training or its equivalent that is comprehensive and sustained. One of the 2 years shall take place after receiving the doctoral degree. It is desirable that 1 year be spent in a broadly defined clinical training program (e.g., an internship in clinical psychology).
3. The equivalent of 1 year of full-time training in clinical sleep disorders under the supervision of a diplomate of the American Board of Sleep Medicine working in a sleep disorders center. The candidate shall receive satisfactory ratings by the Board-certified sleep specialist supervisor on the evaluation form provided by the Board (see **Evaluation by a Board-Certified Sleep Specialist**, next section). This year may overlap the clinical training required in Paragraph 2 above.
4. A fully completed application, including a satisfactory evaluation from a Board-certified sleep specialist, and three letters of reference.

In addition, the applicant shall

a. have evaluated a minimum of 50 patients, under supervision, including both interviewing and polysomnographic testing.
b. have interpreted 75 polysomnograms and 25 Multiple Sleep Latency Tests.
c. have carried out behavioral treatments for a minimum of 10 patients.
d. be familiar with the American Psychological Association's Ethical Standards of Psychologists.

The applicant must submit a letter that specifies how he or she meets Requirements 2 and 3. The applicant's training in clinical sleep disorders and all research conducted during the course of the year must be described in detail.

Evaluation by a Board-Certified Sleep Specialist

All applicants must provide the name of a Board-certified sleep specialist who has personal knowledge of the applicant's abilities in patient interviewing, record scoring, polysomnography interpretation, differential diagnosis, and treatment and follow-up care. The Board will contact the Board-certified sleep specialist and request an evaluation of the applicant's clinical competence in sleep medicine.

Suggested Reading List

Carskadon, M. A. (Ed.). (1992). *Encyclopedia of sleep and dreaming.* New York: Macmillan.

Chokroverty, S. (Ed.). (1994) *Sleep disorders medicine: Basic science, technical considerations, and clinical aspects.* Boston: Butterworth-Heinemann.

Daly, D. D., & Pedley, T. A. (Eds.). (1990) *Current practice of clinical EEG* (2nd ed.). New York: Raven Press.

Ferber, R., & Kryger, M. (1995). *Principles and practice of sleep medicine in the child.* Philadelphia: Saunders.

Hauri, P. (Ed.). (1991). *Case studies in insomnia.* New York: Plenum Press.

Horne, J. A. (1988). *Why we sleep.* Oxford, England: Oxford University Press.

Kryger, M. H., Roth, T., & Dement, W. C. (Eds.). (1994). *Principles and practice of sleep medicine* (2nd ed.). Philadelphia: Saunders.

Lydic, R., & Biebuyck, J. F. (Eds.). (1988). *Clinical physiology of sleep.* New York: Oxford University Press.

Mendelson, W. (1987). *Human sleep: Research and clinical care.* New York: Plenum Press.

Morin, C. M. (1993). *Insomnia: Psychological assessment and management.* New York: Guilford Press.

Shepard, J. W. (Ed.). (1991) *Atlas of sleep medicine.* Mount Kisco, NY: Futura.

Thorpy, M. J. (Ed.). (1991). *Handbook of sleep disorders.* Mount Kisco, NY: Futura.

Tyner, F., Knott, J. R., & Mayer, W. B. (1983). *Fundamentals of EEG technology: Vol. 1. Basic concepts and methods.* New York: Raven Press.

Author Index

Aaron, J., 389, *397*
Abbrecht, P. H., 286, *296*
Åberg, H., 453, *459*
Abramowitz, J. S., 470, *479*
Abramsky, O., 89, *107*
Abramson, H. S., 379, *381*
Acres, J. C., 286, *295*
Adams, H. P., *382*
Agnew, H., 237, *246*
Agnew, H. W., 39, *56*, 97, 98, 99, *105*, 467, *478*
Agnew, H. W., Jr., 92, 94, *110*
Aguglia, U., 261, *280*
Ahmed, S., 49, *54*
Åkerstedt, T., 47, *52*, 88, *105*, *109*, 251, 254, 257, *263*, *264*, 404, 406, *420*, *422*
Albers, H. E., *54*
Albertario, C. A., *478*
Aldaz, J. A., 327, *336*
Aldhous, M., 51, *52*
Aldrich, M. S., 65, 66, *70*, *71*, 378, *380*
Alexander, S. D., 328, *334*
Allan, J. S., *32*, *53*, 239, 245, *246*, 263
Allegretta, A., *380*
Allen, K. M., *279*
Allen, R., *159*
Allen, R. P., *295*
Allen, T., 326, *335*
Almqvist, M., 452, *461*
Altaescu, G., 388, *400*
Alvarez, B., 232, *245*
Alvarez, W. A., 309, *312*
Ameabe, Y., 378, *383*
American Hospital Association, 386, *397*
American Psychiatric Association, 61, *70*, 133, 134, 144, 148, 154, *158*, 484, *499*
American Psychiatric Association Task Force on Benzodiazepine Dependency, 341, *353*

American Sleep Disorders Association, 60, *70*, 113, *121*, 135, 136, 142, 144, 146, 148, 152, 154, *158*, 229, 232, 233, 235, 239, 240, 241, 243, *246*, 290, *295*, 316, *333*
Anand, V. K., 301, *312*
Anch, A. M., 19, 28, *32*, 85, 86, *105*, 284, *296*
Ancoli-Israel, S., 25, *32*, 65, *70*, 118, *121*, 185, 188, *189*, 375, *380*, 449, 450, 451, 452, *459*, *461*
Anderer, P., *354*
Anders, T. F., *174*
Anderson, M., 48, *53*
Anderson, M. W., 148, *158*, 317, *334*
Anlauer, P., *265*
Antic, R., 103, *106*, 287, *295*
Antony-Baas, V., 19, *34*
Antrobus, J. S., 21, *33*
Arand, D. C., 323, *334*
Arand, D. L., 77, 103, *105*
Arce, C., *106*
Arendt, J., 51, *52*, *56*, 67, *71*
Argentino, C., 374, *380*
Arkin, A. M., 495, *499*
Armington, J. C., 85, *105*
Armstrong, P., 289, *297*
Arnold, J. L., 188, *190*
Asberg, M., 346, *353*
Aschoff, J., 35, 39, 41, 47, 51, *52*, *53*, 249, 254, *263*
Aserinsky, E., 21, *32*, 111, *121*, 493, *499*
Ashkenasy, J. J., 378, *380*
Askenasy, J. J., 496, *501*
Askenasy, J. J. M., 98, *107*
Asplund, R., 453, *459*
Association of Sleep Disorders Centers, 60, *70*, 112, *121*
Atkins, J., 470, *478*
Atkinson, R. L., 289, *297*

Attanasio, R., 68, 70
Aubert, G., 392, 400
Aurell, J., 386, 397
Avery, D. H., 452, 463

Bach, V., 94, 105
Backman, L., 83, 109
Bad, S., 72
Badia, P., 103, 107, 452, 462
Badr, S., 122, 281
Baekeland, R., 25, 33
Baele, P., 392, 400
Baker, D. I., 453, 462
Baker, T., 84, 106
Balfours, E. M., 375, 381
Ballinger, C. B., 452, 459
Balsano, F., 380
Balter, M. B., 125, 159, 329, 338, 344, 353, 488, 501
Bamford, J., 384
Barnes, C. D., 28, 34
Barocka, A., 87, 106
Baron, R., 386, 397
Barry, T., 125, 127, 159, 492, 501
Barthlen, G. M., 379, 381
Bartle, E. J., 108
Bartlett, D., 88, 108, 394, 399
Bartnicke, B., 422
Baskett, J. J., 390, 397
Bates, D., 383
Batista, A., 380, 383
Bauer, M. S., 399
Baumgartner, A., 89, 90, 95, 105
Becker, C. E., 92, 108
Beckman, B., 166, 174
Beersma, D. G., 48, 52, 53, 54
Belenky, G., 108
Bell, J. S., 324, 334
Benca, R. M., 171, 173, 345, 353, 413, 420, 457, 460, 483, 499
Benich, J. J., 286, 295
Benkert, R. E., 458, 460
Benoit, O., 253, 264
Bensimon, G., 255, 264
Benson, A. J., 241, 247
Benson, H., 336, 492, 500
Benson, K. L., 493, 503

Bentley, S., 389, 397
Benz, R. L., 372, 373, 374, 381, 383
Berger, H., 12, 32
Bergmann, B., 412, 421
Bergmann, B. M., 29, 34, 96, 109, 260, 265, 395, 400, 414, 415, 420, 421, 422, 423
Bergofsky, E., 372, 382
Berkman, L. F., 29, 34
Berlin, R. M., 393, 397, 473, 477
Berman, S. R., 446, 462, 499, 502
Bernstein, D. A., 322, 334
Berry, D. T. R., 270, 279, 451, 460, 463
Berry, R. B., 103, 105, 346, 353
Berry, T., 327, 337
Berthon-Jones, M., 88, 110, 112, 122, 291, 297, 300, 313, 364, 369
Bettinardi, O., 324, 337
Bidwell, T., 462
Bikelman, A., 268, 279
Biller, J., 382
Bird, H. A., 452, 462
Bisson, R. U., 214, 224
Bittman, E. L., 54
Bixler, E., 204, 207
Bixler, E. O., 57, 70, 488, 500
Blachy, P. H., 395, 397
Black, J., 335
Blake, R. L., 476, 477
Bledsoe, T. A., 392, 397
Bleecker, E. R., 295
Blevins, W. L., 296
Bliwise, D., 207, 443, 458, 460
Bliwise, D. L., 186, 188, 301, 313, 321, 333, 378, 381, 443, 446, 447, 448, 449, 453, 454, 455, 458, 459, 460, 461, 462, 484, 499
Bliwise, N. G., 47, 53, 242, 246, 449, 455, 456, 459, 460, 461
Block, A. J., 270, 279, 285, 295
Blood, M., 51, 55
Blumenthal, S. J., 475, 477
Blunt, V. A., 470, 478
Boecker, M. R., 452, 462
Bohlman, M. E., 295
Bokan, J., 463
Bokan, J. A., 463

Bonnet, M. H., 77, 78, 81, 100, 101, 102, 103, *105*, *106*, 323, *334*, 486, *502*
Bonora, M., 392, *397*
Boomkamp, A., *207*
Bootzin, R. R., 131, 135, 150, 152, *158*, 315, 318, 319, 320, 321, 322, 323, 326, *334*, *337*, *338*
Borbely, A. A., 52, *53*, 94, *96*, 186, *189*
Borgeson, S. E., 375, *381*, 392, *399*
Borkovec, T. D., 322, 323, *334*, *338*, 487, 490, *499*, *500*
Borland, R. G., 79, *106*
Boulos, Z., 70, *247*
Bourdeleau, P., *265*
Bourdin, H., *108*
Bowes, G., 394, *397*
Bowman, T. O., *398*
Boyd, M., *110*
Boylan, M. B., 323, 324, *337*
Boys, R., *33*
Bradley, C., 349, *354*
Bradlow, H., *247*
Bragdon, A. C., 188, *190*
Branconnier, R., 77, *107*
Branham, G. H., 301, *312*
Branum, J. P., 346, *353*
Bredle, D. L., 390, *398*
Brendel, D. H., 77, *106*
Breuninger, W., *478*
Brink, D., 331, *337*
Brocklehurst, J. C., 453, *461*
Brodan, V., 403, *422*
Brodanová, M., 403, *422*
Brooks, D. N., 322, 329, 330, *335*
Brooks, J. O., III, 186, *189*, 443, *461*
Broughton, R., 82, *107*, 206, *207*, 211, 214, 217, 218, *223*, *224*, *225*, 326, *397*
Broughton, R. J., 41, *54*, 163, *173*, 185, 186, *189*, *190*
Browman, C. P., 19, *32*, 85, 86, *105*, 166, *175*, 180, *190*, 216, 219, 220, *224*, 283, *295*
Browman, K. E., *461*
Brown, C. F., 88, *108*
Brown, E., 65, *70*

Brown, E. D., 103, *106*, 447, *461*
Brown, E. N., 36, *53*, *263*
Brown, F. W., *503*
Brown, J. M., 245, *246*
Brown, L. W., 116, *122*
Brown, P., 30, *33*
Brown, R., 297, 412, 413, *421*
Brownell, L. G., 286, *295*, 470, *477*
Bruder, S., *264*
Brugge, K. L., 452, *461*
Brunner, D. P., 94, *106*
Bryan, A. C., *296*
Buchan, W., 483, *499*
Buchanan, R. T., 278, *280*
Buchsbaum, M. S., *110*
Buck, A., 178, *189*
Budzynski, T. H., 324, *332*
Buffenstein, A., 341, *355*
Bundlie, S., 201, *208*
Bundlie, S. R., 69, 71, 112, *122*
Bunney, W. E., 87, *110*, 497, *503*
Bünning, E., 38, *53*
Burden, S., 372, *381*
Burgio, K. L., 453, *461*
Burke, T. V., 88, *109*, 394, *399*
Buruera, J. A., 378, *383*
Burwell, C., 268, *279*
Busis, N. A., 451, *464*
Buton, B. H., *478*
Buysse, D. J., 70, *159*, 448, *461*, *462*, *463*, 498, *499*
Bye, P. T., 364, *369*
Byerley, W., 63, *71*
Byerley, W. F., 342, *353*

Cadieux, R. J., 392, *399*
Cahalane, J. F., 491, *503*
Caldwell, A. B., 130, *159*, 455, *462*, 488, *500*
Campbell, D. E., *421*
Campbell, P. I., *502*
Campbell, S., 48, *53*, 454, *463*
Campbell, S. S., 40, 41, 42, 43, *53*, 70, 148, *158*, 317, *334*
Campell, S., *247*
Campell-Grossman, C., 390, *398*
Campos-Barros, A., *105*

Canet, E., 94, *106*
Cantell, K., *422*
Caplan, H. J., *383*
Caplan, L. R., *382*
Carey, E., 458, *460*
Carlsson-Nordlander, B., 290, *296*
Carpenter, G, *502*
Carroll, P., 99, *107*
Carskadon, M., 65, *70*, 206, *207*, 211,
    224, 389, *397*
Carskadon, M. A., 14, 19, 22, 26, 32,
    47, *53*, 92, 93, 103, *106*, 115, *121*,
    161, 162, 163, *174*, *175*, 177, 178,
    180, 185, 186, *188*, *190*, *191*, 206,
    207, 209, 210, 213, 215, 219, 220,
    223, 224, 242, *246*, 310, *312*, 447,
    458, *459*, *460*, 461, 484, *499*
Cartwright, R. D., 287, 288, *295*
Caruso, L., 63, *71*
Caruso, L. S., 128, 129, *160*
Case, W. G., 330, *337*
Casey, K. R., *400*
Caverly, C. B., 470, *479*
Cerami, A., 417, *423*
Cervinka, R., 256, *265*
Chambers, G., 301, *312*
Chambers, H. F., 417, *422*
Chambers, M. J., 328, *334*
Charbonneau, M., 470, *477*
Charlton, P. D., *398*
Charney, D. S., *500*
Chavagnat, J. J., *313*
Chediak, A. D., 419, *422*
Chedid, L., 403, *422*
Chen, H., 88, *106*, 394, *397*
Cherniak, N. S., 285, *295*
Chernik, D., 491, *500*
Cheshire, K. E., 311, *312*
Chevalier, A., 430, *449*
Cinque, J., *246*
Cirignotta, F., 268, 269, *280*
Claman, D., *335*
Clark, G., 480, *478*
Clark, G. L., *382*
Clark, M., 67, *71*
Cleary, P. D., 251, *264*
Clerk, A., *335*

Clift, A. D., 394, *398*
Cobarrubias, M., 450, *459*
Cobert, B., *503*
Coble, P., 493, *501*
Coble, P. A., *159*, 215, 225, 487, *502*
Cockrem, J. F., 390, *397*
Cohen, H., 487, *500*
Cohen, S. A., 47, *53*, 242, *246*
Cohn, M. A., *246*, 419, *422*
Cole, R. J., 186, *190*, 218, *223*, 251,
    255, *263*
Cole, W. E., 32, *34*, 116, *122*
Colecchi, C. A., 331, *337*
Coleman, R., *160*, 203, 206, *207*
Coleman, R. M., 72, 230, 232, *246*,
    248, 254, *263*
Colligan, M. J., 251, 257, 260, *263*, *266*
Collins, K. J., 452, *461*
Colquhoun, W. P., 75, *106*, 251, 256,
    263, *265*
Comi, G., *381*
Commella, C. L., 378, *381*, 465, *461*
Connel, L. J., 243, *246*
Connell, L. J., 47, *54*, 215, *224*
Conner, R., 496, *501*
Connolly, L. A., 391, 392, 393, *398*
Connolly, S. J., 375, *381*, 392, *398*
Conroy, R. T., 35, *53*
Conway, W., 270, *280*, 375, *381*, 392,
    398
Conway, W. A., *224*
Cook, B. L., 330, *337*
Cook, W. R., 286, *295*
Cook, Y. R., *460*
Cooper, K. R., 88, *109*, 394, *399*
Coppola, M., *190*
Corsi-Cabrera, M., 85, *106*
Corson, W. A., *190*
Cosio, M. G., 470, *477*
Cote, L., *462*
Coulson, A. H., *313*
Coursey, R. D., 324, *334*
Cox, K., 393, *398*
Coy, T., 118, *121*
Coyle, K., 327, *336*
Coyne, L., 326, *335*
Crile, G. W., 412, *421*

Criner, G. J., 396, *399*
Crocker, B. D., 264, *279*
Cromwell, R. I., 495, *502*
Cropp, A. J., 390, *398*
Culbert, J. P., 317, 318, 321, 333, *337*
Curless, R. H., *383*
Curzon, G., *478*
Czeisler, C., *160*
Czeisler, C. A., 28, *32*, 36, *43*, 48, *53*, *54*, *52*, 84, *106*, 135, *159*, *174*, 209, 224, 239, 244, 245, *246*, *247*, *248*, 251, 254, 258, 261, *263*, *264*, *265*

Daan, S., 48, 52, *53*, *54*
Dahl, R. E., 115, *121*
Dahlitz, M. J., 232, *245*
D'Allest, A. M., 94, *106*
D'Alonzo, G. E., 396, *399*
Daughaday, W., 28, *34*
Davenne, D., *108*, 411, *422*
Davenport, Y., *55*
Davidson, J. R., 403, *422*
Davies, D. R., 330, 331, *334*
Davies, H., *461*
Davis, A. W., 88, *107*
Davis, D. M., 494, *500*
Davis, J. E., 389, *400*
Davis, N. S., 430, *439*
Davison, G. C., 332, *334*
Dawson, D., 43, 48, *53*, 148, *158*, 316, 317, *334*, *337*
Deary, I. J., 308, 311, *312*
DeBehnke, R. D., 276, *280*
deBruyn, L., *207*
de Candolle, A. P., 38, *53*
Decker, M. J., 188, *190*
Decoster, F., *264*
Dee, P., 289, *297*
deGroot, W. J., 272, *281*, 284, *296*
Dehan, M., 94, *106*
De Joseph, J. F., 466, *478*
de la Torre, B., 89, *105*, 406, *420*
Del Conte, A., *478*
DeLisser, E. A., 393, *400*
De Los Santos, L., *478*
de Mairan, J., 38, *53*
DeMartino, M. F., 495, *499*

Dement, W., 27, *32*, 65, *70*, *72*, 80, 94, *106*, *107*, *174*, 204, 206, *207*, 211, 213, 223, 224, 443, *460*, 496, *501*
Dement, W. C., 22, 25, 26, 30, *32*, *33*, *34*, 47, *53*, *54*, 57, 58, *71*, 93, 94, 103, *106*, *109*, 112, 113, 116, *122*, *160*, 161, 162, 163, 164, 165, *174*, *175*, 177, 186, *190*, 209, 210, 213, 215, 220, 223, 224, 225, 236, 242, *246*, *248*, 273, *279*, 285, 295, 301, 313, 376, *382*, 395, *400*, 443, 447, 454, 455, 458, *459*, *460*, *461*, 499
Dempsey, J., *72*, *122*, *281*, *462*
Dennis, M., *384*
DePrins, J., *265*
Derderian, S. S., *296*
Derk-Jan, D., *247*
DeRoshia, C. W., 48, *56*
Desa, M. M., 346, *353*
Devinsky, O., 379, *381*
Dew, M. A., *462*
de Wall, L. P., *383*
Dewan, E., 31, *32*
Dexter, J., 100, *106*
Diagnostic Classification Steering Committee, 212, 220, 224, *465*, 477
Diaz-Guerrero, R., 237, *246*
Dickel, M. J., 451, *461*
Dickins, Q. S., *110*
Dietzel, M., *105*
Dijk, D., 84, *106*
Dijk, D. J., 43, 48, *54*, 66, *70*, 94, *106*, 247
DiMatteo, M. R., 306, 308, *312*, *313*
Dinarello, C. A., 403, *422*
Dinges, D., *382*
Dinges, D. F., 41, *54*, *174*, 209, 215, 224, 260, *263*, 303, 308, *312*, *313*, 403, 404, 405, 406, *421*
Doerr, P., *52*
Doghramji, K., *478*
Dohno, S., 386, *398*
Dollinger, S. L., 430, *439*
Dolly, F. R., 285, *295*
Domar, A. D., *336*
Donnell, J. M., 81, *106*

Doran, B. R. H., 392, *400*
Dore, C., 452, *461*
Dore, P., *313*
Douglas, J., 318, *337*
Douglas, N. J., 309, 311, *312*, 365, 366, *369*, 394, *400*
Douglas, S. D., 260, *263*, *421*
Downey, R., 100, 101, 103, *106*
Dozier, J. E., 495, *502*
Drake, M. E., 379, *382*
Driver, H. S., 468, 475, *477*
Drucker-Colin, R., 30, *33*
Dudley, H., 381, *397*
Dudley, H. A. F., 386, *399*
Duffy, J. F., *53*, 245, *246*, *263*
Duke, P., *174*
Dunham, D. W., 218, *224*
Dunham, W., *223*
Dunleavy, D. L. F., 30, *33*
Duron, B., 112, *121*, 268, *280*
Durrer, D, 104, *110*
Duschesne, P., *223*
Dyken, M. E., 376, *381*

Eastman, C. I., 48, *54*, *70*, 244, *246*, *247*, 251, *253*
Ebert, D., 87, *106*
Edelman, N. H., 87, *109*, 394, *400*
Edinger, J. D., 127, *159*, 219, *224*, 321, 328, *334*, 488, *500*
Edwards, S. A., 494, *500*
Egan, P., 386, *399*
Ehlers, C. L., 475, *478*
Ehrenberg, B., 379, *381*
Ehrenpreis, A. B., 488, *500*
Ehrhart, J., 19, *34*
Eichler, V. B., 45, *55*
Eiken, T., 195, *190*
Eisen, J., 405, *422*
Eisenstein, R. B., 393, *399*
Ekblad, U. U., 473, *477*
Ekbom, K., 471, *477*
Ekbom, K. A., 64, *71*
Ekholm, E. M., 473, *477*
Eldridge, F., 162, *174*
Eldridge, F. L., 285, *295*
Ellman, S. J., 21, *33*, 99, *107*

Elmqvist, D., 386, *397*
Emsellem, H. A., 188, *190*
Endo, S., 47, *55*, 243, *247*
Engle-Friedman, M., 320, 321, *334*
Engleman, H. M., 309, 311, *312*
Eno, E. N., 324, *338*
Epstein, D., 3, *334*
Epstein, D. R., 328, *325*
Eriksson, B., 346, *333*
Erman, M., 33, 217, *224*
Erman, M. K., 166, 169, *174*, *175*, 368, *369*, *502*
Erwin, C. W., 218, *224*
Eschenbach, K., 415, *421*
Espie, C. A., 152, *158*, 322, 329, 330, *335*
Espinoza, H., 103, *106*, 287, *295*
Ettinger, M., 101, *208*
Ettinger, M. G., 69, *71*, 112, *122*
Eveloff, S. E., *399*
Everson, C. A., 29, *34*, 36, *109*, 395, *398*, *400*, 412, 414, 415, 416, 417, *420*, *421*, *422*, *423*
Eves, L., 112, *122*, 291, *297*, 300, *313*
Eveslage, J., 291, *296*
Exton-Smith, A. N., 452, *461*
Eyland, E. A., 452, *462*

Fahn, S., *462*
Fahrion, S. L., 326, *335*
Falcone, T., 470, *477*
Fang, V. S., 415, *420*, *421*, *422*
Färkkilä, M., *483*
Farr, L. A., 390, *398*
Farrell, P., 372, *381*
Fasiczka, A. L., *461*, *501*, *502*
Fassbender, K., *421*, *423*
Fast, A., 474, *477*, *478*
Fatranska, M., *52*
Fein, A. M., *478*
Feinberg, I., 84, *106*
Feinberg, R., 217, *224*
Feinsilver, S. H., 470, *477*, *478*
Feinstein, B., 324, *335*
Feistel, H., 87, *106*
Feldman, D. E, *460*
Fell, R., *62*, *121*, 380, *459*

Fenollosa, B., 378, *383*
Fenton, G., *478*
Ferber, R., 113, *122*, 188, *190*, 494, *500*
Ferguson, P. W., 301, *312*
Ferini-Stambi, L., 379, *381*
Fertig, J., *108*
FICSIT Group, 453, *462*
Fieschi, P., *390*
Figueroa, W. G., *383*, *463*
Filippi, M., *381*
Findley, L., 161, *174*
Findley, L. J., 267, 270, 271, *279*, *280*
Fine, J., 494, *500*
Fiorica, V., 88, *107*
Fireman, M. J., *55*
Fischman, M. W., 79, *107*
Fish, D., *383*
Fisher, C., 112, *122*, 494, *500*
Fisher, J., 26, *33*, 130, *159*, 488, *500*
Fixley, M. S., 270, *280*
Flagg, W., *175*, *207*
Fleetham, J., *190*
Fletcher, E. C., 276, *280*
Fogg, L. F., 242, *246*
Folkard, S., 67, *71*, 251, 254, 256, 257, 261, *263*, *264*, *265*
Folkerts, M., *109*
Follingstad, D. R., 323, *335*
Ford, D., 57, 59, *71*
Ford, D. E., 114, *121*, 489, *500*
Foret, J., 255, *264*
Fortier, J., *109*
Foster, F. G., 484, *501*
Foulkes, M. A., *382*
Fouque, D., 374, *382*
Frank, E., *463*, 475, 477, *478*, *501*, *502*
Frank, K. A., *398*
Frankel, B. L., 324, *334*
Franklin, K. A., 375, *381*
Franklin Writings, 395, *398*
Fredrickson, P. A., 170, *174*, 396, *353*
Freedman, R. F., 323, 324, *335*
Freedman, R. R., 323, *335*
Freeman, C. R., 211, *224*
Freinhar, J. P., 309, *312*
Freitag, W. D., *263*
Freitag, W. O., *32*

French, J., 214, *224*
French, J. M., *383*
Freud, S., 21, *33*
Frey, R., *354*
Friberg, Y., 89, *105*
Friedman, L., 186, *189*, 321, 322, *335*, 443, 456, *461*, 484, *499*
Friedman, L. F., 453, *461*
Friedman, R., *336*, 492, *500*
Friedmann, J., 92, *107*
Fröberg, J., 89, *109*, 422
Froberg, J. E., 89, *105*
Frommlet, M. S., 454, *463*
Fry, J., 453, *461*
Fry, J. M., 116, *122*
Fuchs, D., *423*
Fujita, S., 289, *295*
Fukumasu, H., *478*
Fuller, C. A., 27, *33*, 39, 44, 43, *54*, *55*
Funch, D. P., 494, *500*
Fyhrquist, F., *463*

Gaarder, K. R., 324, *334*
Gadbois, C., 258, *264*
Gaillard, J., 201, *207*
Gaillard, R. C., *108*
Galanos, C., *423*
Gale, E. N., 494, *500*
Gallagher, K., *478*
Gallup Organization, 125, *158*, 348, *363*
Gander, P. H., 47, 243, *246*
Garamoni, G. L., *501*, *502*
Gardner, D., 166, *174*
Garfinkel, L., 29, *33*, 260, *265*, 452, *461*
Garnett, D., 265, *296*
Garnier, A., *108*
Garvey, M. J., 330, *337*
Gaspar, T., 390, *398*
Gastaut, H., 112, *121*, 268, *280*
Gaulier, B., 125, *159*
Gaultier, C., 94, *106*
Gay, C., 472, 475, *479*
Gay, T. J. A., 386, *399*
Gee, J. B., 285, *296*
Gelber, D., 376, *381*

Genser, S. G., 88, *107*
Georgi, K., *110*
Gerard, P., 452, 453, *461*
Gerber, C., *463*
Getsy, J. E., 308, 310, 311, *312*, *382*
Ghanem, Q., *223*
Ghata, J. N., 251, *265*
Gibbons, P., *110*
Gibson, M., *54*
Gidro-Frank, S., 206, *207*, *462*
Giedke, H., *52*
Gilbert, A., 331, *335*
Giles, D. E., *502*
Gillberg, M., 89, *105*, 406, *420*
Gilliland, M., 415, *421*
Gilliland, M. A., 29, *34*, 96, *109*, 260, *265*, 395, *400*, 414, 415, *421*, *423*
Gillin, J., 63, *71*
Gillin, J. C., *55*, *108*, *110*, 135, *158*, 186, *190*, 218, *223*, 239, *247*, 285, *296*, 342, 347, *353*, 457, *460*, 483, 497, *499*, *492*
Gilmore, R. L., *460*
Gimbel, K. S., 386, *398*
Gislason, T., 462, *461*
Gitlin, D. A., *400*
Gladstone, W. R., *54*
Glaros, A. G., 332, *334*
Glazer, G., 89, *107*
Gleich, G. J., *296*
Glenville, M., 82, 83, *107*
Globus, G., *107*
Glovinsky, P., 63, *71*, 232, *247*
Glovinsky, P. B., 99, *107*, 126, 128, 129, 130, 146, *159*, *160*, 232, *248*, 322, *335*
Godbout, R., 372, 373, *382*
Goldberg, J., 376, *381*
Goldman, M. D., *400*
Goldman, S. M., *295*
Gomez, S. A., 211, *224*
Gong, H., *313*
Good, D. C., 376, *381*
Good, R., 323, *335*
Goodenough, D. R., 487, 493, 495, *500*
Goodnow, J. J., 81, *110*
Goodrich, C. A., 409, *422*

Goodwin, F. K., 48, *59*, *55*, 142, *159*, 255, *266*
Gorczynski, R., 403, *422*
Gorczynski, R. M., 405, *422*
Gordon, D. L., *382*
Gordon, N. P., 251, 257, *264*
Gordon, S. H., 396, *398*
Gorin, A. B., 276, *280*
Gothe, B., 285, *295*
Gottlieb, J. S., 237, *246*
Gould, D., *190*
Graeber, R. C., 47, *54*, 174, 209, 215, 224, 242, 243, *246*
Graf, K. J., *105*
Graham, P. J., 430, *439*
Gramling, S. E., 488, *501*
Granström, M., *422*
Grayson, J. B., 322, *334*
Green, L., 495, *302*
Green, R. L., 243, *247*
Greenberg, H. E., 372, *382*
Greenblatt, D. J., *175*, 329, 330, *337*, *338*, 341, *353*
Greenfield, B., *296*
Greenspon, L. W., *463*
Greenwood, K. M., 317, 332, 335, *337*
Gregory, K. B., 243, *246*
Gresham, S., 237, *246*
Griffiths, L., 453, *461*
Griffiths, R. R., 344, *353*
Groos, G., 45, *55*
Gross, R. T., 417, *500*
Gruen, W., 196, *190*, 218, *223*
Grunberger, J., *354*
Grunstein, R. R., 286, *293*
Gudewill, S., 410, *421*, *423*
Guevara, M. A., *106*
Guilleminault, C., 162, 170, *174*, *175*, 188, *191*, 204, 205, 207, 211, *224*, 225, *246*, 267, 269, 290, 285, 290, 295, *296*, 301, *313*, 317, *335*, 375, 376, *381*, *382*, *383*, 392, *398*, *399*, *461*, *499*
Guillet, P., *265*
Gujavarty, K., 372, *382*
Gujavarty, K. S., 166, *175*, 180, *190*, 295

Gujavarty, S., 216, 219, 220, *224*
Gulevich, G., 80, *107*
Gundel, A., *56*
Gupta, M. A., 474, 475, *477*
Gyulay, S., 188, *190*
Gyulay, S. G., *279*

Hackett, S., *190*
Haefely, W., 340, *353*
Hagen, J. H., 396, *399*
Hahn, P. M., *295*, 449, *462*
Haider, M., *265*
Hairston, L. E., 272, *281*
Hajdukovic, R., 217, *224*
Hajdukovic, R. M., 169, *175*, 449, *462*
Halberg, F., 35, 36, *54*, *55*
Halfens, R., 393, 394, *398*
Hall, C. S., 21, *33*
Hall, W. V., *336*
Hallett, M., 272, *281*, 372, *381*
Halpin, D., *462*
Hamilton, C. R., 22, *33*
Hammond, E. C., 29, *33*, 240, *265*
Hanley, J., *33*
Hanninen, O., 251, *264*
Hanning, C. D., 392, *398*
Hansell, H. N., 389, 396, *398*
Hanson, B. S., 452, *461*
Haponik, E. F., 289, *295*
Harbison, L., 451, *463*
Hardin, J. M., *461*
Harma, M. I., 251, *264*
Harper, R. M., 272, *280*
Harrington, M. E., 235, *246*
Harris, D. L., 477, *478*
Harris, P. D., *398*
Harris, R. B., 443, *460*
Hartman, P. G., 98, *110*, 135, *160*, 215, *225*
Hartmann, E., 25, 30, *33*, 77, *107*, 324, *335*
Hartse, K., *225*
Hartse, K. M., 166, *174*, 217, *224*
Harvey, E. N., 12, *33*
Harvey, K., *174*
Haskell, W. L., 443, *460*
Hastie, S. J., 470, *478*

Hathaway, S. R., 133, *159*
Hauri, P., 26, *33*, 213, *224*, 324, 325, *335*, *336*
Hauri, P. J., 130, 136, 152, *159*, 186, *190*, 257, *264*, 317, *335*, 488, 490, 491, *500*
Hausfeld, J. N., *190*
Hawkins, D., 491, *500*
Hayes, A. J., *159*
Hayes, B., 84, *106*
Haynes, S. N., 323, 324, *335*
Hays, M. B., 288, *297*
Hays, R. D., 306, *313*
Hazlett, E., *110*
Hazlewood, L., 320, 321, *334*
He, J., 270, *280*, 375, *381*, 392, *398*
Healey, D. W., 451, *462*
Healey, P. J., 451, *462*
Healey, S., *70*, 130, *159*, 455, *462*
Heaton, S., *108*
Hedemark, L. L., 285, *295*
Heffler, D., 322, *336*
Heitmann, A., 214, *225*
Hellekson, C., 324, *335*
Heller, S. S., 396, *398*
Helton, M. C., 390, *398*
Hening, W. A., 451, *462*
Henkle, J. Q., 376, *381*
Henley, K., 495, *500*
Hennessey, A., 341, *355*
Henriet, M. T., *108*
Henry, J. N., *313*, *382*
Hensley, M. J., 272, *279*, *281*, 286, *296*, *297*
Henson, D., 356, *369*
Henton, C. L., 493, *500*
Herman, J. H., 21, *33*
Hershey, T., *110*
Hershko, C., 388, *400*
Hertel, A., *110*
Hertz, G., 466, 467, 469, 470, 471, 474, 475, 477, *478*
Hertzman, P. A., 286, *296*
Herz, L., 454, *463*
Heuser, G., 31, *33*
Hier, D. B., *382*
Higgins, E. A., 88, *107*

Hildebrandt, G., 255, *264*
Hill, M. W., 285, *296*
Hill, N. S., *399*
Hill, T., 389, *396*
Hiller, F. C., 215, *225*
Hilton, B. A., 386, 388, *398*
Hindmarch, I., 452, *462*
Hirsch, N. P., *383*
Hirshkowitz, M., 22, 25, 33, 185, *190*
Hishikawa, Y., *223, 246, 462*
Hla, K. M., 450, *462*
Ho, A., 475, *478*
Ho, S., *175*
Hoban, T. M., 48, *54*
Hobart, G. A., 12, *33*
Hobson, J. A., 21, *33*
Hoch, C. C., 456, 446, 448, *462, 463,*
    499, 502
Hoddes, E., 164, 165, *174,* 211, 213, *224*
Hoehler, K., 468, *478*
Hoelscher, T. J., 127, *159,* 188, *190,*
    321, *334,* 488, *500*
Hofeldt, F., *296*
Hoff, J. I., *383*
Hoffman, K., 249, *263*
Hoffstein, V., 273, *280, 296*
Holley, D. C., 48, *56*
Holley, J. L., 371, *381*
Hollon, S. D., 331, *336*
Holsboer, F., *421, 423*
Holtzman, P., 415, *423*
Holzer, B. C., 215, *225,* 349, *353*
Hood, E. M., 322, *333*
Hor, G., *110*
Hori, H., *462*
Horne, J., 31, *33,* 402, *421*
Horne, J. A., 82, 85, 86, 95, *107,* 168,
    174, 255, *264,* 395, *398*
Hosboer, F., *423*
Houck, P. R., 456, *462, 463, 499, 402*
Howard, R. S., *383*
Howe, R. C., 324, *338*
Hozumi, S., *462*
Hughes, H. H., 324, *336*
Hughes, L., 236, *246*
Hughes, M., *381, 461*
Hughes, R. C., 324, *336*

Hulbert, J. R., *382*
Humm, T. M., *110*
Humphrey, F. J., *500*
Hunt, H., 310, *336*
Huntley, A., *107*
Hursch, C. J., 22, *34,* 485, *503*
Hurwitz, L. F., 456, *463*
Husband, A. J., 412, 413, *421*

Iampietro, P. F., 88, *106*
Iber, C., *190*
Icaza, E., *421*
Iijima, S., 237, *247*
Ilan, Y., 89, *107,* 388, *400*
Ilmarinen, J., 251, *266*
Imanaka, M., *478*
Imes, N. K., 271, 276, 273, *280, 281,*
    286, *296*
Inamorato, E., 380, *381*
Ingham, R. H., 458, *460*
Ingram, R. H., Jr., 272, *281, 297*
Ingrand, P., *313*
Innes, J. M., 331, *335*
Inouye, S. T., 45, *54*
International Classification of Diseases,
    9th revision, 60, *71*
International Classification of Diseases,
    9th revision, Clinical Modification,
    60, *71*
International Classification of Sleep
    Disorders, 113, *122*
Ionescou-Pioggia, M., 321, *334*
Irbe, D., *381,* 454, *461, 462*
Irwin, M., 347, *353*
Issa, F., 364, *369*
Issa, F. G., 88, *110,* 112, *122,* 289, 291,
    296, 287, 300, *313,* 375, *381*
Ives, D. G., *461*
Iwanaga, K., *478*

Jabbari, B., 286, *296*
Jabour, E. R., 161, *174*
Jacklet, J. W., 235, *246*
Jackson, J. M., 49, *54*
Jacob, M., 475, *476*
Jacobs, E. A., 488, *500*
Jacobs, G. D., 328, *336,* 492, *500*

Jacobsen, F. M., 48, *54*, *56*
Jacobson, A., 31, *33*
Jacobson, E., 322, *336*
Jacquier, M. C., *108*
Jakubowski, G., *463*
James, O. F., *383*
Jamieson, A., 375, *383*
Jarrett, D. B., 475, *477*
Jasinski, D. R., 393, *399*
Jasper, H. H., 181, *190*
Jennings, J. R., *501*, *502*
Jennum, P., 375, *381*, 392, *399*
Jeong, D., *175*
Jewett, M. E., *53*
Jilbert, A. R., 476, *478*
Jimbo, M., 112, *122*
Joel-Cohen, S. H., 470, *478*
Johns, M. W., 165, *174*, 213, 214, 224,
    386, 396, *399*
Johnson, F. H., 215, *225*
Johnson, L., 80, *107*
Johnson, L. C., 19, *34*, 80, 97, 98, *105*,
    107, *108*, 135, *158*, 211, *224*
Johnson, M. P., 245, *246*, *263*
Johnson, R. S., 331, *336*
Johnston, S. H., *159*
Jones, R., 185, *190*
Jones, S., 329, *337*, 492, *501*
Jonsson, B. G., 251, *264*
Jordan, J. B., 325, *336*
Joseph-Vanderpool, J. R., *159*
Jung, R., 104, *122*
Juvela, S., 366, *382*

Kaendler, S. H., *110*
Kahn, A., *463*
Kahn, E., 494, *500*
Kahn, R. L., 446, *463*
Kahn, R. M., *54*
Kalbfleish, J., *296*
Kales, A., 12, 14, 15, 17, 19, 22, 31, *33*,
    34, *70*, 111, *122*, 130, 132, 133,
    159, 184, *191*, *207*, 392, *399*, 455,
    462, 488, 494, *500*, *502*
Kales, J. D., *33*, *70*, 130, 133, *159*, 455,
    462, 488, 494, *500*, *502*
Kalski, R., *420*

Kalton, G., 453, *461*
Kamami, Y., 290, *296*
Kamei, R., 236, 237, *246*
Kamerow, D., 57, 59, *71*
Kamerow, D. B., 114, *121*, 489, *500*
Kamgar-Parsi, B., 239, *247*
Kamphuisen, H. A., *383*
Kant, G. J., 88, *107*
Kantameneni, B. D., *478*
Kantelip, J. P., *108*
Kapen, S., 376, *381*
Kaplan, J., 346, *353*
Kaplan, O., *70*, *121*, *380*, *459*
Kapoor, S. C., *421*
Karacan, I., 22, *33*, *34*, *246*, 371, *381*,
    448, *463*, 467, 475, *478*,485, *503*
Karadzic, V., 496, *501*
Karetsky, M., 387, *399*
Karlsson, C. -G., *422*
Karlsson, T., 83, *109*
Karni, A., 98, *107*, 496, *501*
Karnovsky, M. L., 409, 410, 411, *422*
Kaste, M., 374, *382*
Katsantonis, G. P., 301, *312*
Katsching, H., *265*
Katsuki, Y., 374, *384*
Kaukiainen, A., *463*
Kavey, N., 206, 207, *462*
Kawamura, H., 45, *54*
Kay, D. C., 393, *399*
Keamy, M. F., 392, *399*
Keenan, S., *190*, *223*
Keene, A., 390, *399*
Keener, T. M., *460*
Kehlet, H., 392, *400*
Kelly, K. A., *159*
Kelman, H. R., 489, *501*
Kendrick-Mohamed, J., *463*
Kennedy, G. J., 489, *501*
Kennedy, S. J., *246*
Kerkhof, G. A., *383*
Keystone, E., 405, *422*
Khuder, S., *336*
Kiel, M., 419, *422*
Kiesswetter, E., *264*
Kimmel, P. L., 371, 372, *381*, *382*, 492,
    462

King, A. C., 443, *460*
King, M. G., 412, 417, *421*
Kipnis, D., 28, *34*
Kirby, D. A., 361, *369*
Klauber, M. R., *70, 121, 380*, 450, *459*
Klein, T., 239, *247*
Kleitman, N., 21, 30, *32, 33*, 59, *71*,
    75, *107*, 111, *121*, 177, *190*, 402,
    403, 404, 412, *421*, 496, *501*
Klerman, E. B., 43, *54*
Kline, L. R., 302, 304, 307, 310, 311,
    313, 382
Klocke, R. A., 303, *313*
Kluger, M. J., 417, *422*
Knauth, P., 251, 254, 256, *264, 265*
Knott, J. R., 237, *246*
Knuth, S. L., 88, *108*, 394, *399*
Knutsson, A., 251, 259, *264*
Koella, W. P., 367, *369*
Kofke, W. A., 392, *399*
Kogi, K., 257, *264*
Kokkoris, C. P., 237, 240, *247*
Kollar, E. J., 85, 87, *107, 107*
Koller, M., 231, 256, *265*
Komiya, K., 379, *382*
Koob, G. F., 66, *71*
Korczyn, A. D., *225*
Korman, E., 232, *248*
Kornfeld, D. S., *398*
Koshorek, G., *225*, 345, *354*
Kostis, J. B., 349, *353*, 451, *462*
Koulack, D., 487, *500*
Kovar, S., 412, *421*
Kowall, J., 470, *478*
Kowall, J. P., 135, *160*
Kowatch, R., 327, *337*
Kowatch, R. A., 125, 127, *159*, 492,
    501
Koziol, J. A., 169, *175*, 217, *224*
Krachman, S. L., 396, *399*
Kraemer, H., *225, 460*
Kramer, M., 486, *502*
Kravitz, H., 288, *295*
Kravitz, R. L., 306, *313*
Kribbs, N. B., 100, *108*, 260, *263*, 302,
    303, 304, 307, 308, 310, 311, *312,*
    313, 374, *382*

Krieg, J. C., *423*
Krieger, J., 302, *313*
Krill, R. L., 387, *399*
Kripke, D. F., 25, 29, *32, 33*, 70, *121*,
    186, 188, *189, 190*, 218, *223*, 251,
    260, *263, 265*, 347, *353, 380*, 449,
    450, 452, *459, 461, 462*
Kronauer, R. E., *32*, 43, *53, 54*, 247,
    263
Kronauer, R. F., 245, *246*
Kronenberg, R. S., 285, *295*
Krueger, B. R., 170, *174*
Krueger, J. M., 403, 409, 410, 411,
    418, 419, *422, 423*
Krupka, M., *354*
Kryger, M. H., 58, *71*, 112, 113, *122*,
    270, *280*, 283, 286, *295, 296*, 375,
    381, 392, *398*, 470, *477*
Krystal, A. D., 218, *224*
Kubillus, S., 411, *422*
Kufferle, B., *265*
Kuhlo, W., 112, *122*
Kuhn, E., 403, 404, *422*
Kulkosky, P. J., 326, *337*
Kuller, L., *461*
Kuna, S. T., 272, *280*
Kundi, M., 256, *265*
Kupfer, D. J., 148, *159*, 215, *225*, 246,
    446, *461, 462, 463*, 475, *478*, 484,
    485, 487, 488, 493, 498, *499, 500,*
    501, 502
Kuppen-van Merwijk, A., 393, *398*
Kurihara, E., 379, *382*
Kurosaki, Y., 47, *55*, 243, *247*
Kurten, I., *105*
Kurtz, D., 302, *313*
Kushida, C. A., 29, *34*, 96, *109*, 395,
    400, 414, *420, 421, 422, 423*
Kutner, N. G., 453, *462*

Labanowski, M., *335*
Lack, L., 316, 317, *336, 337*
Lacks, P., 150, *159*, 318, *336*
LaDou, J., 255, *265*
Lake, C. R., 346, *353*
Lamphere, J., 103, *109*, 221, *224*
Lane, T. W., 323, *338*

Langevin, B., 374, *382*
Lansdown, R., 318, *337*
Lantz, D. L., 326, *336*
Lapierre, O., 64, *71*
Lapp, L., 31, *34*
Large, A. A., 386, *399*
Larsson, H., 271, *281*
Larsson, L. H., 290, *296*
Lategola, M. T., 88, *107*
Lauber, J. K., 47, *64*, 243, *246*
Lavie, P., 89, *107*, 163, *179*
Lazarus, H. R., 396, *399*
Lazarus, J. M., 373, *383*
Lee, J. K., 36, *55*
Lee, K. A., 391, *500*, 466, 468, *478*
Leger, D., 117, *122*
Leger, P., 374, *382*
Lehman, M. N., 45, *54*
Leibenluft, E., 497, *501*
Leigh, T. J., 432, *462*
Leitch, C. A., *420*
Leiter, J. C., 88, *108*, 394, *399*
Lemmi, H., *246*
Lenn, N. J., 45, *55*
Lenzi, P., *105*
Lenzi, P. L., 269, *280*
Leung, L., 92, *108*
Levendosky, A. A., *159*
Levere, R., 318, *337*
Levey, A. B., 327, *336*
Levi, L., *422*
Levine, B., 93, 103, *108*
Levine, N. S., 278, *280*
Levine, R. J., 303, *313*
Levine, S., 364, *369*, 496, *501*
Levinson, P. D., 375, *382*, 392, *399*
Levy, S., 364, *369*
Lew, N. L., 373, *383*
Lewy, A. J., 48, 49, 51, *54*, *55*, *70*, 142, *159*, *247*
Li, V., *313*
Libert, J. P., *105*
Lichstein, K. L., 322, 331, *336*
Lick, J. R., 322, *336*
Light, A. I., 82, *108*
Light, R. W., 346, *353*

Lilie, J., 288, *295*
Linde, S., 213, *224*
Lindsay, W. R., 322, 329, 330, *335*
Lineback, W., 455, *463*, 488, *502*
Lipke-Molby, T., 451, *463*
Lipper, S., 321, *334*
Lisansky, E. J., 89, *109*, *110*
Litt, I. F., *174*
Liu, L., 244, *246*
Lloyd, S., 288, *295*
Lobban, M. C., 254, *264*
Locher, J. L., *461*
Lockwood, G., 323, *335*
Loewenfeld, I. E., 217, *224*
Loh, L., *400*
Loomis, A. L., 12, *33*
Loosen, P. T., 331, *336*
Lorenzo, I., *106*
Louden, M. B., 378, *382*
Love, B. B., *382*
Lovin, P. A., 488, *500*
Loving, R. T., 261, *263*
Lovoi, M. S., 276, *280*
Lowenstein, O., 217, *224*
Lowrie, E. G., 373, *383*
Lowry, S. F., 417, *423*
Lozoff, B., 440, *439*
Lubin, A., 81, 82, 97, *107*, *108*, *110*
Luciano, D., 379, *381*
Lue, F. A., 403, 405, *422*
Lugaresi, E., 268, 269, *280*
Lutley, K., *223*
Lydic, R., *54*
Lynch, J. J., 386, *398*

Maasen, A., 256, *265*
McAbee, R. S., *503*
McAvay, G., 489, *502*
McCabe, T. G., 323, 324, *337*
McCall, V., *190*
McCall, W. V., 188, *190*, 218, *224*
McCann, C. C., 301, *313*
McCann, V. D., 87, *108*
McCarley, R., 495, *501*
McCarley, R. W., 17, 21, *33*
McClusky, H. Y., 331, *336*
McCool, C., *108*

McDonald, C. S., 452, *464*
McDonald, K., 329, *337*, 492, *501*
Macdonald, L. R., 324, *335*, *338*
McEnany, G., 468, *478*
McEvoy, R. D, 103, *106*, 287, *295*
McGeary, J., 491, *503*
McGill, T., *336*
McGowan, W. T., 323, *335*
McGuire, J., 391, *400*
Machen, M., *463*
Machen, M. A., *159*, *462*
Mack, J. M., 390, *398*
McKeon, J. L., *279*
McKinley, J. C., 133, *159*
McLoughlin, Q., 258, *265*
McMann, J. M., *421*
McMurray, R. G., 88, *108*
McNicholas, W., *296*
McPartland, R. J., 493, *501*
Maglio, R., *462*
Magnin, P., *108*
Mahan, R. P., 256, *266*
Mahoney, M. P., 244, *246*
Mahowald, M., 201, *208*
Mahowald, M. W., 69, *71*, 112, *122*
Maingourd, Y., *105*
Maislin, G., 100, *108*
Majde, J. A., 409, 410, 411, *422*
Malbecq, W., *265*
Males, J. L., 277, *281*
Malm, J. R., *398*
Manber, R., 315, *334*
Mann, F. C., 258, *265*
Mann, L. D., *502*
Mannsmann, U., *105*
Manogue, K., 417, *423*
Mant, A., *190*, 452, *462*
Marana, R., 89, *105*, 506, *420*
Marchione, K., 331, *336*
Markey, S. P., 48, *54*, 142, *159*
Markley, C. L., 48, *56*
Marks, V., 31, *52*
Marler, J. R., 374, *382*
Maron, L., 342, *356*
Marsh, E. E., 374, *382*
Marsh, G. R., 188, *190*, 218, *224*, 321, *334*

Marshall, J., 374, *382*
Martens, H., *247*
Martensson, B., 346, *353*
Martin, E. D., *500*, *502*
Martin, R., 278, *281*
Martin, R. J., 271, 273, *280*, 286, *296*
Martin, S. E., 309, *312*
Martinelli, V., *381*
Martinez, A. P., 393, *400*
Martinowitz, G., 89, *107*
Martins, A., 380, *383*
Martins, P., 380, *383*
Masand, P., 69, *71*
Masny, J., 188, *190*
Mason, W., 25, *32*, 188, *189*
Mason, W. J., *70*, *121*, 380, *459*
Masterton, J. P., 386, *399*
Matheson, J., *336*
Matsumoto, M., *478*
Matsuo, S., *478*
Maul, F., *110*
Mayer, J., *296*
Mazar, M. E., 394, *400*
Mazar, M. F., 86, *109*
Mazumdar, S., *463*
Meade, T. E., 288, *297*
Meck, R., 309, *313*
Meddis, R., 30, *33*
Meers, A., 256, *265*
Melander, A., 89, *109*
Mellinger, G. D., 125, *159*, 344, *353*, 488, *501*
Mellor, E. F., 249, *265*
Mendels, J., 491, *500*
Mendelson, W. B., 28, *33*, 285, *296*, 349, *353*, 372, 374, *381*, *382*, 452, *462*
Menn, M., *207*
Menn, S. J., 368, *369*
Menza, M. A., 378, *382*
Merlotti, L., 84, *109*, 344, 348, *354*, 451, *462*
Messin, S., 25, *32*, 188, *189*
Meurice, J. C., 310, *317*
Meyer, T., 389, *397*
Meyer, T. J., 388, 389, *399*
Michael-Jacoby, A., 390, *398*

Michelson, L. K., 331, *336*
Middelkoop, H. A., *383*
Midkiff, K., 256, *266*
Miescke, K. J., 48, *54*
Mikami, A., 237, *247*
Milby, J. B., 331, *336*
Miles, L., 236, *246*
Miles, L. E., 25, *33*, 185, *190*, *225*, 239, 247
Miles, L. E. M., 239, *247*
Miller, D. H., *383*
Miller, G., 364, *381*, 452, *462*
Miller, L. S., 48, *54*
Miller, M. H., 349, *353*
Miller, T. B., 409, *422*
Millman, R., *190*, 389, *397*
Millman, R. P., 371, 372, 375, *382*, 392, *399*
Mills, G. H., 469, *478*
Mills, J. N., 35, *53*
Minatti-Hannuch, S. N., 380, *381*
Mindell, J. A., 116, *122*
Miner, J. D., 258, *265*
Minter, K., 341, *355*
Mishima, K., *462*
Mistlberger, R. E., 235, *246*
Mistleberger, R., 45, 46, *55*
Mistleberger, R. E., 45, *54*
Mitcha, J., 214, 224
Mitchell, G., 496, *501*
Mitchell, S., 112, *122*
Mitler, M., 206, *207*, 499
Mitler, M. M., 19, *32*, 66, *71*, 85, 86, 105, 161, 163, 166, 169, *175*, 180, *190*, 209, 216, 217, 219, 220, *233*, *234*, 235, 295, 368, *369*, 449, *462*
Mitnick, L. L., 85, *105*
Miyajima, T., 379, *382*
Mizanu, Y., 379, *382*
Mohr, J. P., *382*
Mohsenin, V., 376, *382*
Moldofsky, H., 236, 237, *247*, 403, 405, 406, 407, 410, *422*, 474, *470*, 488, *493*
Moline, M. L., 116, *122*
Möller, A. A., *423*
Mondini, S., 269, *280*

Monk, T. H., 75, 76, *108*, 138, *159*, 251, 252, 253, 254, 257, 258, 261, *264*, *265*, *461*, *462*
Monroe, L. J., 323, *336*
Montagna, P., 69, *71*, 268, *280*
Monti, J. M., 392, *353*
Montplaisir, J., 64, 65, *71*, 372, 373, 382
Moorad, P. J., *503*
Moore, C. A., 22, *33*, 185, *190*
Moore, R. Y., 45, *55*, 229, *247*, 249, 265
Moore, S. E., 291, *296*
Moore-Ede, M. C., 27, *33*, 39, 44, 45, 46, *54*, *55*, 135, *159*, *246*, 254, *263*
Moote, C. A., 387, *399*
Moran, W. B., 270, *280*
Morawetz, D., 328, *336*
Morden, B., 496, *501*
Morehead, M. A., 378, *382*
Morgan, K., 451, *462*
Mori, A., 47, *55*, 243, *257*
Morin, C. M., 121, *122*, 125, 127, 136, 150, *159*, 317, 318, 321, 327, 328, 329, 331, 332, 333, *336*, *337*, 488, 492, *501*
Morlock, H. C., 217, *225*
Morris, D. L., 417, *422*
Morris, M., 316, *337*
Morris, M. G., 417, *422*
Morrison, A. R., 495, *500*
Moses, J. M., 97, 98, *107*, *108*
Mosko, S. S., 451, *461*
Mosley, I. F., *383*
Mott, D. E., 324, *334*
Mott, P. E., 258, *265*
Motta, H., 376, *382*
Mougey, E. H., 88, *107*
Mougin, C., *108*
Mougin, F., 95, *108*
Mowrer, O. H., 437, *439*
Mowrer, W. M., 437, *439*
Moyer, N. J., 217, *225*
Muehlbach, M. J., *110*, 214, *225*, 251, 266
Mueller, P. S., *55*
Muir, K. R., *400*

Mullaney, D., *107*
Mullaney, D. J., 186, *190*, 218, *223*
Muller, J. E., *382*
Munn, D., 390, *398*
Murdy, J. M., *383*
Murphy, F., 389, *397*
Murphy, P. J., 452, *462*
Murray, C. F., *190*
Murtagh, D. R. R., 318, 332, 333, *337*
Musisi, S., 236, *247*
Muzet, A., 19, *34*, *105*
Muzio, J. N., 25, *34*
Myers, B. L., 452, *462*

Nagamine, H., *247*
Nahmias, J., 387, *399*
Naitoh, P., 19, *34*, 81, 85, 87, 88, 97,
    98, *97*, *108*
Nakai, Y., *478*
Namerow, N., 85, *107*
Nanami, T., *247*
National Commission on Sleep
    Disorders Research, 31, *34*, 114,
    116, 117, 118, *122*, 125, *159*
National Institute of Mental Health,
    Consensus Development
    Conference, 340, 332, *354*
Naumann, M., *56*
Neau, J. P., *313*
Neilly, J. B., 100, *108*
Nekich, J., 443, *460*
Nekich, J. C., 459, *460*
Nelson, W., 36, *55*
Nespor, S., 371, *381*
Neville, K. J., 214, *224*
Nevsimalova, S., *223*
Newell, S. A., 379, *382*
Newhouse, P. A., 77, *108*
Newman, A. B., *461*
Newman, J., 218, 223, *224*
Newsome, D. A., 48, *54*, *55*, 152, *159*
Newton, T. F., 487, *502*
Nicassio, P., 318, 323, 324, *334*
Nicassio, P. M., 131, 135, 150, 152,
    158, 32, 323, *337*
Nicholson, A. N., 47, *54*, 79, *106*, *109*,
    241, 242, 243, *247*, 349, *334*

Nicolai, A., *265*
Nides, M., *313*
Nilsson, L. G., 83, *109*
Nino-Marcia, G., 470, *478*
Nino-Murcia, G., *190*, 301, *313*
Nishimura, A., 374, *384*
Nofzinger, E., *502*
Nofzinger, E. A., 171, *175*, 491, 493,
    501, *502*
Norman, S. E., 419, *422*
North, C. S., *460*
Noyes, R., Jr., 330, *337*
Nunnery, S. L., 396, *398*

Obermeyer, W., 415, *423*
Obermeyer, W. H., 457, *460*, 483, *499*
O'Brian, P. C., 346, *353*
O'Brien, G. T., 322, *334*
Office of Technology Assessment,
    249, 250, 259, 260, *265*
Ogita, S., 469, *478*
Ogle, K. N., 217, *225*
Okawa, M., 239, *247*, 454, *462*
Oldani, A., *381*
Oliver, R., *478*
Olmstead, E., 257, *264*
Olson, L. G., *279*
Orav, E. J., 163, *175*
Ordway, L., 306, *313*
Orem, J., 28, *34*
Orne, E. C., *421*
Orne, M. T., *421*
Orr, W. C., 185, *190*, 246, 270, 271,
    272, 273, 276, 277, 278, *280*, *281*,
    286, *296*, 386, 387, 388, *399*
Orr, W. F., 495, *502*
Orth-Gomer, K., 251, 261, *264*, *265*
Ory, M. G., 453, *462*
Orzack, M. H., 77, *107*
Osborn, L. M., 477, *478*
Ostberg, O., 255, *264*
Ostberg, O. A., 168, *174*
Ostergren, P. O., 452, *461*
Oswald, I., 30, *32*, *33*, 474, *502*
Oudart, H., *105*
Owen, N., 331, *335*
Owen, W. F., 373, *373*

Pack, A. I., 100, *108*, 302, 303, 304, 307, 310, 311, *312, 313*
Palmblad, J., 89, *105, 109*, 404, 406, *420, 422*
Palomaki, H., 269, *281*, 374, *382, 383*, 392, *399*
Palta, M., *72, 132, 281*, 462
Pang, G., 412, *421*
Pappenheimer, J. R., 409, *422*
Papper, S., 371, *382*
Papsdorf, J. D., 323, 324, *335*
Paquereau, J., *313*
Park, R., *175*
Parker, C. E., 251, *264*
Parker, L., 450, *459*
Parkes, J. D., 232, *245*, 472, *479*
Parmeggiani, P. L., 25, 26, *34*
Partinen, M., 269, *281*, 374, 375, 376, *382, 383*, 392, *399*, 453, *460, 463*
Pascoe, P. A., *79, 106*, 241, 243, *247*, 349, *354*
Paskewitz, D. A., 386, *398*
Pasnau, R. O., 85, 87, *107, 108*
Pasternak, R. E., 457, *463*
Patel, R., *460*
Patte, F., *313*
Paulson, M. M., *33*
Pavia, T., 380, *383*
Paynter, D., 317, *336*
Peake, G. T., 89, *109, 110*
Pearson, H. E., 395, *399*
Peavy, G. M., *336*
Pedersen, M. H., 392, *400*
Pedrosi, B., 344, *354*
Pegram, V., 185, *190*
Peiser, L., *33*
Pelayo, R., *335*
Pelayo, R. P., 232, *247*
Pelletier, G., 64, *71*
Penetar, D. M., *108*
Peniston, E. G., 326, *337*
Pennock, B. E., 273, *280*
Percy, L., 324, *335*
Perks, W. H., 470, *478*
Perlis, M. L., 315, *334*
Perry, P. J., 330, *337*
Perry, S. W., 394, *399*

Peskind, E., *463*
Peterson, D. D., 372, 373, 374, *381, 383, 463*
Petrie, S. R., *159*
Petrini, B., 404, *422*
Petta, D., 443, 458, *460*
Petta, D. E., *461*
Petta, D. F., *460*
Pettitt, A. N., 82, *107*
Pfalser, J. L., 88, *107*
Pflug, B., *110*
Phelps, P. J., 325, *336*
Phillips, B. A., 88, *109*, 394, *399*, 451, *460, 463*
Phillips, E. R., *246*
Phillips, R., 164, *174*, 211, *224*
Phillipson, E. A., 236, *247*, 394, *397*
Picket, C., *296*
Pickett, C. K., 394, *400*
Piercy, M., 95, *109*
Pilsher, J. J., 415, *421, 422*
Pittard, J. T., *503*
Poceta, J. S., 166, 169, *174, 175*
Poceta, S., 368, *369*
Pohl, H., 249, *263*
Poiasek, J., 254, *266*
Polasek, J., 48, *56*
Pollak, C. P., *72, 160*, 217, 225, *247, 248*
Pollard, B. J., 392, *400*
Pollmächer, T., 410, *421, 423*
Polman, C. H., *383*
Polo, O., 473, *477*
Polzella, D. J., 496, *502*
Ponce-deLeon, M., *106*
Pond, D., *190*
Popli, A. P., 69, *71*
Popp, W., 276, *281*, 301, *313*
Powell, J. W., 215, *224*
Powell, N., 470, *478*
Powell, N. P., 290, *296*
Prather, M. B., 477, *478*
Pressman, M., *190*
Pressman, M. R., 217, *225*, 372, 373, 374, 375, *381, 383*, 453, *463*
Preston, T. A., 130, *159*
Preston, T. Z., 455, *462*

Prete, F. R., 415, *423*
Price, R. J., 413, *426*
Price, T. R., *382*
Prinz, P. N., 452, 454, *463*
Prosser, R. A., 45, *55*
Prowse, K., 470, *478*
Pursley, A. M., *460, 461*

Qualls, C. R., 89, *109, 110*
Quant, J. P., 85, *109*
Quintans, J., 412, *421*
Quirk, R. S., 346, *353*

Radomski, M. W., 89, *110*
Radtke, R. A., 188, *190*
Rafferty, T. D., 285, *296*
Rajagopal, K. R., 286, *296*
Rajna, P., 379, *383*
Ramos, J., *106*
Ramsing, T., 392, *400*
Rand, C., *313*
Rand, C. S., 302, 303, 306, 308, *313*
Rando, K. C., 22, *33*
Randolph, C., 349, *353*
Raney, D., 390, *398*
Rappaport, B. A., *190*
Raskind, M., *463*
Rasura, M., *380*
Rauhala, E. R., 473, *477*
Rault, R., 371, *381*
Rauscher, H., 276, *281*, 301, *313*
Raynal, D. M., 239, *247*
Reading, J. C., 477, *478*
Rechtschaffen, A., 12, 14, 15, 17, 19,
    22, 29, 30, *32, 34*, 45, *54*, 96, *109,*
    111, 112, *122*, 184, 185, *190, 191,*
    260, *265*, 346, *354*, 395, *400*, 412,
    414, 415, *420, 421, 422, 423*
Record, C., *478*
Redline, S., 188, *190*, 313, *382*
Reed, H. L., 415, 417, *421*
Reeder, M. K., 392, *300*
Reeves-Hoche, M. K., 309, *313*
Refetoff, S., 415, *420, 421, 422*
Reiher, J., 375, *383*
Reilly, C., 256, *266*
Reilly, T., 95, *109*

Reiman, J., 476, *477*
Reinberg, A., 255, *265*
Reiter, R. J., 46, *55*
Remmers, J. E., 272, *281*, 284, *296*
Ren, Z., 376, *381*
Renaud, A., *108*
Renaux, S. A., 334, *363*
Rennotte, M., 392, 393, *400*
Reppert, S., 46, *55*
Resor, S., 206, *207*
Reynolds, C. F., 63, *70, 77, 106*, 148,
    159, 171, 175, 215, 225, 446, 457,
    462, 463, 485, 487, 488, 497, 498,
    499, 500, 506, 502
Reynolds, C. F., III., *159*, 457, *461,*
    462, 463, 502
Richardson, G., *72, 160*, 206, *207, 248*
Richardson, G. S., *32*, 135, *159*, 161,
    163, 166, *174, 175*, 213, 215 223,
    246, 258, 265, 265
Richman, N., 318, *337*, 430, 431, *439*
Richter, C. P., 43, *55*
Rickels, K., 330, *337*
Riedel, B. W., 322, *336*
Ries, R. K., 454, *463*
Riley, R. W., 290, *296*
Rios, C. D., *32, 263*
Ristanovic, R. K., 378, *381*, 455, *461*
Ritenour, A. M., *159*
Rivers, M., *223*
Rivest, R., 375, *383*
Rivkees, S., 46, *55*
Rivlin, J., 289, *296*
Roache, J. D., 344, *353*
Roberston, T., *382*
Robert, D., 374, *382*
Robin, E., 268, *279*
Rodenstein, D. O., 392, *400*
Rodin, J., 489, *502*
Roehrs, T., 93, 103, *108, 109*, 168, *175,*
    201, *208*, 215, 224, 225, 229, 233,
    236, 243, *247*, 341, 342, 343, 344,
    354, 347, 348, *354*, 455, *463*, 488,
    502
Roehrs, T. A., 83, 84, *109*, 344, *354,*
    462
Roffwarg, H., 166, *174*

Roffwarg, H. P., 25, *33, 34, 246, 502*
Rogers, A. S., 79, *106*
Rogers, R. M., 64, *71,* 271, 273, 276, *280*
Rohrbaugh, M., 396, *338*
Rolletto, T., 324, *337*
Romberg, H. P., *264*
Ronda, J. M., *32, 53, 263*
Roos, R. A., *383*
Rosa, R. R., 77, *106,* 257, 260, *263,* 486, *502*
Rose, C., *478*
Rose, E. A., 387, *399*
Rosekind, M., 32, *34,* 116, *122*
Rosekind, M. R., 215, *224*
Rosen, A., 83, *109*
Rosen, G., 494, *502*
Rosen, J., 457, *463*
Rosen, R. C., 32, *34,* 116, *122,* 349, *353,* 378, *382,* 451, *462*
Rosenberg, J., 492, *400*
Rosenberg, P. A., *336*
Rosenthal, L., 83, 84, 98, *109,* 344, *354*
Rosenthal, L. D., 344, *354, 462*
Rosenthal, N. E., 48, *54, 55, 56,* 127, 142, *159*
Rosenthal, R., 326, *338*
Rosevear, C., 32, 116, *122*
Ross, J. J., 85, *109,* 467, *478*
Ross, V., 464, *463*
Roth, B., *223*
Roth, R., 203, *208*
Roth, T., 58, *71,* 83, 93, 103, *108, 109,* 112, 113, *122,* 166, 168, *154, 175, 190,* 215, 217, *223, 224, 225,* 229, 233, 236, 243, 246, 247, 270, *280,* 341, 342, 343, 344, 345, 348, *364, 375, 381,* 492, *398,* 453, *462, 463,* 488, *502*
Rovaris, M., *381*
Rowe, J. W., 446, *463*
Rubenstein, A. E., *225*
Rubenstein, B. S., 98, *107,* 496, *501*
Rubio, P., 378, *383*
Rugh, J. D., 494, *502, 503*
Rundall, O. H., 185, *190*
Rusak, B., 45, 46, *55,* 235, *246*

Rush, A. J., 491, *502*
Ruskis, A., 285, *296*
Russ, D., 324, *335*
Rutenfranz, J., 251, 254, *264, 265*
Rye, D. B., *381,* 494, *461, 462*
Rysnek, K., 403, *422*

Sacchetti, M. L., *380*
Sack, D. A., 48, *54, 55, 56*
Sack, R. L., 48, 49, 51, *54, 55*
Sadeh, A., 186, *191*
Sagi, D., 98, *107,* 496, *501*
Saijonmaa, O., *443*
St. John, W. M., 392, *397*
Sajben, N., *207*
Saletu, B., *105,* 347, *354*
Salia, P. J., 371, *381*
Salmi, T., *463*
Salom, S. R., 321, *335,* 453, *461*
Saltzman, S., 494, *502*
Salvio, M., 315, *334*
Salzarulo, P., 430, *439*
Samel, A., *56*
Sampson, M. G., *295*
Samson, D., 390, *398*
Sanavio, E., 323, 324, 328, *337,* 490, *502*
Sanchez, R., *32, 263*
Sande, M. A., 427, *422*
Sandercock, P., *384*
Sanders, M., *190*
Sanders, M. H., 273, *280,* 291, *296*
Sandyk, R., 379, *383*
Sangal, R. B., 166, *175*
Sansom, L., 331, *335*
Sant'Ambrogio, G., 272, *280*
Sasaki, C., 285, *296*
Sasaki, H., *247*
Sasaki, M., 47, *54, 55,* 243, *247*
Saskin, P., 121, *122,* 127, 146, *160,* 321, *338*
Sassin, J. F., 19, *34, 246*
Satinoff, E., 45, *55*
Sattin, A., 454, 455, *463*
Sattler, H. L., 323, *335*
Sauerland, E. K., 272, *280,* 281, 284, *296*

Saunders, N. A., 88, *110*, *190*, 272, *279*, *281*, 286, 296, 297
Sawyer, B., *190*
Scarisbrick, P., 496, *501*
Schaefer, M., 215, *225*
Schaie, K. W., 446, *463*
Scharf, S. M., *297*
Schechtman, K. B., 453, *462*
Schenck, C., 201, 206, *208*
Schenck, C. H., 69, 71, 112, *122*
Schetman, W. R., 375, *383*
Schiffman, P. L., 87, *109*, 394, *400*
Schilgen, B., 94, *109*
Schleifer, C. R., 374, *383*
Schlernitzauer, M., *463*
Schlesser, M. A., *502*
Schmidt, H. S., *246*, 287, 296, 378, *382*
Schmidt-Nowara, W. W., 288, *297*
Schmitt, F. A., 451, *460*, *463*
Schoeller, D. A., *420*
Schoen, L. S., 301, *312*
Schoenfeld, A., 470, *478*
Schork, N. J., 474, 475, *477*
Schreiber, W., *421*, *423*
Schroeder, J. S., 376, *382*
Schubert, N. M., *313*, *382*
Schuckit, M., 347, *353*
Schuett, J. S., *313*
Schulman, H., *478*
Schultz, P. M., *159*
Schulz, H., *264*
Schuster, C. R., 79, *107*
Schutte, S., 471, *478*
Schwartz, A. R., 303, *312*, *313*, *382*
Schwartz, E., *56*
Schwartz, R. M., *502*
Schwartz, S. M., 317, 318, 321, 333, *337*
Schwartz, W. A., *399*
Schweiger, M. S., 466, 474, *479*
Schweitzer, E., 330, *337*
Schweitzer, P. K., 98, *110*, 214, *225*, 251, *266*, 301, *312*, *500*
Scott, A. J., 255, *265*
Scrima, L., 215, *215*
See, W. R., *354*

Seely, E. W., *247*
Seidel, W., 443, *460*
Seidel, W. F., 47, *53*, *175*, 242, *246*, 459, *460*
Sessler, D. I., 391, *400*
Sforza, E., 268, *280*
Shader, R. I., 329, *338*, 341, *353*
Shafer, R., 449, *462*
Shaham, Y., *108*
Shahani, B. T., 451, *464*
Shapiro, C. M., 57, *71*, 468, 475, *477*
Sharkey, K. M., 186, *191*
Sharp, D., 103, *106*
Shaw, D. H., 487, *502*
Sheilesh, P., 474, *487*
Shelton, R. C., 331, *336*
Shepard, J. W., 286, *281*, 375, *383*
Shepard, J. W., Jr., 104, *109*
Sher, A., 289, *297*
Sherbourne, C. D., 306, *313*
Shere, D. M., 470, *479*
Shimizu, T., *247*
Shoham, S., 411, *422*
Shoham, V., 326, *338*
Shoham-Salomon, V., 326, *338*
Shore, E. T., 371, *382*
Shouse, M., 206, *208*
Sicklesteel, J., *109*, *225*
Sicotte, N., *110*
Sides, H., 323, *335*
Silver, R., *54*
Simmons, F., 162, *174*
Simmons, F. B., 285, *295*, *297*
Simmons, M., *313*
Simon-Rigaud, M. L., *108*
Simons, A. D., 491, *503*
Simons, R. N., 29, *33*, 260, *263*
Sing, H. C., *108*
Sing, T. C., *108*
Singer, C. M., 48, *54*, *55*
Singh, J., 387, *399*
Skatrud, J., 72, *122*, *281*
Skatrud, J. B., *462*
Skinner, M. I., 387, *399*
Skwerer, R. A., 48, *54*
Slattery, J., *384*
Sleep Research Society, 27, *34*

Sloan, J., *422*
Sloan, K., *110*
Slutsky, A. S., 273, *280*
Smirne, S., *381*
Smith, B. M., *463*
Smith, C., 31, *34*
Smith, C. B., 417, *421*
Smith, C. S., 256, *266*
Smith, J. R., 448, *462*
Smith, L. G., *190*
Smith, P. L., *295*, 302, 303, 304, 307, *312*, *313*, *382*
Smith, R. O., 276, *280*
Smith, T. L., 347, *353*
Smythe, H., 164, *174*, 211, *224*
Snoek, F. J., *383*
Snyder, S., 472, *479*
Sobrino, R., 378, *383*
Sokoloff, L., 417, *421*
Solberg, W. K., 494, *502*
Soldatos, C. R., 70, *207*, 488, 494, *500*, *502*
Soltani, K., *422*
Somers, V. K., 376, *381*
Sood, R., 331, *337*
Soutre, E., *159*
Spencer, M. B., 79, *106*, 241, 243, *247*
Spiegel, R., *499*
Spielman, A., 63, *71*
Spielman, A. J., *72*, 99, *107*, 121, *122*, 126, 127, 128, 129, 130, 144, 146, *159*, *160*, 217, *225*, 232, *247*, *248*, 321, 322, *335*, *338*
Spinweber, C. L., 135, *158*, 211, *224*
Spriggs, D. A., 374, *383*
Stack, J. A., *499*, *502*
Stahl, M. L., 271, *280*, 386, 387, 388, *399*
Stakes, J. W., 451, *464*
Stamm, D., *52*
Stampi, C., 214, 218, *224*, *225*
Standards of Practice Committee, American Sleep Disorders Association, 136, *160*, 188, *191*
Starr, A., 395, *397*
Starz, K. E., *159*

Stepanski, E., 103, *108*, *109*, 343, 344, *354*
Stepanski, E. J., 344, *354*
Stephan, F. K., 45, *55*
Steriades, M., 17, *34*
Sterman, M. B., 324, 326, *335*, *336*, *338*
Stevenson, J. E., 430, *439*
Stewart, D., 372, *381*
Stewart, K. T., 244, *246*
Stone, B. M., 79, *109*, 243, *247*
Stone, J., 329, 331, *337*, 492, *501*
Stoohs, A., 395, *400*
Stoohs, R., 188, *191*, 205, *207*
Stoohs, R. A., 94, *109*
Stopa, E., 46, *55*
Storm, W. F., 214, *224*
Stout, A. L., 488, *500*
Strander, H., *422*
Strassman, R. J., 89, *109*, *110*
Stratmann, I., 255, *265*
Strijers, R. L., *383*
Strogatz, S. H., 37, *243*
Strohl, K., *190*
Strohl, K. P., 188, *190*, 272, *281*, 286, *296*
Strollo, P. J., 64, *71*
Strong, J. A., *33*
Struthers, G., *478*
Sugerman, J. L., *110*, 251, *266*
Sugita, Y., 233, *237*, *247*
Sullivan, C. E., 88, *110*, 112, *122*, 286, 289, 291, *295*, *296*, 297, 300, *313*, 372, *381*, 394, *397*
Sullivan, C. F., 364, *369*
Sulzman, F. M., 27, *33*, 39, 44, *54*, *55*
Sun, J. H., *108*
Suratt, P. M., 270, *280*, 289, *297*
Suthipinittharm, P., *422*
Svanborg, E., 271, *281*, 290, *296*, 395, *399*
Sved Williams, A. E., 476, *478*
Swaab, D. F., *383*
Swartz, M. N., 416, *423*
Sweatman, P., 286, *295*
Switzer, D. A., 270, *279*
Switzer, P. K., 331, *336*
Symons, J. D., 89, *110*

Tachibana, N., 379, *383*
Tadmor, B., 388, *400*
Takahashi, K., *247, 462*
Takahashi, Y., 28, *34*, 122, *122*
Takebayashi, T., *478*
Tamagawa, K., 379, *382*
Tamarkin, L., *56*
Tan, T. L., 492, *502*
Tanaka, B., *478*
Tank, Y., 394, *397*
Tanke, E. D., 453, *461*
Tanne, D., 98, *107*, 496, *501*
Tanner, C. M., 378, *381*, 455, *461*
Taphoorn, M. J., 379, *383*
Tashkin, D. P., 302, *313*
Taska, L. S., 349, *353*
Tassinari, C., 112, *121*
Tassinari, C. A., 268, *280*
Tasto, D. L., 251, 257, *266*
Taylor, M. E., *33*
Telakivi, T., *463*
Tellis, C., *296*
Tepas, D. I., 217, *225*, 256, *266*
Tepper, B., *54*
Terman, J., 45, *55*
Terman, M., 45, *55*, 70, 244, *247*
Teshima, Y., 237, *247*
Thaller, J. L., 494, *502*
Thase, M. E., 171, *175*, 491, 493, *501,
    502, 503*
Thawley, S. E., 263, *281*
Thisted, R. A., 457, *460*, 483, *499*
Thomas, C., 489, *501*
Thomas, E. H., 215, *225*
Thomas, L., 166, *175*
Thomas, M., *109*
Thomas, M. A., *109*
Thomas, M. L., *109*
Thomas, S. A., 386, *398*
Thompson, L., *108*
Thorne, D., *108*
Thorne, D. R., 88, *108*
Thornton, A. T., 103, *106*, 287, *295*
Thorpy, M. J., 60, *71*, 121, *122*, 127,
    146, *160*, 166, 169, 170, *175*, 215,
    216, 219, *225*, 232, 233, 235, *247*,
    248, 321, *338*

Thrummed, A. J., *503*
Thurmond, A., *110*
Tierney, N. M., 392, *400*
Tilkian, A., 285, *295*
Timko, C., 489, *502*
Timms, R. M., *175*
Timms, V., 85, *109*
Ting, M., *296*
Tinklenberg, J., 454, *461*
Tobler, I., 41, *53*, 94, *106*, 186, *189*
Todd, M. A., 390, *397*
Tolle, R., 94, *109*
Tolley, E. A., 418, *423*
Tong, Y. L., 36, *55*
Toni, D., *380*
Topf, M., 389, *400*
Toth, L. A., 418, 419, *423*
Townsend, R. E., 81, *108*
Tracey, K. J., 417, *423*
Trachsel, L., *423*
Traskman-Bendz, L., 346, *353*
Trontell, M. C., 87, *109*, 394, *400*
Tsao, C., 321, *334*
Tsujimoto, R. N., 332, *334*
Turvey, T., 322, *335*
Tusji, Y., 374, *384*
Tyler, D. B., 81, *110*
Tyre, E., *460*

Uhlenhuth, E. H., 125, *159*, 344, *353*,
    488, *501*
Ulrich, R. F., 493, *501*
Unger, P., *422*
Urry, H., 326, *338*
U. S. Environmental Protection
    Agency, 389, *400*

Valley, V., 214, *224*
Valor, R., 376, *382*
van Decar, D. H., 393, *400*
Van den Hoed, J., *175*, 206, 207, 215,
    217, *225*
VanderPlate, C., 324, *338*
van der Velde, E. A., *383*
Vandiver, R., *55*
VanHelder, T., 89, *110*
Van Hilten, B., 378, *383*

Van Loon, J. H., 258, *266*
Van Oot, P. H., 333, *338*
van Someren, E., *383*
Van Vitert, B., *383*
Vasavada, N., *502*
Vaughn, L. K., 417, *422*
Vedder, H., *421, 423*
Vejvoda, M., *56*
Vela-Bueno, A., *207*
Veres, J., 379, *383*
Verhaegen, P., 276, *265*
Verhulst, S., 376, *381*
Vermeulen, A., 104, *110*
Vernallis, F. F., 494, *503*
Verrier, R. L., 361, *369*
Vidotto, G., 324, *337*
Vieux, N., 255, *264, 265*
Vignau, J., 232, *245*
Violi, R., *380*
Visscher, F., *383*
Vitaliano, P. P., 454, *463*
Vitiello, M. V., 452, 454, *463*
Vogel, F., *503*
Vogel, G., 344, *354*
Vogel, G. W., 99, *110,* 341, 342, *355,* 491, *503*
Volicer, L., 454, *463*
Volk, S., 87, *110*
von Schenck, H., 89, *109*
Votteri, B., *190*

Wachter, H., *423*
Wada, S., *247*
Wadhwa, N. K., 372, *382*
Wagner, A., 346, *353*
Wagner, D. R., 232, 233, 235, 242, *248*
Walker, J. M., 257, *266*
Walker, M., *110*
Walsh, J. K., 19, *32,* 79, 85, 86, 98, *105, 110,* 135, *160,* 214, *225,* 251, *266,* 301, *312*
Walsleben, J. A., *295*
Walter, J., 403, *422*
Walters, A., *462*
Walters, E. D., 326, *335*
Walton, E., 127, *159,* 327, *337,* 492, *501*

Wanke, T., 301, *313*
Ware, J. C., 491, 493, 494, *503*
Warlow, C., *384*
Warnes, H., 64, *71*
Warwick, D. P., 258, *265*
Wasserman, J., 404, *422*
Wasserstein, A. G., 371, *382*
Watts, F. N., 327, *336*
Watts, N., *381, 461*
Watts, R. L., *381, 461*
Wauquier, A., *383*
Weaver, D., 46, *55*
Webb, W. B., 25, 27, 30, 31, *34,* 39, *56,* 77, 92, 94, 97, 99, *85, 110,* 270, *279,* 467, *478*
Weber, R., *110*
Weber, S., 72, 122, *281*
Wechsler, L. R., 451, *464*
Wedderburn, A. A. I., 254, *266*
Weerts, T. C., 322, *334*
Weerts, T. D., 490, *499*
Wegmann, H. M., 47, *54, 56*
Wehr, T., 154, *160*
Wehr, T. A., 48, *54, 55, 56,* 142, *159,* 239, *247,* 255, *266,* 414, 415, 417, *421, 497, 501*
Weil, J. V., 394, *400*
Weilburg, J. B., 69, *71*
Weiler, S. J., *295*
Weinberg, A. N., 416, *423*
Weinstein, L., 99, *107*
Weiss, J. W., 161, *174*
Weiss, L., 474, *477*
Weitzman, E. D., 41, *56,* 67, *72,* 127, 142, 144, *160,* 217, *225,* 232, 233, 235, 244, *246, 247, 248*
Wellens, H. J. J., 104, *110*
Welsh, J., 376, *381*
West, P., 286, *295,* 470, *477*
Westbrook, P. R., *190, 223*
Wetterberg, L., 89, *105*
Wever, R., 39, 53, 229, *248*
Wever, R. A., 39, 40, 48, *56,* 249, 254, *263, 266*
Whaley, R., 268, *279*
White, D. M., *55*
White, D. P., 394, *400*

Whitehouse, W. G., *421*
Whyte, J., 206, *207*
Widrow, L., *461*
Wiedemann, K., *423*
Wiegand, M., 419, *423*
Wildgruber, C. M., 48, *56*, 254, *266*
Wilhoit, S. C., 270, *280*, 289, 297
Wilkinson, R. T., 82, 83, 92, *107*, *110*, 214, *225*, 251, 254, *266*
Williams, A., *190*
Williams, D. E., 454, *463*
Williams, H. L., 81, 82, *110*, 217, *225*
Williams, L., 285, *295*
Williams, R., 237, *246*, 371, *381*
Williams, R. L., 22, 25, 34, 97, 99, *105*, 467, *478*, 485, *503*
Williams, V., 331, *336*
Williams, W. H., 385, *340*
Wilms, D., 100, *106*
Wilson, M. A., 239, *248*
Wing, A. M., 82, *108*
Wingard, D. L., 29, *34*
Winget, C. M., 48, *56*
Winkle, R. A., 375, *381*, 392, *398*
Winter, J. B., 260, *265*
Wisbey, J., 186, *190*
Wise, R., *313*
Wise, R. A., 302, 306, 308, *312*
Wisser, H., *52*
Witkin, H. A., 487, *500*
Wittels, E., 270, *280*
Wittig, R., 224, *225*, 341, *354*
Wittig, R. M., *462*
Wold, L., 415, *421*
Wolf, A. W., 430, *439*
Wolf, P. A., *382*
Wolf, R., *105*
Wolff, S. M., 403, *422*
Wollmann, R., 415, *421*
Wolpe, J., 327, *338*
Wolpert, E., 112, *122*
Wood, A. M., 386, *400*
Wood, J. M., 319, *334*
Woods, L. A., 390, *398*
Woolf, G. M., 394, *397*
Wooten, S. A., 286, *295*
Wooten, V., 331, *336*

Wright, E. C., 308, *313*
Wright, H., 316, 317, *336*
Wright, K. P., Jr., 452, *462*
Wright, V., 452, *462*
Wroe, S. J., 374, *384*
Wu, A., 394, *399*
Wu, J. C., 87, 88, *110*, 497, *503*
Wyatt, J. K., 315, *334*
Wynter, J., 376, *381*

Yamada, T., 376, *381*
Yang, M., 448, *463*
Yan Liu, S. M., 373, *383*
Yasuda, T., 374, *384*
Yeager, A. L., 457, *463*
Yesavage, J. A., 186, *189*, 321, *335*, 443, 453, 454, *461*, 484, *499*
Yinnon, A. M., 388, *400*
Yolles, S. F., *295*
Yoss, R. E., 217, *225*
Youakim, J., *478*
Young, T., 64, *72*, 118, *122*, 270, 271, *281*
Young, T. B., *462*

Zaffke, M. E., 468, *478*
Zamel, N., *296*
Zammit, G. K., 452, *464*
Zarcone, V., 211, *224*
Zarcone, V. P., 66, *75*, 164, *174*, *225*, 347, *355*, *461*, 493, *499*, *495*
Zaugg, L., 260, *263*, 421
Zauli, C., 269, *280*
Zendell, S. M., *110*, *122*
Zentella, A., 417, *423*
Zepelin, H., 447, *502*, *464*
Zeplin, H., 30, *34*
Zimmer, B., *502*
Zimmerman, J., *160*
Zimmerman, J. C, *72*, *246*, *248*
Zimmerman, M. B., 376, *381*
Zorick, F., 93, 103, *108*, *109*, 215, *224*, 225, 341, 343, *354*, 348, *334*, 455, *463*, 488, *502*
Zorick, F. J., 166, *174*, 217, *224*, 270, *280*, 375, *381*, 392, *398*
Zorzi, M., 324, *337*

Zucconi, M., 269, *280*, *381*
Zucker, I., 45, *55*
Zukerman, E., 380, *381*
Zulley, J., 40, 41, 42, 43, *44*
Zweizig, J. R., *33*

Zwick, H., 268, *281*, 301, *313*
Zwillich, C. W., *296*, 309, *313*, 394, *400*
Zwilling, G., 25, *33*
Zwyghuizen-Doorenbos, A., 93, *109*, 215, *225*

Subject Index

Accidents, 117. *See also* Traffic
  accidents
Acrophase, 37
Actigraphy
  children, 430
  in excessive sleepiness
    assessment, 218
  and polysomnography, 186–187
Actillume recording, 186–187
"Activation-synthesis hypothesis," 21
Active-NREM sleep, 427–430
Acute sleep deprivation, 92
Adaptive theory, sleep function, 30
Addition tasks, 81–82
Adeno-tonsillar hypertrophy, 278
Adjustment sleep disorder, 432
Adolescence
  excessive daytime sleepiness,
    432–435
  sleep disorders prevalence, 115
Advanced sleep phase syndrome,
    235–237
  case illustration, 146–148
  description of, 68, 231, 235–237
  light therapy, 316–317
  polysomnography, 203, 237
  sleep log, 147
Affective disorders, 483–503
Aging, 441–464. *See also* Elderly
  advanced sleep phase disorder, 146
  arousal threshold differences,
    101–102
  and circadian rhythms, 75–76
  National Commission report, 116
  normative sleep changes, 446–447
  recovery sleep, 77–78
  shift work effects, 255–257
  sleep deprivation effects, 75, 77
  sleep fragmentation sensitivity, 101
  sleep pattern changes, 22, 24–25,
    446–448

Aircrew members, 242–243
Airway occlusion. *See* Upper airway
  obstruction
Alcohol avoidance, 285, 347
Alcohol use/abuse
  cardiopulmonary effects, 367
  hypnotic drug contraindication,
    343–344
  insomnia role, 347–348
  REM sleep effects, 347
  in self medication, insomnia,
    347–348
Alertness cycle, 163
Alpha adrenoreceptor agonists,
    349–350
Alpha rhythm
  characteristics, 12
  elderly, 447
  and sleep deprivation, 85, 94
  and sleep onset, 12–13
Alzheimer's disease, 454–455
Ambien (zolpidem), 330, 341
Ambulatory polysomnography,
    1–189
Ambulatory twenty-four-hour
  monitoring, 217–218
American Board of Sleep Medicine
  certification by, 515–520
  history, 515–516
American Sleep Disorders
  Association, 113
Amnesia, and hypnotic drugs, 344
Amphetamines, 77, 79, 346
Amplitude (core body temperature),
    37
Amplitude (EEG)
  age-related changes, 448
  definition, 12
Anesthesia, 391–393
Animal models, 2
Anterograde amnesia, 344

Antibody response, animals, 412–414
Antidepressants
 hypnotic effects, 344
 insomnia cause, 346–347
 sleep latency, 490–491
Antihistamines, 345
Antihypertensive drugs, 3, 11
Anxiety, 483–503
 cross sectional/longitudinal data, 484–490
 versus depression, sleep markers, 484–485
 and dreams, 495
 elderly, 456–457
 and insomnia, 485–488
 sleep disturbances, 484–490
 tailored behavioral interventions, 490
 treatment effects, 490
Anxiety attack, 495
Apnea. See Sleep apnea
Apnea-hypopnea index, 270–271
Arousal
 and anxiety treatment, 490
 insomnia relationship, 323
 relaxation training, 323, 490
Arousal thresholds, age differences, 101–102
Articulatory suppression, 327
"As needed" medication, 352
Association of Sleep Disorders Centers, 60
Asthma, 364–365
Atenolol, 349
Atrial natriuretic factor, 453
Automobile accidents. See Traffic accidents
Autonomic balance, 25–26
Autonomic effects, sleep deprivation, 87–88, 496–497
Average evoked response, 217
Awakenings, and polysomnography, 201

B lymphocytes, 404, 413
Backache, in pregnancy, 474

Bacteremia, sleep-deprived rats, 416
Bacterial infection, 418–419
Barbiturates, 349
Basal sleep need, 93
Basophils, 403
Bay Area Sleep Cohort, 444–445, 458–459
Bed and bedroom cues, 318–320
Bedtime problems, children, 4
Bed-wetting, 437–438
Behavioral observations, 212
Behavioral techniques, 315–338
 cardiopulmonary function improvement, 368
 children, 432, 437–439
 insomnia, 315–338
 pharmacological treatment combination, 329–332
 REM sleep effect, depression, 491
Bell-and-pad system, 437
Benadryl (diphenhydramine), 431
Benzodiazepine receptor agonists, 340–345
 addiction liability, 344
 administration and dosage, 351–352
 behavioral techniques combination, 329–332
 children, 436
 contraindications, 344–345
 and hospitalization, 393–394
 indications for, 342–343, 350–351
 nightly versus intermittent use, 352
 obstructive sleep apnea risk, 285
 pharmacokinetics and metabolism, 341–342
 and respiration, 366
 in shift work adjustment, 251
 side effects, 343–344
 sleep stage effects, 341–342
 tolerance, 341
 withdrawal, 330, 348
Bereavement, 457–458
Beta blockers, 349, 367, 451
Bilevel airway pressure, 293

Biofeedback
    and anxiety, 490
    effectiveness, 324–325
    insomnia, 323–324, 490
Biological rhythms, 35–56. See also
        Circadian rhythms
Blind persons, 239
Blood culture, and sleep
        deprivation, 416
Blood pressure
    apnea episode effect, stroke,
        375–376
    elderly, medication role, 450–451
    fragmented sleep effect, 103
Board certification, 515–520
Body core temperature
    circadian rhythm marker, 27–28,
        36–37
    long-term sleep deprivation, rats,
        415–416
    polysomnography interpretation,
        203
    sleep-wake cycle relationship,
        39–43
    in time-free environments, 39–43
    total sleep deprivation effects, 87
Breathing control, 362–364. See also
        Sleep apnea
Bright light exposure. See Light
        exposure/therapy
Bruxism, 69, 493–494

Caffeine, 79, 345–346
Cancer growth, sleep deprivation, 412
Candida albicans infection, 418
Carbon dioxide laser treatment, 290
Cardiac arrhythmias, 114, 361
Cardiac death, 114, 361, 449
Cardiac function, 359–360, 362
Cardiovascular disease, 359–369
    circadian influences, 362
    mortality, 449–450
    and obstructive sleep apnea, 271,
        276
        elderly, 449–451
    and sleep disorders, treatment, 368
    and snoring, 268–269

Cardiovascular medication, 450–451
Cataplexy, 65–66. See also
        Narcolepsy
Catecholamines, and sleep
        deprivation, 86–87
CD4 cells, 404
Cell-mediated immunity, 404–408
Central sleep apnea
    definition, 65
    and end-stage renal disease,
        372–373
Cerebral blood flow, and apnea, 375
Cerebrovascular disorders. See Stroke
Cheyne-Stokes respiration, 360–361
Children, 427–439
    assessment, 429–430
    sleep disorders, 430–439
    sleep pattern, 427–430
Chronic fatigue syndrome, 275
Chronic obstructive pulmonary
        disease, 365–366
Chronotherapy
    children and adolescents, 433–434
    delayed sleep phase syndrome,
        144, 244, 433–434
Circadian rhythm disorders, 60,
        66–68
Circadian rhythms, 27–28, 35–56
    and aging, 75
    basic features, 27, 35–56
    biological basis, 43–46
    cardiopulmonary function
        influence, 362
    and excessive daytime sleepiness,
        163
    free-running period, 39–40
    hospitalization effects, 390–391
    and jet lag, 241–242
    measurement and terminology,
        36–38
    polysomnography, 201, 203
    shift work factor, 253–256
    and sleep deprivation, 75–76
    sleep-wake system influence, 39–43
    in temporal isolation conditions,
        39–43
    timing factors, 46–51

Classical conditioning, 26
Classifications, sleep disorders, 59–62
Claustrophobia, nasal CPAP reaction, 309
Cleft palate, 278
Clinical interview. *See* Diagnostic interview
Clonidine, 349–350
Cocaine, 79
Cognitive-behavioral therapy
  benzodiazepine combination, 329–332
  in benzodiazepine withdrawal, 330
  in depression, and REM sleep, 491
  insomnia treatment, 326–329, 492
    depression/anxiety effects, 492
Cognitive performance, and sleep deprivation, 402
Cognitive restructuring, 327–329
Commuting time, shift workers, 258
Compliance problems. *See* Treatment compliance
Computerized polysomnography, 184–185
Conditioning, 26
Congestive heart failure
  and obstructive sleep apnea, 276, 360–361
  sleep effects on, 360
Continuous positive airway pressure. *See* Nasal continuous positive airway pressure
Core body temperature. *See* Body core temperature
"Core sleep," 95
Cortisol levels, 28, 88–90, 415
CPT codes, 513
Cytokines, 406–407, 410, 417
Cytotoxic T cells, 404

Daily diary. *See* Sleep log
Dalmane (flurazepam), 285, 341
Daytime sleepiness. *See* Excessive daytime sleepiness
Death rate, 29. *See also* Mortality

Delayed sleep phase syndrome, 229–235
  adaptation to, 232
  case illustration, 142–144
  characteristics, 67–68, 229–235
  children and adolescents, 433–434
  chronotherapy, 244
  depression association, 233, 235
  incidence, 232
  insomnia distinction, 233
  light therapy, 234–235, 316–317
  pathophysiology, 235
  polysomnography, 235
  sleep log, 143, 233–234
Delta activity
  elderly, 448
  sleep deprivation effects, 85, 94
  slow wave sleep characteristics, 15–17
Demand positive airway pressure, 293–294
Denial, and treatment compliance, 308
Dental appliances, 288–289
Depression, 483–503
  and anxiety, sleep markers, 484–487
  cross sectional/longitudinal data, 484–490
  and delayed sleep phase syndrome, 233, 235
  DSM-IV criteria, 486
  early morning awakening, 148
  elderly, 456–457, 489
  and excessive daytime sleepiness, 171
  and insomnia, 487–490, 492
  jet lag association, 243
  pregnancy, 475
  REM density, 493
  REM deprivation effects, 99–100
  REM latency, 484–487, 491
  shift workers, 255
  sleep disturbance, 484–490
  total sleep deprivation treatment, 87, 497
  treatment effects, 490–491
Dermatoses, 414, 416–417

Desmopressin, 438
Desynchronization, jet lag, 241–242
Diagnostic interview
   excessive daytime sleepiness,
      166–168
   insomnia, 125–158
Dialysis patients, 371–374
Diary record. *See* Sleep log
Diazepam (Valium), 494
Diphenhydramine (Benadryl), 431
Diuretics, 367, 453
L-dopa, 373, 455
Dream reorganization technique, 437
Dreaming
   anxiety link, 495
   elderly, 447
   neurophysiological theory, 21
   in pregnancy, 476
   REM deprivation studies, 96–97
   REM sleep association, discovery,
      21
Drug-induced insomnia. *See*
   Medication-induced sleep
   disturbance
Drug therapy. *See* Medication
DSM-IV, 60–61, 511–512
Dyssomnias, 61–62
Dysthymia, 171

Early morning awakening, 236–237,
   489
Eastward travel, 241–242
Edentrace, 188
Educational level, and compliance,
   308
EEG biofeedback, 323–326
EEG sleep. *See also specific sleep stages*
   in polysomnography, 178–179, 183
   sleep and wakefulness correlates,
      11–13
   sleep stage characteristics, 14–22
Elderly, 441–464
   arousal thresholds, 101–102
   circadian rhythm changes, 75–76
   depression, 489
   dreaming, 447
   insomnia, 452, 455–457, 489

National Commission report,
   118–119
nocturia, 452–454
normative sleep changes, 446–448
psychological factors, 455–458
recovery sleep, 77–78
REM sleep, 447–448
sleep apnea, 448–451
   mortality, 449–450
sleep deprivation effects, 75, 77
sleep fragmentation sensitivity,
   101–103
snoring prevalence, 443
Electrode placement,
   polysomnography, 181, 183
Electroencephalography. *See* EEG
   sleep
Electromyography, 14–18, 20, 178,
   183
Electrooculography, 14–18, 20, 178,
   183
EMG biofeedback, 323–326, 490
End-stage renal disease, 371–374
Endocrine factors, sleep deprivation,
   88–90
Endotoxin, 410–411
Energy conservation theory, 30
Energy expenditure, sleep
   deprivation, rats, 414–415
Entrainment
   light exposure role, 48–50
   melatonin role, 49, 51
   and non-24-hour sleep-wake
      syndrome, 239–240
   zeitgebers in, 47–48
Enuresis, 437–438
Eosinophils, 403
Ephedrine, 346
Epilepsy, 378–379
Epinephrine levels, 88, 415
Epochs, 14
Epworth Sleepiness Scale, 165,
   213–214
Escherichia coli infection, 418
Estrogen therapy, 450–451
Ethanol, 347
Ethics, nasal CPAP monitoring, 303

Excessive daytime sleepiness,
    161–175
  associated clinical conditions,
    169–173
  children and adolescents, 432–435
  circadian factors, 163
  clinical interview, 166–168
  definition, 163–164
  fatigue difference, 164
  history taking, 212–213
  introspective measures, 164–165,
    213–214
  measurement, 209–223
  objective estimates, 165–166
  performance measures, 214–215
  physiological measures, 214–222
  polysomnography, 195–196
  self-report assessment, 164–165,
    213–214
  treatment outcome assessment,
    219–222
Exercise performance
  partial sleep deprivation, 94–95
  total sleep deprivation, 88
Extroverts, sleep requirements, 25
Eye movements, 12–22. See also REM
    sleep

Factor S, 409
Fatigue, 164
Fetal complications, 470–471
Fever, 411
"First night effect," 487
Fluoxetine (Prozac), 491
Flurazepam (Dalmane), 285, 341
Follicle-stimulating hormone, 89–90
Forced vital capacity, 87
Free-running rhythms, 38–40
Frequency (EEG), 12
Frontalis EMG biofeedback, 490

Gastrointestinal illness, 452
Gender differences. See Sex
    differences
Generalized anxiety disorder,
    485–488
Genioglossus muscle, 88, 272, 394

Germany, shift work regulation, 250
Governmental regulations, shift
    work, 249–250, 252
Granulocytes, 403
Growth hormone
  sleep deprivation effects, 88–90
  sleep-state dependence, 28

H_1 antihistamines, 345
Halcion (triazolam), 341
Hallucinations, 80–81
Head banging, 438
Headaches, 380
Heart failure. See Congestive heart
    failure
Heart rate
  polysomnography recordings, 183
  and total sleep deprivation, 87
Hemodialysis, 371–374
Hertz (EEG), 12
History-taking considerations
  excessive sleepiness, 212–213
  insomnia, 127–139
HIV infection, 419
Holocaust survivors, 457
Homeostasis, 26–27
Hospitalization, 385–387
  biological rhythm disturbances,
    390–391
  hypnotic medication use, 393–394
  ICU setting, 386–390
  and sleep apnea, 392–393
  sleep deprivation effects, 394–396
Humeral immunity, 404, 407–409
Hypercatabolism, 415–417
Hypernycthemeral syndrome, 237
Hypersomnia, 64–66, 170
Hypertension, 276, 375
Hypnagogic hallucinations
  description of, 65–66, 69
  in narcolepsy versus sleep apnea,
    274–275
Hypnotic drugs, 340–345. See also
    Benzodiazepine receptor
    agonists
  administration and dosage,
    351–352

behavioral techniques
    combination, 329–332
cardiopulmonary effects, 366–367
contraindications, 344–345
and hospitalization, 393–394
indications for, 342–343, 350–351
obstructive sleep apnea risk, 285
in shift work adjustment, 251
side effects, 343–344
Hypopnea
    diagnosis and treatment, 64–65
    stroke link, 374–377
Hypothalamus, and circadian
    rhythms, 43–45
Hypothermia, 417
Hypothyroidism, and sleep apnea,
    277–278, 286
Hypoxemia, 375
Hypoxia, 363, 366

ICD-9-CM, 60, 62, 509
ICU psychosis, 395–396
Idiopathic hypersomnia, 170
Imipramine, enuresis treatment,
    438
Immune system, 401–424
    animal studies, 412–418
    and infection, sleep response,
        418–420
    sleep deprivation effects, 401–424
        hospitalized patients, 395
    and sleep loss, 260
Immunomodulators, sleep
    promotion, 409–411
Immunosuppression, 411–417
Incentives, and task performance, 82
Incontinence, 453
Infancy, sleep pattern, 22, 24,
    427–429
Infection
    and sleep deprivation, rats,
        416–417
    sleep response, 418–420
Information processing, REM sleep
    function, 97–98
Infradian rhythms, 36
Inhibited personality style, 133–134

Insomnia
    assessment, 127–141
    behavioral techniques, 315–338
        medication combination,
            329–332
    benzodiazepine treatment,
        340–345
    biofeedback, 323–326
    bright light effects, 316–317
    case illustrations, 141–158
    children, 430–432
    classification systems, 60–62
    cognitive therapy, 326–328
    course of, 127–131
    depression/anxiety link, 487–490,
        492
        temporal relationship, 489–490
        treatment effects, 492
    drug causes, 345–350
    DSM-IV, 134
    elderly, 452, 455–457, 488
        and psychopathology, 488
    history taking considerations,
        127–139
    medical factors, 134–135
    National Commission report, 114,
        118
    perpetuating factors, 130–131
    polysomnography, 185, 198
    precipitating factors, 130
    predisposing factors, 130
    psychological functioning,
        133–134, 487–488
    sleep hygiene information,
        316–317
    sleep-restriction therapy, 321–322
    stimulus control instructions,
        318–321
Inspiratory effort, physiology, 272
Intelligence, and sleep requirements,
    25
Intensive care units, 386–390
    lighting in, 388–389
    noise levels, 389–390
    psychotic reactions, 395–396
    REM sleep effects, 387
    and sleep apnea, 387

Interferons, 406–407
Interhemispheric coupling, 85
Interleukins, 403, 407, 410–411, 413
International Classification of
    Diseases-9-CM, 60, 62, 509
International Classification of Sleep
    Disorders, 60–62, 505–508
Interview assessment
    excessive daytime sleepiness,
        166–168
    insomnia, 125–158
Introverts, sleep requirements, 25
Irregular sleep-wake pattern,
    240–241
Irritability, 496

Japan, shift work regulation, 250
Jet lag syndrome, 241–243
    description of, 66–67, 241–243
    eastward travel effects, 241–242
    mood changes, 243
    polysomnography, 243
    and reentrainment, 47, 43
    westward travel effects, 241

K complexes, 17–19
Kidney failure, 371–374
Kidney transplantation, 374
Knowledge transfer, 116–117

Laser-assisted surgery, 290
Lawsuits, shift workers, 260–261
Leg cramps, in pregnancy, 474–475
Leg movements, 203–204. See also
    Periodic limb movement
    disorder
Legislative regulation, shift work,
    249–250, 252
Leukocytes
    interferon production, 408
    sleep deprivation response, 403,
        412
Life stress, elderly, 457
"Light boxes," 251
Light exposure/therapy
    advanced sleep phase syndrome,
        148, 245

circadian rhythm influence, 28
delayed sleep phase syndrome,
    142, 244–245
entrainment effects, 48–49
insomnia effect, 316–317
phase response curve, 49–50
shift work adjustment, 251
Lighting, intensive care units,
    388–389
Long sleepers
    longevity, 260
    personality characteristics, 25
Longevity, 260. See also Mortality
Luteinizing hormone, 88–90
Lymphocytes, 403–405, 413

Macrophages, 403, 408
Maintenance of Wakefulness Test,
    216–217
    and excessive daytime sleepiness,
        166
    goals of, 220–221
    indications for, 217
    Multiple Sleep Latency Test
        relationship, 220–221
    and polysomnography, 180
    in treatment outcome assessment,
        219–221
Major depression. See Depression
"Masked depression," 499
Maxillomandibular advancement,
    290
Medical disorders. See also specific
        disorders
    and excessive daytime sleepiness,
        171–172
    insomnia role, 134–135
    and sleep disorder classification,
        61–62
Medical school training, 116
Medication
    behavioral treatment combination,
        329–332
    children, 436
    evaluation for, 350–351
Medication-induced sleep disorders
    apnea, 450–451

elderly, 456
insomnia, 135, 345–350
Medilog/Respitrace system, 188
Meditation, 322–323
Medroxyprogesterone acetate, 286
Melatonin
   bright light effects, 49
   circadian rhythms role, 46
   hospitalization effects, 390–391
   phase response curve effect, 49, 51
   shift work adjustment use, 251
   and sleep deprivation, 88–89
Memory, 98, 496
Mental disorders, classification,
      61–62
MESAM system, 188
Mesor, 37
Microsleeps
   characteristics, 12, 14
   and sleep deprivation, 85–86
Migraine, 380
Mimosa pudica, 38
MMPI profiles, 133, 455–456, 488
Monitoring. See Patient monitoring
Monoamine oxidase inhibitors,
      490–491
Moonlighting, 258
"Morningness" trait, 255–256
Mortality
   and obstructive sleep apnea,
      270–271, 392–393
      elderly, 448–450
   sleep habits relationship, 29
Multiple sclerosis, 379
Multiple Sleep Latency Test
   goals of, 220–221
   indications for, 216
   pathological sleepiness measure,
      165–166, 215–216
   physiological sleepiness measure,
      83–84, 180
   and polysomnography, 206
   stimulant drug effects, 77–78
   in treatment outcome assessment,
      219–221
Muramyl peptides, 411, 413
Muscular dystrophy, 363–364

Myocardial infarction
   circadian influences, 361
   and obstructive sleep apnea, 271
Myopia, 85
Myxedema, 277–278

Nadir (body core temperature), 37
Napping
   and biological rhythms, 41–43
   infants and children, 428–429
   in narcolepsy versus sleep apnea,
      274
Narcolepsy
   children and adolescents, 434–435
   description of, 65–66
   and excessive daytime sleepiness,
      169–170
   historical perspective, 112
   National Commission findings,
      117–118
   obstructive sleep apnea
      differentiation, 274–276
   polysomnography indication,
      195–197
   portable polysomnography, 183,
      188
   in pregnancy, 471–472
Narcoleptic tetrad, 65–66
Narcotics, 285–286
Nasal bilevel pressure, 293
Nasal continuous positive airway
      pressure
   adaptation to, 293
   adherence rate, 302, 305–306
   claustrophobic reactions, 309
   compliance, 300–311
   efficacy, 310–311
   instrumentation, 300–301
   intermittent use, 311
   in obstructive sleep apnea,
      291–294, 300–311
   patient monitoring, 302–307
   patterns of use, 303–307
   side effects, 309
   surgery complications prevention,
      393
   withdrawal from, 311

National Commission on Sleep
Disorders Research, 113–121
Natural killer cells, 404–406, 408
Neuroendocrine rhythms, 28
Neuromuscular disease, 363–364
Neuroticism, 256
Neutrophil levels, 403, 412
Newborn infants, 427–428
Night-shift workers, 254, 258
Night terrors, 435–436
  children, 435–436
  in pregnancy, 472–473
  and psychopathology, 494
Night wakings, children, 431–432
Nightmares
  and anxiety, 495
  children, 436–437
Nocturia, 452–454
Nocturnal backache, pregnancy, 474
Nocturnal penile tumescence, 493
Nocturnal polysomnography, 136.
    See also Polysomnography
Nocturnal seizures, 69
Noise levels, intensive care units,
    389–390
Nonsteroidal anti-inflammatory
    drugs, 452
Non-REM sleep. See NREM sleep
Non-24-hour sleep-wake syndrome,
    237–240
  in blind persons, 239–240
  pathophysiology, 239–240
  Raster plot, 238
Norephedrine, 346
Norepinephrine levels, 88, 348
NREM deprivation, 96–100
NREM sleep
  endotoxin enhancement of,
    410–411
  infants and children, 427–430
  normal pattern, 22–23
  polysomnography, 13–22, 178–179
Nystagmus, 85

Obesity, and pregnancy, 470
Obstructive sleep apnea syndrome,
    267–279

age of symptom onset, 274
and anesthesia, 391–393
cardiovascular complications, 271,
    276, 449–450
and Cheyne–Stokes respiration,
    360–361
children and adolescents, 434
cleft palate link, 278
clinical presentation, 64–65,
    267–279
elderly, 448–451
  mortality, 449–450
and excessive daytime sleepiness,
    169
historical perspective, 268
and hypothyroidism, 277–278,
    286
insomnia role, 135–136
mortality, 270–271, 392–393,
    449–450
napping response, 274
narcolepsy distinction, 273–276
nasal CPAP treatment, 291–294
natural history, 270–271
pharmacological treatments,
    286–287
polysomnography, 205
in pregnancy, 469–470
sleep position effects, 287–288
and snoring, 268–271
stroke link, 374–377
surgical treatment, 289–291
treatment, 283–312
  compliance, 299–312
treatment outcome assessment,
    221
Open heart surgery, 387
Optimal sleep concept, 95
Oxygen desaturation, saturation
  and back pain, pregnancy, 474
  cardiovascular events, elderly, 449
  polysomnography interpretation,
    204–205
  postsurgical monitoring, 393
  in pregnancy, 470
  respiratory effects, 363
  and sleep apnea, stroke, 375–376

Pacing effects, task performance, 82
Pain, chronic, 452
Pain sensitivity, 496
Paradoxical intention, 326–327
Paranoia, 80–81
Parasomnias, 68–69
  children and adolescents, 435–439
  classification, 60–62
  description, 68–69
  in pregnancy, 472–473
Parasympathetic-sympathetic
    balance, 25–26
Parkinsonism, 378
Parkinson's disease, 454–455
Partial sleep deprivation, 91–96
  antidepressant effects of, 497
  behavioral-psychological effects, 92
  hospitalized patients, 394–396
  physiology, 92–96
Pasteurella multocida infection, 418
Patient monitoring
  continuous positive airway
      pressure, 302–311
  ethics, 303
Penile tumescence,
    polysomnography, 184, 493
Performance tasks, 79–83
  difficulty level, 81–82
  duration effects, 81
  and partial sleep deprivation, 82
  sleep fragmentation effects,
      100–101
  in sleepiness assessment, 214–215
  and total sleep deprivation, 80–83
Periodic limb movement disorder
  benzodiazepine indication, 343
  description of, 65
  elderly, 448–449, 451
  and end-stage renal disease,
      372–373
    mortality relationship, 373
  and excessive daytime sleepiness,
      170
  insomnia assessment, 136
  polysomnography, 197, 202–204
  in pregnancy, 471
Personality disorders, 148–150

Personality traits
  insomnia, 133–134
  short- versus long-sleepers, 25
Pharmacological treatment. See also
    Benzodiazepine receptor
    agonists
  behavioral treatment combination,
      329–332
  evaluation for, 350–351
Pharyngeal surgery, 278, 289–290
Phase-advanced rhythms, 37, 49–50.
    See also Advanced sleep phase
    syndrome
Phase-delayed rhythms, 37, 49–51.
    See also Delayed sleep phase
    syndrome
Phase response curve, 49–50
Phasic REM behaviors, 180
Physiological sleepiness
  and sleep deprivation, 83–84,
      92–93, 98–99
  sleep fragmentation effects, 103
"Pickwickian" syndrome, 268
Pindolol, 349
Pineal gland, 46
Plants, circadian rhythm, 38
Polygraph, 178
Polymorphonuclear neutrophils, 403
Polysomnography, 177–191, 193–207
  basic methods, 181, 183–184
  circadian rhythms, 201, 203
  computerization, 184–185
  costs, 185
  delayed sleep phase syndrome, 235
  electrode placement, 181, 183
  indications for, 185–198
  insomnia assessment, 136
  interpretation, 193–207
  periodic movements
      interpretation, 203–204
  pregnancy studies, 467–468
  sleep stage characteristics, 14–22,
      178–179, 199–202
  sleep stage interpretation, 199–202
  and subjective reports, 199
  test conditions, 198–199
  video recording, behaviors, 205–206

Portable polysomnography,
185–189
Positional re-training, 288
Positron emission tomography, 88
Postnatal psychosis, 476
Postpartum women, 466–468,
475–476
Predisposing factors, insomnia,
128–130
Preeclampsia, 473–474
Pregnancy, 465–479
    affective changes, 475–476
    breathing difficulties, 469–471
    and dreaming, 476
    polysomnography, 467–468
    sleep disorders, 469–477
    sleeping positions, 468–469
    subjective sleep complaints,
    466–467
Productivity, shift workers, 260
Progesterone augmentation
    obstructive sleep apnea, 286
    and periodic leg movements, 451
Programming-reprogramming
    hypothesis, 31
Progressive relaxation, 322
Prolactin, 89–90
Prone sleeping position, 469
Propranolol, 349, 367
Protriptyline, 286
Prozac (fluoxetine), 491
Pseudodementia, 498
Pseudoephedrine, 346
Psychoanalytic theory, dreams, 21
Psychological factors. See Anxiety;
    Depression
Psychophysiological insomnia, 322,
343
Public policy, 111–122
Pulmonary function. See Respiration
Pupillometry, 217

Quiet-NREM sleep, 427–430

R & K system, 14–15
Rapid rotating shift systems, 254
Rating scales, 164–165, 213–214

Rats
    long-term sleep deprivation,
    414–418
    short-term sleep deprivation,
    412–414
Rebound sleep. See REM rebound
Recovery sleep
    age-related differences, 77, 84–85
    EEG measures, 84
    and partial sleep deprivation,
    92–94
    and REM deprivation, 99
    replacement times, 84
    sleep fragmentation effects, 103
    and slow-wave sleep deprivation,
    99
    and total sleep deprivation,
    84–85
Recrudescence, 348
Reentrainment
    jet lag adjustment, 47, 243
    non-24-hour sleep-work
    syndrome, 239
    and zeitgeber shift, 47–48
Relaxation training
    effectiveness, 322–323
    hypnotic use reduction, 331
    insomnia treatment, 322–323
REM behavior disorder
    description, 69
    and parkinsonism, 378
REM debt, 27
REM density
    and depression, 493
    elderly, 447
REM deprivation, 96–100
    and depression, 99, 497
    and dreaming, 96–97
    physiology, 98–100
    recovery sleep, 99
REM latency
    in depression, 484–487
    versus anxiety, 485–487
    elderly, 447
    and recovery sleep, age
    differences, 77–78, 84
REM pressure, 99

REM rebound, 103
    age differences, 77
    alcohol effects, 347
    and benzodiazepines, 348
    intensive care unit setting, 387
REM sleep
    age-related changes, 22, 24–25, 77
    and bereavement, 457–458
    in depression, 484–485, 491
    dreaming association, 21
    elderly, 447–448, 457–458
    infants and children, 427–430
    information processing theory,
        47–98
    normal pattern, 22–23
    phasic behaviors in, 180
    polysomnography, 19–21,
        178–180, 201–202
    in pregnancy, 467–468, 475
    and recovery sleep, 77–78, 84, 94,
        93
    respiration effects, 364
    restorative hypothesis, 31
REM sleep behavior disorder, 112
REM suppression, antidepressants,
    341–342
Renal dialysis, 371–374
Renal transplantation, 374
Repeated Test of Sustained
    Wakefulness, 216–217
Resident physicians, 92
Respiration. See also Sleep apnea
    circadian influences, 362
    drug effects, 366–367
    and partial sleep deprivation, 94
    polysomnography, 183, 204–205
    restrictive lung disease effects,
        363–364
    sleep effects, 362–363
Respiration rate, sleep deprivation, 87
Respiratory disease, 359–369, 452
Restless legs syndrome
    benzodiazepine indication, 343
    description of, 64
    and end-stage renal disease,
        371–373
    insomnia role, 135

polysomnography, 197
    in pregnancy, 471
Restorative sleep
    function of, 30
    sleep fragmentation studies,
        100–101
Restrictive lung disease, 363–364
Retinal pacemaker, 45
Rocking, 438, 494
Rotating shift systems, 254

Sedative medication
    cardiopulmonary effects, 366–367
    obstructive sleep apnea risk, 285
Seizure threshold, 87
Seizures, 69, 379
Selective serotonergic reuptake
    inhibitors, 346–347, 491
Selective sleep deprivation, 96–100,
    497
Selegiline, 378
Self-paced tasks, 82
Self-report measures, 164–165,
    213–214
"Self-soothers," 432
Sensorimotor rhythm biofeedback,
    324–326, 490
Serial reaction time tasks, 82
Serotonin reuptake inhibitors,
    346–347, 491
Sertraline (Zoloft), 491
Sex differences
    and aging, 25
    sleep pattern, 465
Sexual arousal, 493
Shift work, 249–266
    adjustment to, 67, 251
    age factors, 255
    circadian factors, 253–256, 261
    coping remedies, 251–252
    deleterious effects, 249, 251
    employee counseling, 261–262
    employer counseling, 260–261
    and excessive daytime sleepiness,
        167–168
    mental health, 255
    protective legislation, 249–250, 252

research initiatives, 259–260
sleep factors, 256–257
social and domestic factors,
    257–260
three-factor model, 252–259
Short sleepers
longevity, 260
personality characteristics, 25
Short-term memory performance, 83
"Signalers," 432
Simulations, 214
Skin dermatoses, 414, 416–417
Sleep apnea. *See also* Central sleep
    apnea; Obstructive sleep
    apnea syndrome
and Alzheimer's disease, 454
and anesthesia, 391–393
children and adolescents, 434
controlled studies need, 442
elderly, 440–443, 453–454
and end-stage renal disease,
    372–374
historical perspective, 112
intensive care unit setting, 387
mortality, 270–271, 392–393,
    449–450
National Commission report, 114,
    117–118
and nocturia, 453
polysomnography, 186, 188,
    195–196, 202, 204–205
in pregnancy, 469–470
prevalence, 114
seizures relationship, 379
Sleep apnea rate, 204
Sleep architecture, 179
Sleep debt
and daytime sleepiness, 162
and homeostasis, 26–27
Sleep deprivation, 73–75. *See also*
    Partial sleep deprivation;
    Total sleep deprivation
aging effects, 75, 77–78
animal studies, immune response,
    412–418
antibody response effects, 412–414
as antidepressant, 87, 497–499

children and adolescents, 432–434
and circadian rhythms, 75
cognitive performance effects, 402,
    496
diagnostic utility, 497–498
hospitalized patients, 394–395
and ICU psychosis, 396
immune system effects, 395,
    401–424
immunosuppression, rats,
    416–417
lethality, rats, 414–418
mood change, 497–498
performance task measures,
    79–83, 402, 496
psychophysiology, 74–105,
    496–498
stimulant drug interactions, 77, 78
Sleep diary. *See* Sleep log
Sleep efficiency
elderly, 447
normative values,
    polysomnography, 198–200
Sleep fragmentation, 100–104
and aging, 25
behavioral-psychological effects,
    100–102
physiology, 103–104
Sleep habits
and excessive daytime sleepiness,
    167
insomnia evaluation, 138
Sleep hygiene
efficacy of, 317
in insomnia, 316–317
and shift workers, 257
Sleep latency, normative values,
    198–200
Sleep log
case illustrations, 141–158
delayed sleep phase syndrome,
    233–234
in drug use evaluation, 350
insomnia assessment, 139–158
and polysomnography, 203
sample of, 140
sleepiness assessment, 213

Sleep-maintenance insomnia. *See also* Advanced sleep phase syndrome
  elderly, 442
  light therapy, 316–317
  stimulus control instructions, 319
Sleep need, shift workers, 256–257
Sleep onset, EEG correlates, 12–13
Sleep-onset insomnia. *See also* Delayed sleep phase syndrome
  case illustration, 150–152
  light therapy, 316–317
  sleep log, 151
  stimulus control instructions, 319
Sleep onset REM period, 274–275
Sleep paralysis, 65–66, 69
Sleep phase advance. *See* Advanced sleep phase syndrome
Sleep phase delay. *See* Delayed sleep phase syndrome
Sleep requirements, 25
Sleep-restriction therapy, 146, 321–322, 328–329
Sleep spindles
  characteristics, 17–108
  infants, 429
Sleep stages
  classification standards, 14–15
  polysomnography, 14–23
  smoothing rules, 22
Sleep starts, 170
Sleep talking, 435–436, 495
Sleep tendency, 210
Sleep terrors, 68–69
Sleepiness, 209–223. *See also* Excessive daytime sleepiness
Sleeping position
  and obstructive sleep apnea, 287–288
  in pregnancy, 468–469
Sleepwalking
  children and adolescents, 435–436
  description of, 68–69
  in pregnancy, 472–473
  and psychopathology, 494
Slow-eye movements, 12–13, 21–22

Slow rotating shift systems, 254
Slow wave sleep
  age-related changes, 24–25, 77
  delta activity, 15–17
  deprivation of, 98–99, 103
  elderly, 448
  endotoxin effects, 410–411
  infection response, 418–420
  normal pattern, 22–23, 178, 200
  polysomnograph interpretation, 200–202
  in pregnancy, 467–468
  in recovery sleep, 77–78, 94, 103
  tissue restitution function, 30–31
Smoothing rules, 22
SMR biofeedback, 324–326
Snoring
  cardiovascular complications, 268–269
  decibel level, 269
  elderly, 443
  epidemiology, 269–270
  medical aspects, 268–270
  pregnancy risk factor, 470–471
  stroke risk factor, 374
  surgical interventions, 289–291
  upper airway occlusion, 269–271
Social cues, 51
Somatoform disorders, 173
Somnogen, 403
Split sleep pattern, 154
Spousal bereavement, 457
Stage 1 sleep
  age-related changes, 24, 447
  polysomnography, 19–22, 178, 200–202
Stage 2 sleep, 24, 178
Stage 3 sleep. *See* Slow wave sleep
Stage 4 sleep. *See also* Slow wave sleep
  delta activity, 17
  deprivation of, 99
  in pregnancy, and depression, 475
Standard shift work index, 256
Stanford Sleepiness Scale, 164–165, 213
Staphylococcus aureus infection, 418

Stimulant drugs
  insomnia cause, 345–346
  sleep deprivation interactions, 77,
    78
Stimulus control instructions,
    318–321, 328–329
  compliance, 320–321
  effectiveness, 318
  hypnotic drug combination,
    331–332
  in multicomponent packages,
    328–329
Streptococcus pyogenes infection, 418
Stroke, 374–377
  mortality, and sleep apnea, 376
  risk factors, 374
  sleep apnea link, 374–376
Structured interview. See Diagnostic
    interview
Subjective insomnia, 322
Substance abuse, shift workers, 257
Substance-induced sleep disorders, 61
Sudden cardiac death, 204, 361, 449
Sudden infant death syndrome
  National Commission report, 115,
    118
  prevalence, 115
Sundowning, 454
Supine sleep position
  obstructive sleep apnea, 287–288
  in pregnancy, 479
Suprachiasmatic nuclei, 44–45
Supraventricular tachycardia, 361
Surgery, 385–387
  biological rhythm disturbances, 390
  intensive care unit factors, 386–390
  REM sleep effects, 386–387
  and sleep apnea, 391–393
Systematic desensitization, 437

T lymphocytes, 405, 407, 413
Task performance. See Performance
    tasks
Tau
  definition, 38
  flexibility of, 43
  in temporal isolation conditions, 40

Temazepam, 331–332, 341
Temperature rhythm. See Body core
    temperature
Temporal isolation, 39–43
10–20 electrode placement, 181, 183
Testosterone levels, 28
Thalidomide, 466
Theophylline
  and insomnia, 346, 441
  obstructive sleep apnea treatment,
    287
Theta activity
  in REM sleep, 20
  sleep deprivation effects, 85, 94
Theta EEG biofeedback, 324
Thought stopping, 327
Thyroid hormones, 88–90, 415, 417
Thyroid-stimulating hormone, 88–90
Time-lapse video somnography, 430
Time zone change. See Jet lag
Tissue restitutive theory, 30–31, 395
Tonsillar hypertrophy, 278
Tonsillectomy, 434
Total sleep deprivation, 80–81
  antidepressant effect, 87, 497
  autonomic effects, 87–88
  behavioral-psychological effects,
    80–83
  physiology, 83–85
  recovery sleep time, 84
Tracheostomy, 289
Traffic accidents
  obstructive sleep apnea, 271
  shift workers, 258
Transient ischemic attacks, 375
Treatment compliance
  behavioral techniques, insomnia,
    320
  nasal CPAP, 300–309
Treatment monitoring. See Patient
    monitoring
Triazolam (Halcion), 331, 341
Tricyclic antidepressants
  and cardiopulmonary disease, 367
  enuresis treatment, 438
  REM latency, 490–491
L-tryptophan, 287

Tumor necrosis factor, 410
Tumor response, sleep deprivation,
    412

Ultradian rhythms, 36
Upper airway obstruction
    pathogenesis, 271–273
    and total sleep deprivation, 88
Urge incontinence, 453
Uvulopalatopharyngoplasty, 288–290

Valium (diazepam), 494
Ventilatory drive response
    fragmented sleep effects, 103
    selective sleep deprivation, 99–100
    total sleep deprivation, 87–88

Ventricular arrhythmias, 104, 361
Videorecordings, children, 430
Vigilance. *See* Performance tasks
Vision, and sleep deprivation, 85
Visual Analogue Scale, 213
Vitalog system, 188

Weight loss, 283–284
Westward travel, 241–242
White blood cells, 402–403, 412
Wilkinson Vigilance Test, 214
Wrist-worn devices. *See* Actigraphy

Zeitgebers, 47–48
Zoloft (sertraline), 491
Zolpidem (Ambien), 330, 341

About the Editors

Mark R. Pressman has been involved in the diagnosis and treatment of sleep disorders as well as human sleep research for the past 19 years. In the last 16 years he has worked in this field full-time. Dr. Pressman received his master's and PhD in experimental psychology from Ferkauf Graduate School of Psychology, Yeshiva University, New York. Dr. Pressman was founding co-director of the Sleep Disorders Center, Department of Neurology, the Medical College of Pennsylvania at Eastern Pennsylvania Psychiatric Institute in Philadelphia and served as Assistant Professor of Neurology and Psychiatry at the medical school. He is currently Associate Director and Administrator of the Sleep Disorders Center, Lankenau Hospital and Medical Research Center, Wynnewood, Pennsylvania. In addition, he is Clinical Associate Professor of Medicine at the Jefferson Medical College in Philadelphia. Dr. Pressman is an active researcher who has published over 60 articles on the topics of the pathophysiology and treatment of clinical sleep disorders as well as the psychophysiology and neurophysiology of human sleep and alertness. Dr. Pressman is a licensed psychologist and Diplomate of the American Board of Sleep Medicine. He is a frequent peer reviewer for sleep related journal manuscripts, a member of the faculty of American Sleep Disorders Association annual National Sleep Medicine Course, and frequent lecturer on sleep-related topics.

William C. Orr graduated from the University of Delaware and completed his graduate training at Washington University, St. Louis. After spending three years at the Walter Reed Army Institute of Research, Dr. Orr accepted a position at the University of Oklahoma College of Medicine. Dr. Orr remains in Oklahoma City and is currently the President and Chief Operating Officer of the Institute for Healthcare Research at Baptist Medical Center of Oklahoma in Oklahoma City. He has done extensive research on both sleep disorders and gastrointestinal disease. He is the author of books on sleep disorders and the diagnosis of esophageal disease. He has published over 200 works on subjects ranging from sleep apnea syndromes and excessive daytime sleepiness to the role of sleep in the pathogenesis of various acid and peptic diseases. Dr. Orr has served as a consultant to the National Institutes of Health and a variety of hospitals throughout the United States, and he serves as a reviewer for numerous medical journals. In addition, he has served on the Research Committee for the American College of Gastroenterology and is a board member of the National Sleep Foundation. He is also Past-President of the Southern Sleep Society and a Diplomate of the American Board of Sleep Medicine.